# Healthcare Systems Engineering

# Healthcare Systems Engineering

Editor: Peter Haddock

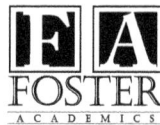

FA
FOSTER
ACADEMICS

www.fosteracademics.com

www.fosteracademics.com

**FA**
**FOSTER**
A C A D E M I C S

Cataloging-in-Publication Data

Healthcare systems engineering / edited by Peter Haddock.
    p. cm.
Includes bibliographical references and index.
ISBN 978-1-63242-546-1
1. Biomedical engineering. 2. Medical care. 3. Health services administration.
4. Systems engineering. I. Haddock, Peter.
R856 .H43 2018
610.28--dc23

Foster Academics,
118-35 Queens Blvd., Suite 400,
Forest Hills, NY 11375, USA

ISBN 978-1-63242-546-1 (Hardback)

# Contents

# Preface

Healthcare engineering is an emerging field developed by amalgamating the concepts of healthcare with the techniques of engineering. It involves the diagnosis, treatment, prevention and management of diseases. Also included in this field is the improvement of mental and physical health. The objective of this book is to give a general view of the different areas of healthcare systems engineering and its applications. It brings forth some of the most innovative concepts and elucidates the unexplored aspects of this field. It is a valuable compilation of topics, ranging from the basic to the most complex advancements in healthcare systems engineering. It aims to equip students and experts with the advanced topics and upcoming concepts in this area.

The researches compiled throughout the book are authentic and of high quality, combining several disciplines and from very diverse regions from around the world. Drawing on the contributions of many researchers from diverse countries, the book's objective is to provide the readers with the latest achievements in the area of research. This book will surely be a source of knowledge to all interested and researching the field.

In the end, I would like to express my deep sense of gratitude to all the authors for meeting the set deadlines in completing and submitting their research chapters. I would also like to thank the publisher for the support offered to us throughout the course of the book. Finally, I extend my sincere thanks to my family for being a constant source of inspiration and encouragement.

**Editor**

# A Systematic Review on Existing Measures for the Subjective Assessment of Rehabilitation and Assistive Robot Devices

**Yiannis Koumpouros**

*Technological Educational Institute of Athens, Department of Informatics, Agiou Spyridonos, Aigaleo, 12243 Athens, Greece*

Correspondence should be addressed to Yiannis Koumpouros; ykoump@teiath.gr

Academic Editor: Yinkwee Ng

The objective of the current study is to identify and classify outcome measures currently used for the assessment of rehabilitation or assistive robot devices. We conducted a systematic review of the literature using PubMed, MEDLINE, CIRRIE, and Scopus databases for studies that assessed rehabilitation or assistive robot devices from 1980 through January 2016. In all, 31 articles met all inclusion criteria. Tailor-made questionnaires were the most commonly used tool at 66.7%, while the great majority (93.9%) of the studies used nonvalidated instruments. The study reveals the absence of a standard scale which makes it difficult to compare the results from different researchers. There is a great need, therefore, for a valid and reliable instrument to be available for use by the intended end users for the subjective assessment of robot devices. The study concludes by identifying two scales that have been validated in general assistive technology devices and could support the scope of subjective assessment in rehabilitation or assistive robots (however, with limited coverage) and a new one called PYTHEIA, recently published. The latter intends to close the gap and help researchers and developers to evaluate, assess, and produce products that satisfy the real needs of the end users.

## 1. Introduction

The aging of society along with the lack of caregivers forces innovations to help people in their daily lives. Nowadays, robots come in many forms and can be used in many ways to help people with disabilities. Although much research has been done in the field resulting in several prototypes, few assistive robots exist in common use today. The high costs and the uncertainty regarding the benefits gained are major barriers to their widespread adoption. It is therefore crucial to follow a more multidisciplinary approach during the design phase. For example, an engineering design with only healthy subjects many times leads to a system not appropriate for the target population of persons with a disability. Engineers, therapists, physiatrists, and ergonomics experts as well as the end users (people with disabilities) should be a part of the design team from the beginning of any such effort. To this end, the design team should be able to measure the satisfaction of the end users at any stage of the development phase.

Measuring user satisfaction helps to measure the overall quality of a product or service. Tracking user satisfaction during the development phase can help developers and researchers make sure that the changes they are making improve the product/service for users. In customer relationship management, user (or customer) satisfaction is a measure of the degree to which a product or service meets the user's expectations. Consumer satisfaction is a central concept in many domains (business, research, etc.) and has held a central position in marketing since the 1950s until today, with an increasing interest and importance. The realization of this importance has led to a proliferation of research on consumer satisfaction [1–4]. According to [5] we can distinguish two different types of user satisfaction: the process-oriented approach (equal to the difference between expected satisfaction and achieved satisfaction) and the outcome-oriented approach (as an attribute extracted from a product or service after its consumption). The evaluation of any technology device requires the objective and subjective assessment of the product/service. An objective assessment is one that needs no professional judgment to give a score correctly, while subjective assessment yields many possible answers of varying quality and requires professional judgment to give a score [6]. Subjective assessment records the facts presented by the end user that show his/her perception, understanding, and interpretation of what is happening and therefore measures his/her satisfaction. The next step is to quantify them appropriately.

The evolution of Information and Communication Technologies (ICT) [7] along with nanotechnology and other sciences (e.g., medicine and behavioral science) presents a unique potential for innovative technology products and services that help people in their daily lives. The application of such innovations in healthcare has already driven in products that some years ago belonged to the scientific imagination sphere. For example, robotic technology has provided the opportunity to benefit the lives of people with disabilities (i.e., as a manipulator mounted on a desk or wheelchair or mobile base or body worn; as a mobility or communication assistant; etc.). Many commercial products are available nowadays for mobility and manipulation for people with physical disabilities (e.g., the Tek RMD [8] and the Manus robotic arm [9]), for telepresence purposes, and so forth [10], while others are being developed at research institutions worldwide. To this end, researchers are struggling to collect end users' sentiments towards the technologies developed in order to match the products with the real needs of the end customers.

Rehabilitation robotics is a special branch of robotics which focuses on machines that can be used to help people recover from severe physical trauma or assist them in activities of daily living. Rehabilitation robotics has applications in all areas of physical therapy, presenting a wide range of advancements in robotic prosthesis and other domains. Another important sector is that of assistive robotics, which tries to combine and integrate several technologies in order to meet the needs of people with various disabilities.

Focusing on the healthcare sector, quality of care and patient satisfaction are major issues [11]. Thus, the assessment of any service or device from the perspective of the patient is crucial. The current study is concerned with the question of whether any reliable and valid instruments have been developed to assess assistive or rehabilitation robot devices from the user's perspective. To the best of our knowledge, no such research has previously been carried out or published.

## 2. Materials and Methods

A search of peer-reviewed published literature was conducted in January 2016 for articles related to the subjective assessment of assistive or rehabilitation robot devices. This was performed through the Internet via MEDLINE, PubMed, Scopus, and CIRRIE. The keywords used (employing Boolean phrases) in the searches included the following: *satisfaction, assessment, assess, user, subjective, robot, robotic, assistive, rehabilitation, psychometric, test, scale, metrics, evaluation, usability, acceptability,* and *acceptance.* Articles published after 1980 were considered for further studying. We included only studies published in English and research from peer-reviewed journals. The resulting publications were examined in a first step for potential inclusion based on their title and abstract, while we excluded any duplication. In a second

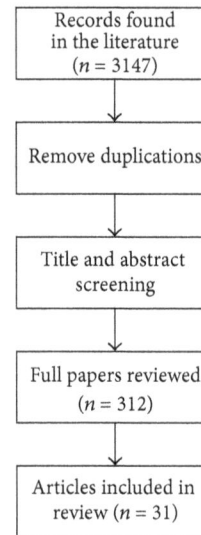

FIGURE 1: Workflow of the selection process for subjective assessment of rehabilitation and assistive robot devices.

step, after reviewing the abstract and title, the remaining publications underwent a full text review. We also manually searched the references lists of these articles for additional relevant sources. The whole process is depicted in Figure 1.

The initial query returned 3147 results. After the initial screening (reviewing the titles and abstracts and removing duplicates), the number was reduced to 312 articles. The eligibility criteria for inclusion were as follows: (i) studies involve assistive or rehabilitation robot devices (e.g., socially assistive robots, robot controlled wheelchairs, and exoskeleton devices), (ii) at least one outcome measure was used in the study, (iii) the study should include formative, process, or summative evaluation that assesses the rehabilitation or assistive robot device, (iv) the study was a peer-reviewed article (published in a journal or conference), and (v) articles are written in the English language. Finally, all articles were evaluated in terms of the clarity of the evidence presented. The second phase included a full text review of the selected articles. The main factors for excluding many articles included the following: (i) article was not written in English, (ii) the study provided a descriptive summary of the evaluation without giving more details (e.g., questionnaire/scale used), (iii) the number of participants in the study was very limited (<3 participants) or undefined, (iv) articles/studies were in the following subject areas: biochemistry, genetics and molecular biology, mathematics, chemical engineering, social sciences, materials science, physics and astronomy, psychology, arts and humanities, immunology and microbiology, agricultural and biological sciences, decision sciences, dentistry, energy, environmental science, business management and accounting, chemistry, earth and planetary science, pharmacology-toxicology and pharmaceutics, and undefined, (v) articles were in books and notes, and (vi) they assessed the technology used through quantitative data only (objective evaluation). For data extraction and analysis purposes we followed the Cochrane research methodology [12].

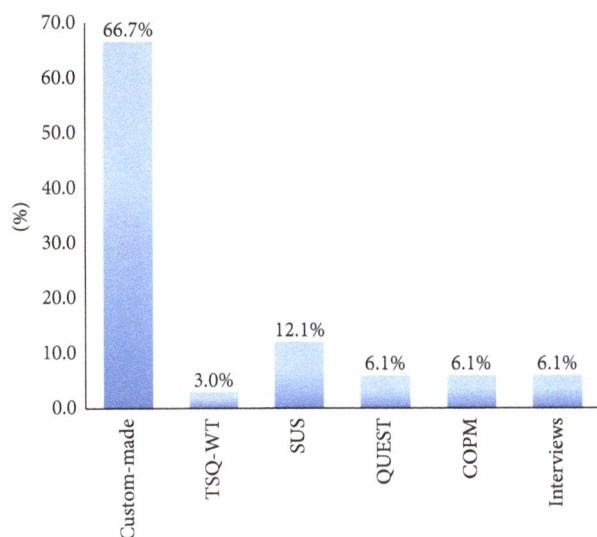

FIGURE 2: Subjective measure used in the studies reviewed (%).

The processing and organization of the articles was made using the MS Excel and EndNote X6.0.2 programs.

## 3. Results

Even though the initial query returned a large number of articles ($n = 3147$), only 312 (9.914% of 3147) underwent a full text review. Finally, 31 articles (9.935% of 312) met the inclusion criteria and were included in the review. Table 1 summarizes the subjective measures used in these studies.

A wide range of rehabilitation and assistive robot devices are reviewed in Table 1 (e.g., wheelchairs, exoskeleton devices, socially assistive robots, therapeutic systems, telepresence systems, and haptic technologies). The majority of the research presented was conducted in the United States of America (15.2%) and Italy (12.1%), followed by Canada (9.1%), Netherlands (9.1%), Japan (9.1%), France (9.1%), Spain (9.1%), the United Kingdom (6.1%), Germany (6.1%), South Korea (3%), Portugal (3%), Israel (3%), and Austria (3%).

In the majority of the studies there were a limited number of patients participating either due to research/pilot testing or due to difficulty finding the right participants fitting in the study. Only one study managed to have 83 patients [13]. Twenty-two out of the thirty-one studies used patients to evaluate the device, while three recruited college or university students, two recruited healthcare professionals, and the remaining four used healthy subjects. Additionally, two of the studies used healthy subjects as control groups. Figure 2 presents the distribution of the subjective measures used in the studies.

The last column of Table 1 presents the number of items (questions) used in each study under the subjective measure used. The question mark "?" in Table 1, when used, means that there is no evidence (at least to the authors' knowledge) that the specific subjective measure/scale is valid or reliable. The authors decided to use this instead of marking the specific measure as not valid or not reliable because the articles report

the scale as valid. However, after searching the literature, we found no evidence on the validity and reliability of the scale in the language used in the specific study; so, we decided to present it as being in question in terms of its validity and reliability in the language used. Moreover, in the last column of the table there may appear two values separated by a comma. This means that the study used two different subjective measures and each value in the column represents the number of items (questions) used for each one of them.

## 4. Discussion

The review of the literature provided a thorough survey of evaluations for rehabilitation or assistive robot devices concerning the satisfaction and the subjective assessment of the end users. The review began with a great number of articles returned ($n = 3147$) but was ultimately narrowed to 312 of which 31 were finally included in the review. The majority of the articles failed to meet the inclusion criteria presented because most of the studies evaluated the devices by using only objective measures (e.g., Fugl-Meyer scale [14], modified Ashworth scale [15], Barthel index [16], and NASA-TLX [16]) and other clinical measurements relevant to the scope and the population of the study.

It is really impressive that the great majority (66.7%) of the research included in the review used custom-made subjective measures to evaluate the satisfaction of the end users and assess the rehabilitation or assistive robot device used subjectively [17–38]. However, this percentage does not reveal the real problem faced. Someone should also consider the following facts:

(i) Two (2) studies [39, 40] used semistructured interviews due to the lack of any valid and reliable subjective measurement instrument.

(ii) Two (2) studies [13, 41] used the Canadian Occupational Performance Measure (COPM) [42] which is a semi-interview that enables an open dialogue between the end user and the therapist on issues of importance to the patient. It is designed to identify occupational performance problems faced by the patient. During the interview, the therapist tries to identify daily occupations of importance that the patient wants to do, needs to do, or is expected to do but is unable to accomplish. Other domains are also covered, like self-care, productivity, or leisure. Due to the nature of COPM, as described above, it cannot be adopted in all kinds of purpose rehabilitation or assistive devices.

(iii) Four (4) studies [30, 43–45] used the System Usability Scale (SUS) [46] which is a "quick and dirty" ten-item scale for administering after usability tests. However, this scale measures only basic issues of the device and does not take into account other very important issues, like the adaptability of the device, the feeling of safety, the social perception of the user when using the device, the individual dimensions of the device, if it fits well in the environment of the end user, and so

TABLE 1: Summary of review results.

| Robot device used | Region/country | Author/organization (year of publication), publisher [ref. number] | Number of patients/end users | Type of end users | Location of the survey | Subjective measure used | Language of scale used | Valid/reliable scale | Number of scale's items |
|---|---|---|---|---|---|---|---|---|---|
| A sensory system and upper limb biomechanical model combined with a graphical interface | Ontario, Canada | Abdullah et al. (2011), J. Neuroeng. Rehabil. [17] | 20 | Patients | Inpatient Stroke Rehabilitation Unit | Unknown (developed by themselves) | English | –/– | 2 |
| Robotic exoskeleton arm | Italy | Ambrosini et al. (2014), Robotica [43] | 14 | 9 patients + 5 healthy | Villa Beretta Rehabilitation Centre | TSQ-WT, SUS | Italian | ?/?, ?/? | TSQ-WT (30), SUS (10) |
| Hand/wrist exoskeleton | United Kingdom, Netherlands, Italy | Amirabdollahian et al (2014), Robotica [44] | 12 | Patients | Not defined | SUS | English | V/R | 10 |
| H2 robotic exoskeleton | Not defined | Bortole et al. (2015), J. Neuroeng. Rehabil. [18] | 3 | Patients | Not defined | Unknown (developed by themselves) | English | –/– | 1 |
| Haptic human-robot partnered stepping | Atlanta, GA, USA | Chen et al. (2015), PLoS ONE [19] | 10 | Healthy | Healthcare Robotics Lab | Unknown (developed by themselves) | English | –/– | 14 |
| Direct physical interface for nursing assistant robots | Atlanta, GA, USA | Chen and Kemp (2010), HRI 2010 [20] | 18 | Healthy (nurses) | Healthcare Robotics Lab | Unknown (developed by themselves) | English | –/– | 11, 10 |
| Robot suit HAL (Hybrid Assistive Limb) | Tokyo, Japan | Chihara et al. (2016), Neurol. Med. Chir. [39] | 15 | Patients | Kyoto University Hospital | Interviews | | | |
| Robot "El-E" | Atlanta, GA, USA | Choi et al. (2008), ASSETS '08 [21] | 8 | Patients | Healthcare Robotics Lab | Unknown (developed by themselves) | English | –/– | 8 |
| SAM robotic aid system (a mobile Neobotix base equipped with a semiautomatic vision interface and a Manus robotic arm) | France | Coignard et al. (2013), Annals of Phys. and Rehab. Med. [22] | 29 + 34 | 29 patients + 34 healthy (control group) | Hopale Foundation in Berck-sur-Mer and the Kerpape Rehabilitation Centre in Ploemeur | Unknown (developed by themselves) | French | –/– | 9 (technical aspects), 7 (acceptability and usage) |
| Hybrid FES-robot (exoskeleton) | Spain | del-Ama et al. (2014), J. Neuroeng. Rehabil. [48] | 4 | Patients | Not defined | QUEST | English | V/R | 7 from 12 |
| Wheelchair mounted robotic assisted transfer device | Pittsburgh, USA | Grindle et al. (2015), BioMed Res. Int. 2015 [23] | 18 | Patients | 2011 National Veteran Wheelchair Games | Unknown (developed by themselves) | English | –/– | 4, 7 |
| iCat robot | Netherlands | Heerink et al. (2010), Int. J. Soc. Robot. [24] | 30 | Healthy | Not defined | Unknown (based on the UTAUT questionnaire) | English | –/– | 41 |
| ARM, HEXAR-KR40P | South Korea | Kim et al. (2014), Int. J. Precis. Eng. Man. [25] | 80 | Patients | Not defined | Unknown (developed by themselves) | English | –/– | 1 |
| A-gear: wearable dynamic arm support | Netherlands | Kooren et al. (2015), J. Neuroeng. Rehabil. [26] | 4 | 3 patients + 1 healthy | Radboud UMC Outpatient Clinic | Unknown (developed by themselves) | Not defined | –/– | Not defined |
| Grasping robot | France | Laffont et al. (2009), Arch. Phys. Med. Rehabil. [27] | 20 + 24 | 20 patients + 24 healthy (control group) | Four French departments of physical and rehabilitation medicine | Unknown (developed by themselves) | French | –/– | 3 |
| Haptic-robotic platform for upper limb | Canada | Lam et al. (2008), J. Neuroeng. Rehabil. [28] | 8 | Healthy (physical and occup. therapists) | Not defined | Unknown (developed by themselves) | English | –/– | 9 |
| Teleoperated robot system Telenoid R3 | Japan | Liu et al. (2015), HRI 2015 [29] | 20 | Healthy (college students) | ATR Intelligent Robotics and Communication Labs, Kyoto | Unknown (developed by themselves) | Japanese | –/– | 2 |

TABLE 1: Continued.

| Robot device used | Region/country | Author/organization (year of publication), publisher [ref. number] | Number of patients/end users | Type of end users | Location of the survey | Subjective measure used | Language of scale used | Valid/reliable scale | Number of scale's items |
|---|---|---|---|---|---|---|---|---|---|
| LEGO robot | Spain | López-Samaniego et al. (2014), Bio-Med. Mater. Eng. [30] | 9 | Patients | Not defined | Unknown (developed by themselves), SUS | Spanish | –/–, ?/? | Not defined, SUS (10) |
| InMotion 2 robotic system | Italy | Mazzoleni et al. (2014), Comput. Methods Programs Biomed. [31] | 34 | Patients | Not defined | Unknown (developed by themselves) | Italian | –/– | 7 |
| Personal Transport Assistance Robot (PTAR) | Japan | Ozaki et al. (2013), Arch. Phys. Med. Rehabil. [32] | 8 | Patients | Fujita Health University | Unknown (developed by themselves) | Japanese | –/– | 2 |
| Rehabilitation robot | Canada | Pineau et al. (2010), Advances in Intelligent and Soft Computing [33] | 7 | Healthy (university students) | Not defined | Unknown (developed by themselves) | Not defined | –/– | Not defined |
| Amadeo robot | Italy | Sale et al. (2012), Stroke Res. Treat. [41] | 7 | Patients | Department of Neurorehabilitation, IRCCS San Raffaele Pisana | COPM | | | |
| Robot-enhanced repetitive treadmill therapy (ROBERT) | Germany | Schroeder et al. (2014), Dev. Med. Child Neurol. [13] | 83 | Patients | Not defined | COPM | | | |
| Robot companion (artificial health advisor) | Germany | von der Pütten et al. (2011), ICMI '11 [40] | 6 | Healthy | University of Duisburg-Essen | Semistructured interviews | | | |
| Personal Mobility and Manipulation Appliance (PerMMA) | USA | Wang et al. (2013), Med. Eng. Phys. [34] | 15 | Patients | Center for Assistive Technology, University of Pittsburgh | Unknown (developed by themselves) | English | –/– | 12 |
| Kompaï (indoor assistive robot) | France | Wu et al. (2014), Clin. Interv. Aging [35] | 11 | Patients | Living lab | Unknown (developed by themselves) | English | –/– | 25 |
| ASIBOT (portable robot to aid patients) | Spain | Jardón et al. (2011), Disabil. Rehabil. Assist. Technol. [49] | 6 | Patients | Not defined | QUEST | Spanish | V/R | 12 |
| Intelligent wheelchair | Portugal | Mónica Faria et al. (2013), Assist. Technol. [45] | 46 | Healthy (students) | School of Allied Health Sciences of Porto | SUS | Portuguese | ?/? | 10 |
| Socially assistive robot (Nao) | Austria | Werner and Krainer (2013), ICSR 2013 [36] | 14 | Healthy | Senior Citizen Centre Schwechat | Unknown (developed by themselves) | German | –/– | Not defined |

TABLE 1: Continued.

| Robot device used | Region/country | Author/organization (year of publication), publisher [ref. number] | Number of patients/end users | Type of end users | Location of the survey | Subjective measure used | Language of scale used | Valid/reliable scale | Number of scale's items |
|---|---|---|---|---|---|---|---|---|---|
| Reo Therapy System | Israel | Treger et al. (2008), Eur. J. Phys. Rehab. Med. [37] | 10 | Patients | Loewenstein Rehabilitation Centre | Unknown (developed by themselves) | Not defined | —/— | 15 |
| Robotic and electrical stimulation therapy | United Kingdom | Hughes et al. (2011), Disabil. Rehabil. Assist. Technol. [38] | 5 | Patients | Not defined | Unknown (developed by themselves) | English | —/— | Not defined |

Note: TSQ-WT = Telehealthcare Satisfaction Questionnaire-Wearable Technology; SUS = System Usability Scale, QUEST = Quebec User Evaluation of Satisfaction with Assistive Technology, UTAUT = Unified Theory of Acceptance and Use of Technology, COPM = Canadian Occupational Performance Measure, ? = unknown value, — = not valid (if it appears in the first position of the column "Valid/reliable scale")/not reliable (if it appears in the second position of the column "Valid/reliable scale"), V = valid scale, and R = reliable scale.

forth. So, this scale can capture only very basic issues of the subjective assessment needed for robot-based devices.

(iv) One (1) study [43] utilized the Telehealthcare Satisfaction Questionnaire-Wearable Technology (TSQ-WT) [47]. There has not yet been published (at least to the authors' knowledge) any article in any language related to the validity and reliability of this questionnaire. Thus, it cannot be considered a reliable and valid instrument for the subjective assessment of a technology device.

(v) Two (2) studies [48, 49] utilized the Quebec User Evaluation of Satisfaction with Assistive Technology (QUEST 2.0) scale [50]. According to Holz et al., QUEST 2.0 is a standardized satisfaction assessment tool designed for assistive technologies [51]. Moreover, it has been tested for its validity and reliability in several applications and languages [52, 53]. Although this scale is used with assistive devices, del-Ama et al. [48] used only 7 of the 12 questions incorporated in the original questionnaire in their study.

According to the previous analysis, it is apparent that finally 93.9% of the reviewed studies used neither valid nor reliable instruments to assess the robot devices. Only 6.1% of them used a validated measure (the QUEST scale), which can assess only a subset of the desired aspects (as described in the next paragraphs).

In the early years of many technical fields, the research community often utilizes a wide range of metrics that are not comparable due to a bias towards application specific measures. The primary difficulty in defining common metrics is the incredibly diverse range of human-robot or robot assisted applications. Thus, although metrics from other fields (HCI, human factors, etc.) can be applied to satisfy specific needs, identifying metrics that can accommodate the entire application space may not be feasible [54].

Attempts to categorize both objective and subjective metrics have been made. According to the USUS Evaluation Framework for Human-Robot Interaction [55] the factors *usability*, *social acceptance*, *user experience*, and *societal impact* are considered the main categories of evaluation factors. Each category is divided into specific metrics, either objectively or subjectively measured:

(i) *Usability*. Effectiveness, efficiency, learnability, flexibility, robustness, and utility.

(ii) *Social Acceptance*. Performance expectancy, effort expectancy, attitude towards using technology, self-efficacy, forms of grouping, attachment, and reciprocity.

(iii) *User Experience*. Embodiment, emotion, human-oriented perception, feeling of security, and coexperience with robots.

(iv) *Societal Impact*. All effects of the introduction of robotic agents' consequences for the social life of a specific community (taking into account cultural differences) in terms of quality of life, working conditions and employment, and education.

Among these, the authors propose that the following could be tested using end-user questionnaires, which means that they could be considered subjective:

(i) *Utility*. It refers to how an interface can be used to reach a certain goal or to perform a certain task. The more the tasks the interface is designed to perform, the more the utility it has.

(ii) *Performance Expectancy*. It is the degree to which an individual believes that using the system will help him or her to attain gains in performance.

(iii) *Effort Expectancy*. It indicates to which extent the user perceives that a system will be easy to use.

(iv) *Attitude towards Using Technology*. It is the sum of all positive or negative feelings and attitudes about solving working tasks supported by a humanoid robot.

(v) *Self-Efficacy*. It relates to a person's perception of their ability to reach a goal.

(vi) *Attachment*. It is an affection-tie that one person forms between themselves and another person or object—a tie that binds them together in space and endures over time.

(vii) *Reciprocity*. It is the positive or negative response of individuals towards the actions of others.

(viii) *Embodiment*. It describes the relationship between a system and its environment and can be measured by investigating the different perturbatory channels like morphology, which has impact on social expectations.

(ix) *Emotion*. An emotion is an essential part in social interaction; it has to be incorporated in the assessment and design of robots.

(x) *Feeling of Security*. It is important to investigate how to design human-robot interactions in a way that humans experience them to be safe.

(xi) *Coexperience*. Coexperience describes experiences with objects regarding how individuals develop their personal experience based on social interaction with others.

(xii) *Societal Impact*. Societal impact describes all effects the introduction of robotic agents results in for the social life of a specific community—taking into account cultural differences—in terms of quality of life, working conditions, employment, and education.

The above categorization is the most full and detailed, including aspects that are rarely taken into account when it comes to evaluating a robotic assistant. Most researchers, however, when evaluating an assistive device/technology tend to use questionnaires that give information on the aforementioned fields. However, as Bartneck et al. mention, due to their naivety and the amount of work necessary to create a valid questionnaire, developers of robots have a tendency to quickly cook up their own questionnaires [56]. This conduct results in two main problems: firstly, the validity and reliability of these questionnaires have often not been evaluated and, secondly, the absence of standard questionnaires makes it difficult to compare the results from different researchers [56]. The findings of our review study support this conclusion. It seems that choosing tailored questionnaires is the rule in robotics assessment. However, the existing variety of questionnaires that could be useful for the assessment of rehabilitation or assistive robot devices is narrow, for the reasons described above.

As derived from the current review, QUEST 2.0 may be one questionnaire that can be used in the examined field. However, a strategy that would target maximum coverage of the subjective measures spectrum would require the combined use of two (or more) questionnaires, since QUEST 2.0 covers only some subjective aspects (mainly: feeling of security, perceived effectiveness, and ease of use). We should therefore look into the literature for other valid and reliable scales that are used in different sectors and may be applicable to the examined domain. Other valuated and relevantly common used questionnaires we found in the bibliography were the Assistive Technology Device Predisposition Assessment- (ATDPA-) Device Form [57, 58] and the Psychosocial Impact of Assistive Devices Scale (PIADS) [59]. The ATDPA-Device Form is more relevant in context than the PIADS, targeting the evaluation of overall user experience with assistive technology, while PIADS only emphasizes the psychosocial impact of assistive devices, without targeting the evaluation of the actual experience of interacting with a robot device, but rather the impact that this interaction has on quality of life (QoL). Other questionnaires such as the USE-IT [60] questionnaire were ruled out from the very beginning, since they were not well valuated or not widely used from researchers in the bibliography. It seems therefore that a combination of the QUEST 2.0 questionnaire and the Assistive Technology Device Predisposition Assessment- (ATDPA-) Device Form covers most of the desirable user-experience aspects, with ensured validity and reliability. However, no scales have been identified yet in the literature that could be adopted well and measure the individual functionalities of rehabilitation or assistive robot devices. To this end, the authors developed and are currently examining a new scale called PYTHEIA in order to fill the identified gap. The first results are very satisfactory in terms of their validity and reliability [61]. More specifically, according to the results from the exploratory factor analysis (EFA) with varimax rotation performed, the PYTHEIA instrument presents a three-factor model (the "Independent Functionalities" factor, the "Fit to Use," and the "Ease of Use" factors). The overall Cronbach $\alpha$ of PYTHEIA was found to be 0.793, indicating sufficient consistency. The ICC was excellent (ICC = 0.992, $p$ = 0.000), indicating that the PYTHEIA total scores were highly consistent between initial assessment and reassessment. The paired-samples $t$-test between the two instances of administration indicated no statistically significant systematic bias ($p$ = 0.059). Pearson's $r$ correlation coefficient indicated stability of participants' responses over time (Pearson's $r$ = 0.984,

$p$ = 0.000). Examination of item convergent validity showed that all item intercorrelations for all item pairings were strong or excellent. Pearson's $r$ ranged from 0.946 to 0.996 for the first factor "Independent Functionalities," from 0.465 to 0.724 for the second "Fit to Use," and from 0.354 to 0.732 for the third factor "Ease of Use." This provides evidence that all subscales' items are related to the same construct.

## 5. Conclusions

In this paper we conducted a systematic review of the literature in order to identify existing scales for the subjective assessment of rehabilitation and assistive robot devices. We found that most of the studies are utilizing either custom-made questionnaires or interviews that are neither valid nor reliable instruments to represent the subjective opinion and perception of the end users. There is therefore a great gap in the subjective assessment of rehabilitation or assistive robot devices. The absence of standard scales/questionnaires for the subjective assessment of robot-based devices makes it difficult to design products that meet exactly the needs of the intended end users, to further improve prototypes, or to compare the results from different researchers. Based on the findings of the review, in order to further improve the subjective assessment of rehabilitation and assistive robot devices it is necessary for each study to (i) select as subjects the appropriate target group based on clear and valid inclusion criteria, (ii) involve a sufficient number of representative subjects, (iii) analyse statistically the collected data, and (iv) select an established methodology in order to enable comparison between results of different studies.

## Competing Interests

The author declares that there are no competing interests regarding the publication of this paper.

## Acknowledgments

The work leading to the presented results has received funding from the European Union under Grant Agreement no. 600796.

## References

[1] B2B International, "Customer Satisfaction Survey: How to Measure Satisfaction," 2016, https://www.b2binternational.com/publications/customer-satisfaction-survey/.

[2] ESOMAR, "Customer satisfaction studies [Internet]. ESOMAR World Research Codes & Guidelines," 2005, https://www.esomar.org/uploads/public/knowledge-and-standards/codes-and-guidelines/ESOMAR_Codes-and-Guidelines_CustomerSatisfaction.pdf.

[3] Mckinsey.com, "The three Cs of customer satisfaction: consistency, consistency, consistency," January 2016, http://www.mckinsey.com/insights/consumer_and_retail/the_three_cs_of_customer_satisfaction_consistency_consistency_consistency.

[4] A. Gustafsson, M. D. Johnson, and I. Roos, "The effects of customer satisfaction, relationship commitment dimensions,

and triggers on customer retention," *Journal of Marketing*, vol. 69, no. 4, pp. 210–218, 2005.

[5] D. de Sá, "Improving user satisfaction in VO through systems usability," in *Encyclopedia of Networked and Virtual Organizations*, pp. 694–699, IGI Global, 2008.

[6] L. Suskie, "What are good assessment practices?" in *Assessing Student Learning: A Common Sense Guide*, L. Suskie, Ed., Anker, Bolton, Mass, USA, 1st edition, 2004.

[7] Y. Koumpouros, *Information and Communication Technologies & Society*, New Technologies, Athens, Greece, 2012.

[8] Matia Robotics, "Matia Robotics," 2016, http://www.matiarobotics.com/.

[9] MIT News, *MIT-Manus Robot Aids Physical Therapy of Stroke Victims*, 2016, http://news.mit.edu/2000/manus-0607.

[10] Y. Koumpouros, *Information and Communication Technologies in Healthcare*, Hellenic Academic Libraries Link, Athens, Greece, 2015.

[11] C. van Campen, H. Sixma, R. D. Friele, J. J. Kerssens, and L. Peters, "Quality of care and patient satisfaction: a review of measuring instruments," *Medical Care Research and Review*, vol. 52, no. 1, pp. 109–133, 1995.

[12] "Cohrane handbook for systematic reviews of interventions 4.2.6," in *The Cochrane Library*, J. P. T. Higgins and S. Green, Eds., no. 4, John Wiley & Sons, Chichester, UK, 2006.

[13] A. S. Schroeder, R. Von Kries, C. Riedel et al., "Patient-specific determinants of responsiveness to robot-enhanced treadmill therapy in children and adolescents with cerebral palsy," *Developmental Medicine and Child Neurology*, vol. 56, no. 12, pp. 1172–1179, 2014.

[14] The Rehabilitation Measures Database, *Rehab Measures: Fugl-Meyer Assessment of Motor Recovery after Stroke*, 2016, http://www.rehabmeasures.org/lists/rehabmeasures/dispform.aspx?ID=908.

[15] B. C. Craven and A. R. Morris, "Modified ashworth scale reliability for measurement of lower extremity spasticity among patients with SCI," *Spinal Cord*, vol. 48, no. 3, pp. 207–213, 2010.

[16] C. Collin, D. T. Wade, S. Davies, and V. Horne, "The Barthel ADL index: a reliability study," *International Disability Studies*, vol. 10, no. 2, pp. 61–63, 1988.

[17] H. A. Abdullah, C. Tarry, C. Lambert, S. Barreca, and B. O. Allen, "Results of clinicians using a therapeutic robotic system in an inpatient stroke rehabilitation unit," *Journal of NeuroEngineering and Rehabilitation*, vol. 8, no. 1, article 50, 2011.

[18] M. Bortole, A. Venkatakrishnan, F. Zhu et al., "The H2 robotic exoskeleton for gait rehabilitation after stroke: early findings from a clinical study," *Journal of NeuroEngineering and Rehabilitation*, vol. 12, no. 1, article 54, 2015.

[19] T. L. Chen, T. Bhattacharjee, J. L. McKay et al., "Evaluation by expert dancers of a robot that performs partnered stepping via haptic interaction," *PLoS ONE*, vol. 10, no. 5, Article ID e0125179, 2015.

[20] T. L. Chen and C. C. Kemp, "Lead me by the hand," in *Proceeding of the 5th ACM/IEEE International Conference on Human-Robot Interaction (HRI '10)*, pp. 367–374, Osaka, Japan, March 2010.

[21] Y. S. Choi, C. D. Anderson, J. D. Glass, and C. C. Kemp, "Laser pointers and a touch screen: intuitive interfaces for autonomous mobile manipulation for the motor impaired," in *Proceedings of the 10th International ACM SIGACCESS Conference on Computers and Accessibility (ASSETS '08)*, pp. 225–232, October 2008.

[22] P. Coignard, J. P. Departe, O. Remy Neris et al., "ANSO study: evaluation in an indoor environment of a mobile assistance robotic grasping arm," *Annals of Physical and Rehabilitation Medicine*, vol. 56, no. 9-10, pp. 621–633, 2013.

[23] G. G. Grindle, H. Wang, H. Jeannis, E. Teodorski, and R. A. Cooper, "Design and user evaluation of a wheelchair mounted robotic assisted transfer device," *BioMed Research International*, vol. 2015, Article ID 198476, 9 pages, 2015.

[24] M. Heerink, B. Kröse, V. Evers, and B. Wielinga, "Assessing acceptance of assistive social agent technology by older adults: the Almere model," *International Journal of Social Robotics*, vol. 2, no. 4, pp. 361–375, 2010.

[25] M. J. Kim, D. H. Lee, T. Kim et al., "Lower extremity exercise of knee osteoarthritis patients using portable assistive robot (HEXAR-KR40P)," *International Journal of Precision Engineering and Manufacturing*, vol. 15, no. 12, pp. 2617–2622, 2014.

[26] P. N. Kooren, A. G. Dunning, M. M. H. P. Janssen et al., "Design and pilot validation of A-gear: a novel wearable dynamic arm support," *Journal of NeuroEngineering and Rehabilitation*, vol. 12, no. 1, article 83, 2015.

[27] I. Laffont, N. Biard, G. Chalubert et al., "Evaluation of a graphic interface to control a robotic grasping arm: a multicenter study," *Archives of Physical Medicine and Rehabilitation*, vol. 90, no. 10, pp. 1740–1748, 2009.

[28] P. Lam, D. Hebert, J. Boger et al., "A haptic-robotic platform for upper-limb reaching stroke therapy: preliminary design and evaluation results," *Journal of NeuroEngineering and Rehabilitation*, vol. 5, no. 1, article 15, 2008.

[29] C. Liu, C. T. Ishi, and H. Ishiguro, "Bringing the Scene Back to the Tele-operator: auditory scene manipulation for telepresence systems," in *Proceedings of the 10th Annual ACM/IEEE International Conference on Human-Robot Interaction (HRI '15)*, pp. 279–286, Portland, Ore, USA, March 2015.

[30] L. Lopez-Samaniego, B. Garcia-Zapirain, and A. Mendez-Zorrilla, "Memory and accurate processing brain rehabilitation for the elderly: LEGO robot and iPad case study," *Bio-Medical Materials and Engineering*, vol. 24, no. 6, pp. 3549–3556, 2014.

[31] S. Mazzoleni, G. Turchetti, I. Palla, F. Posteraro, and P. Dario, "Acceptability of robotic technology in neuro-rehabilitation: preliminary results on chronic stroke patients," *Computer Methods and Programs in Biomedicine*, vol. 116, no. 2, pp. 116–122, 2014.

[32] K. Ozaki, H. Kagaya, S. Hirano et al., "Preliminary trial of postural strategy training using a personal transport assistance robot for patients with central nervous system disorder," *Archives of Physical Medicine and Rehabilitation*, vol. 94, no. 1, pp. 59–66, 2013.

[33] J. Pineau, A. Atrash, R. Kaplow, and J. Villemure, "On the design and validation of an intelligent powered wheelchair: lessons from the SmartWheeler project," *Advances in Intelligent and Soft Computing*, vol. 83, pp. 259–268, 2010.

[34] H. Wang, J. Xu, G. Grindle et al., "Performance evaluation of the personal mobility and manipulation appliance (PerMMA)," *Medical Engineering & Physics*, vol. 35, no. 11, pp. 1613–1619, 2013.

[35] Y.-H. Wu, J. Wrobel, M. Cornuet, H. Kervhé, S. Damnée, and A.-S. Rrigaud, "Acceptance of an assistive robot in older adults: a mixed-method study of human-robot interaction over a 1-month period in the Living Lab setting," *Clinical Interventions in Aging*, vol. 9, pp. 801–811, 2014.

[36] F. Werner and D. Krainer, "A socially assistive robot to support physical training of older people—an end user acceptance

study," in *Proceedings of the 5th International Conference on Social Robotics (ICSR '13)*, pp. 562–563, Springer, Bristol, UK, October 2013.

[37] I. Treger, S. Faran, and H. Ring, "Robot-assisted therapy for neuromuscular training of sub-acute stroke patients. A feasibility study," *European Journal of Physical and Rehabilitation Medicine*, vol. 44, no. 4, pp. 431–435, 2008.

[38] A.-M. Hughes, J. Burridge, C. T. Freeman et al., "Stroke participants' perceptions of robotic and electrical stimulation therapy: a new approach," *Disability and Rehabilitation: Assistive Technology*, vol. 6, no. 2, pp. 130–138, 2011.

[39] H. Chihara, Y. Takagi, K. Nishino et al., "Factors predicting the effects of hybrid assistive limb robot suit during the acute phase of central nervous system injury," *Neurologia Medico-Chirurgica*, vol. 56, no. 1, pp. 33–37, 2016.

[40] A. M. von der Pütten, N. C. Krämer, and S. C. Eimler, "Living with a robot companion: empirical study on the interaction with an artificial health advisor," in *Proceedings of the ACM International Conference on Multimodal Interaction (ICMI '11)*, pp. 327–334, November 2011.

[41] P. Sale, V. Lombardi, and M. Franceschini, "Hand robotics rehabilitation: feasibility and preliminary results of a robotic treatment in patients with hemiparesis," *Stroke Research and Treatment*, vol. 2012, Article ID 820931, 5 pages, 2012.

[42] COPM, "Learn to Use the COPM," 2013, http://www.thecopm.ca/learn/.

[43] E. Ambrosini, S. Ferrante, M. Rossini et al., "Functional and usability assessment of a robotic exoskeleton arm to support activities of daily life," *Robotica*, vol. 32, no. 8, pp. 1213–1224, 2014.

[44] F. Amirabdollahian, S. Ates, A. Basteris et al., "Design, development and deployment of a hand/wrist exoskeleton for home-based rehabilitation after stroke—SCRIPT project," *Robotica*, vol. 32, no. 8, pp. 1331–1346, 2014.

[45] B. Mónica Faria, S. Vasconcelos, L. Paulo Reis, and N. Lau, "Evaluation of distinct input methods of an intelligent wheelchair in simulated and real environments: a performance and usability study," *Assistive Technology*, vol. 25, no. 2, pp. 88–98, 2013.

[46] J. Brooke, "SUS: a "quick and dirty" usability scale," in *Usability Evaluation Industry*, P. W. Jordan, B. Thomas, B. A. Weerdmeester, and A. I. McClelland, Eds., Taylor and Francis, London, UK, 1996.

[47] L. Chiari, R. Van Lummel, C. Becker, K. Pfeiffer, U. Lindemman, and W. Zijlstra, "Classification of the user's needs, characteristics and scenarios—update," Report from the EU Project (6th Framework Program, IST Contract no. 045622) Sensing and Action to support mobility in Ambient Assisted Living, 2009.

[48] A. J. del-Ama, Á. Gil-Agudo, J. L. Pons, and J. C. Moreno, "Hybrid FES-robot cooperative control of ambulatory gait rehabilitation exoskeleton," *Journal of NeuroEngineering and Rehabilitation*, vol. 11, no. 1, article 27, 2014.

[49] A. Jardón, Á. M. Gil, A. I. de la Peña, C. A. Monje, and C. Balaguer, "Usability assessment of ASIBOT: a portable robot to aid patients with spinal cord injury," *Disability and Rehabilitation: Assistive Technology*, vol. 6, no. 4, pp. 320–330, 2011.

[50] L. Demers, R. Weiss-Lambrou, and B. Ska, *Quebec User Evaluation of Satisfaction with Assistive Technology (QUEST Version 2.0): An Outcome Measure for Assistive Technology Devices*, Institute for Matching Person & Technology, Webster, NY, USA, 2000.

[51] E. M. Holz, J. Höhne, P. Staiger-Sälzer, M. Tangermann, and A. Kübler, "Brain-computer interface controlled gaming: evaluation of usability by severely motor restricted end-users," *Artificial Intelligence in Medicine*, vol. 59, no. 2, pp. 111–120, 2013.

[52] L. Demers, M. Monette, Y. Lapierre, D. L. Arnold, and C. Wolfson, "Reliability, validity, and applicability of the quebec user evaluation of satisfaction with assistive technology (QUEST 2.0) for adults with multiple sclerosis," *Disability and Rehabilitation*, vol. 24, no. 1–3, pp. 21–30, 2002.

[53] Y. Koumpouros, A. Karavasili, E. Papageorgiou, and P. Siavelis, "Validation of the greek version of the device subscale of the quebec user evaluation of satisfaction with assistive technology 2.0 (QUEST 2.0)," *Assistive Technology*, 2016.

[54] A. Steinfeld, T. Fong, D. Kaber et al., "Common metrics for human-robot interaction," in *Proceedings of the 1st ACM SIGCHI/SIGART Conference on Human-Robot Interaction (HRI '06)*, ACM Proceedings, pp. 33–40, 2006.

[55] A. Weiss, R. Bernhaupt, M. Lankes, and M. Tscheligi, "The USUS evaluation framework for human-robot interaction," in *Proceedings of the Symposium on New Frontiers in Human-Robot Interaction (AISB '09)*, pp. 158–165, Edinburgh, UK, April 2009.

[56] C. Bartneck, D. Kulić, E. Croft, and S. Zoghbi, "Measurement instruments for the anthropomorphism, animacy, likeability, perceived intelligence, and perceived safety of robots," *International Journal of Social Robotics*, vol. 1, no. 1, pp. 71–81, 2009.

[57] M. J. Scherer, *Matching Person and Technology Process and Accompanying Assessment Instruments*, Revised Edition, The Institute for Matching Person & Technology, Webster, NY, USA, 1998.

[58] Y. Koumpouros, E. Papageorgiou, A. Karavasili, and D. Alexopoulou, "Translation and validation of the assistive technology device predisposition assessment in Greek in order to assess satisfaction with use of the selected assistive device," *Disability and Rehabilitation: Assistive Technology*, 2016.

[59] P. Palmer, C. Thursfield, and S. Judge, "An evaluation of the psychosocial impact of assistive devices scale," in *Assistive Technology: From Virtuality to Reality*, A. Pruski and H. Knops, Eds., pp. 740–744, IOS Press, Nieuwe Hemweg, The Netherlands, 1st edition, 2005.

[60] M. B. Michel-Verkerke and A. M. G. M. Hoogeboom, "Evaluation of the USE IT-questionnaire for the evaluation of the adoption of electronic patient records by healthcare professionals," *Methods of Information in Medicine*, vol. 52, no. 3, pp. 189–198, 2013.

[61] Y. Koumpouros, E. Papageorgiou, and A. Karavasili, "Development of a new psychometric scale (PYTHEIA) to assess the satisfaction of users with any assistive technology," in *Proceedings of the 7th International Conference on Applied Human Factors and Ergonomics*, IEEE, July 2016.

# Participative Facility Planning for Obstetrical and Neonatal Care Processes: Beginning of Life Process

**Jori Reijula,[1] Sauli Karvonen,[2] Hanna Petäjä,[3] Kari Reijula,[4] and Liisa Lehtonen[3]**

[1]*Finnish Institute of Occupational Health, Neulaniementie 4, 70210 Kuopio, Finland*
[2]*SKA-Research Oy, Teollisuustie 9, 02880 Veikkola, Finland*
[3]*Turku University Hospital, Kiinamyllynkatu 4-8, 20520 Turku, Finland*
[4]*University of Helsinki, Yliopistonkatu 4, 00100 Helsinki, Finland*

Correspondence should be addressed to Jori Reijula; jori.reijula@gmail.com

Academic Editor: Emiliano Schena

*Introduction.* Old hospitals may promote inefficient patient care processes and safety. A new, functionally planned hospital presents a chance to create an environment that supports streamlined, patient-centered healthcare processes and adapts to users' needs. This study depicts the phases of a facility planning project for pregnant women and newborn care processes (beginning of life process) at Turku University Hospital. *Materials and Methods.* Project design reports and meeting documents were utilized to assess the beginning of life process as well as the work processes of the Women's and Children's Hospital. *Results.* The main elements of the facility design (FD) project included rigorous preparation for the FD phase, functional planning throughout the FD process, and setting key values: (1) family-centered care, (2) Lean thinking and Lean tools as the framework for the FD process, (3) safety, and (4) cooperation. *Conclusions.* A well-prepared FD project with sufficient insight into functional planning, Lean thinking, and user-centricity seemed to facilitate the actual FD process. Although challenges occurred, the key values were not forgone and were successfully incorporated into the new hospital building.

## 1. Introduction

Hospital patient care processes are often forced to adapt to impractical facilities. The premises used for different functions of the same process can be scattered around the hospital, a far cry from seamless patient care. Planning a new hospital presents a unique opportunity to address this issue [1].

Functional planning should guide the design of a new hospital [2] and aim to create facilities that support efficient, streamlined, and patient-centered healthcare (HC) processes while avoiding silos [3]. Functional planning for a new hospital starts with a critical review of current processes in order to modify and develop them so that they will function effectively in the new facilities [4]. There should also be goals for improving the quality, safety, and cost-efficiency of treatment and the work environment [5], as well as the wellbeing and satisfaction of users [6].

At Turku University Hospital (H1), the need for a new hospital building was identified. The facilities at H1, which was planned in the 1950s and built in 1968, were becoming obsolete: there were operation bottlenecks, problems with the quality of indoor air, frequent sewage breakdowns, and fire safety issues [7]. Renovation of the old facilities would have stipulated a temporary hospital for the duration of the work. In the case of renovation, the existing tall, narrow, outdated building structure would have set many limitations for creating a functional, modern hospital [8]. Therefore, a planning process was launched to build a new hospital called the Women's and Children's Hospital. One of its core processes was to be the care of pregnant women and newborns. As this process combines obstetrical and neonatal care, it was reasonable to locate all gynecologic and pediatric care in the same building. The group responsible for functional planning related to the care of pregnancies, deliveries, and newborns was called The Beginning of Life Group. It included all antenatal and perinatal care, newborn care, neonatal intensive care, the breast milk bank, and the follow-up clinic for

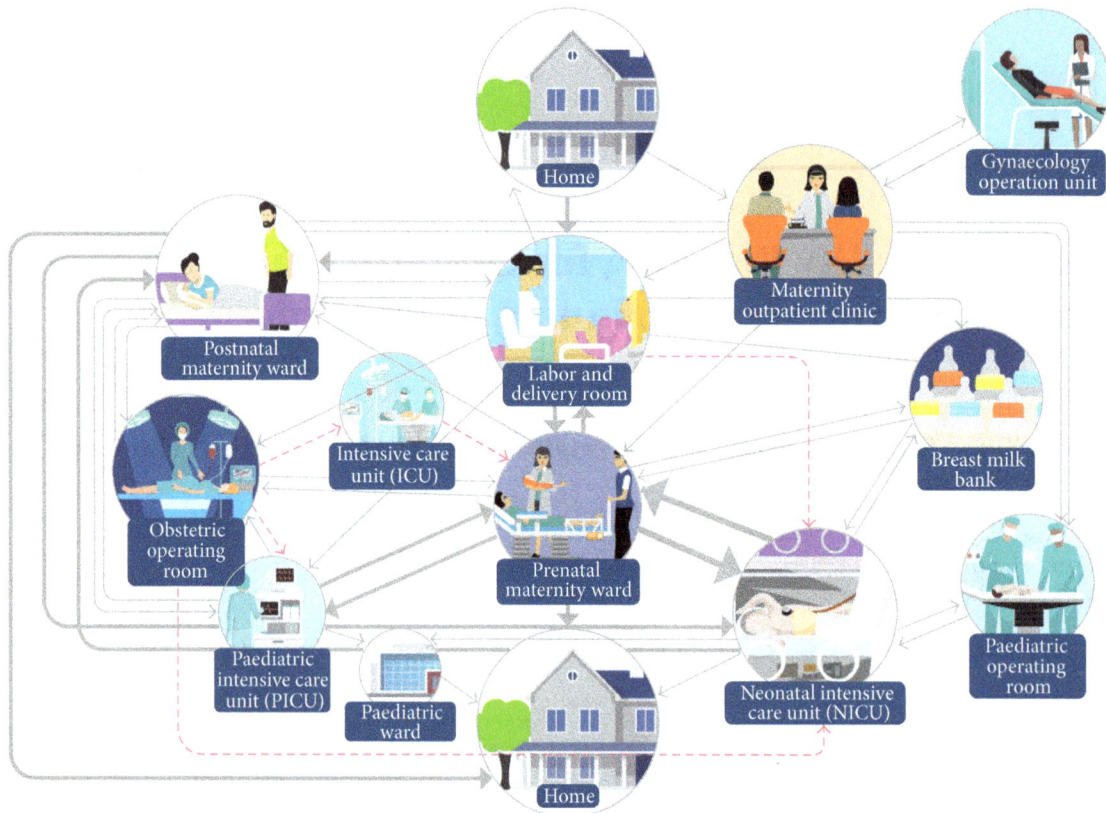

FIGURE 1: The old H1 patient flow process model for the care of pregnant women and newborns. The arrows demonstrate patient transfers between H1 units. The girth of the line delineates the volume of patient flow, with a thick line denoting an intense flow. Critical patient transfers are marked with a dotted red line [15].

very preterm infants. The increasingly popular *Lean thinking* was an integral framework for the functional planning of the process (see [9–11] for more information on Lean HC).

This study aims to depict the formula of functional facility planning carried out by The Beginning of Life Group at H1. The aim is to illuminate the different phases of the facility planning process as well as the most remarkable challenges encountered.

## 2. Materials and Methods

*2.1. Case Hospital.* H1 is one of five university hospitals in Finland and covers a population of approximately one million Finnish citizens. The Beginning of Life Group was led by a pediatrician and included 17 other members: one obstetrician, six midwives, five nurses, one anesthetist, one radiologist, one pharmacist, one patient representative (a parent of two preterm infants, so representing parents and patients), and a project coordinator.

*2.2. Analysis Method.* Three researchers analyzed design reports and meeting documents in order to assess the beginning of life process. The current structure of the process was identified and depicted using a particular patient flow analysis and value stream mapping. The patient flow analysis focuses on describing patients' physical movements in the

hospital [12, 13]. Value stream mapping, a well-known Lean technique, does not describe physical movements of patients precisely but instead focuses on information flow modelling. It also includes lead time information [14]. Thus, the management method used in the planning process is a combination of Lean management and patient flow analysis. Moreover, potentials for synergy, but also bottlenecks, functional problems, and other forms of waste in the process were identified using root cause analysis.

## 3. Results

*3.1. The Current Care Process in the Old Hospital Building.* The structure of H1 was identified as outdated. The hospital layout poorly supported current work processes, which had been revised in the decades since the old hospital was built. Due to the suboptimal hospital layout, work processes were dispersed across several units of the hospital on four different, but not adjacent, floors. In addition, the elevators were commonly sluggish. This caused unnecessary waiting and back-and-forth transfers of patients from one unit to another (see Figure 1). The patient flow in H1 was far from streamlined, as patients were obliged to make several trips between units during a single hospital visit (see Figure 1). Furthermore, the distance (on average approximately 100 meters) from the delivery room to the neonatal intensive care unit (NICU) was

TABLE 1: The key values defined by The Beginning of Life Group.

| Priority | Value | Goal | Example |
|---|---|---|---|
| 1 | Family-centered care | Minimize parent-infant separation | Family rooms |
| 2 | Minimize waste | Create a Lean hospital | Modifiable rooms |
| 3 | Patient and staff safety | Improve hospital safety | Less patient transfers |
| 4 | Cooperation | Improve employee cooperation | Units closer together |

a threat to patient safety as the most ill newborns, after initial resuscitation, had to be transferred seven floors up by elevator and then to the other end of the long building through several doors and over several doorsteps. The reason for the delivery rooms and the NICU not being in close proximity of each other is because there was no modern neonatal intensive care when the old hospital was built.

The insufficient number of patient rooms (12) in the labor and delivery unit caused unnecessary waiting for both mothers and the nursing staff. Only one delivery room in the labor ward had a birth pool, and mothers took turns using the bathing facilities during labor contractions. The lack of space in the delivery rooms and the electric cords lying on the floor presented safety concerns. This was exacerbated by the lack of HC personnel.

The area in the delivery room used for newborn resuscitation and monitoring was small. Therefore, the newborns requiring longer observation or procedures after initial resuscitation were transferred to the NICU, leading to frequent NICU admission.

The mothers of infants cared for at the NICU stayed in the prenatal maternity ward. This caused frequent daily traffic as mothers visited their infants several times a day and returned to their ward for care and meals. After NICU care, as soon as they were stable, over 60% of infants were transferred to the postnatal maternity ward so that mother-infant separation was minimized. Ideally, maternal care and parent beds would be located in the NICU to avoid a large number of within-hospital transfers. In most cases, the limited number of family rooms in the postnatal maternity ward prevented the overnight presence of fathers.

*3.2. Predesign Phase.* The groundwork for the functional design was carried out years before the actual process was initiated. In 2001, a lifecycle decision was made regarding the old H1 Women's and Children's Hospital. It was concluded that the facilities were outdated and needed to be renovated or replaced. However, no official decision was made until 2011, when hospital replacement was agreed upon and the functional design process officially commenced.

Before the actual design process commenced, however, the Department of Pediatrics and the Department of Obstetrics and Gynecology held several joint meetings about their visions for a new hospital. Held between 2005 and 2009, these meetings generated reports about the projected needs of the new hospital space. Key personnel from the Department of Pediatrics and the Department of Obstetrics and Gynecology visited new perinatal centers and centers undergoing renovations or building processes in the United States (e.g., Rainbow Babies and Children's Hospital, Cleveland, Ohio: a three-year

work period in 1997–2000 followed by several visits until 2011), Canada (e.g., Sunnybrook Hospital, Toronto: a visit in 2011), and Sweden (e.g., Uppsala University Hospital: several visits from 2005 and a six-month work period in 2011) to gain insight into state-of-the-art solutions. Key personnel acquainted themselves with the planning processes of these international sites. One crucial observation was that a certain number of key fundamentals should be clearly and thoroughly determined prior to the facility design (FD) process and prioritized during the process. Furthermore, information sharing between hospitals was seen as pertinent. Systematic participation in HC FD forums (e.g., Graven's Conference on the Physical and Developmental Environment of the High Risk Infant) also provided essential knowledge about other hospitals' state-of-the-art innovations and whether they had been good solutions from the users' perspective or nonoptimal solutions which had led to bottlenecks and other unintended functional problems.

*3.3. Design Phase.* A multidisciplinary planning group (n = 17) was founded in 2011 and called The Beginning of Life Group. Its main focus was on developing a functional plan for the beginning of life process including pregnancy, labor, and newborn care. The planning group held approximately 20 design meetings. H1 administration attempted to allocate up to 30% of key personnel's work time for the FD project to cover a six-month period.

The Beginning of Life Group started by discussing the main values that would guide the planning process. Four values were chosen based on the group discussion (Table 1):

(1) Family-centered care was seen as the top priority for the FD. It was operationalized as minimizing parent-infant separation. The new hospital environment was planned to support parents and newborn infants staying together for the entire treatment period. It emphasized the customer point-of-view and attempted to improve user-centricity according to the strategy of the hospital district. Family rooms provide privacy, thereby increasing the comfort of parents and their overnight presence in the hospital.

(2) The group made Lean fundamentals the visible framework for the design phase: eight types of waste in HC (defined in Lean literature) were systematically sought and eliminated. Reducing the number of patient transfers within and between units was an important strategy to eliminate unnecessary work steps (transferring patients and information, signing in and out, and cleaning rooms between patients). Another strategy was to decrease the travel distance

when transferring sick newborns from the delivery room to the NICU. Flexible, modifiable rooms were planned for the NICU that could accommodate the changing needs of a patient throughout their hospital stay (usually beginning with more intensive care and then decreasing in intensity over time).

(3) The group aimed to improve patient and staff safety by various means: effort was made to develop disturbance-free treatment periods, such as fewer transfers within and between units, thereby decreasing communication errors by the staff and minimizing hazards related to the transfer of sick patients. Moreover, single family rooms isolated the patients and their relatives from other patients, decreasing the likelihood of spreading infections.

(4) The group named enhanced cooperation as one method for breaking the boundaries of old silos and reorganizing care based on patient care pathways. This was pursued by creating a single process with a common goal: getting the mother and baby home healthy. The new environment would decrease boundaries between units, even including a stabilization room for newborns in the delivery room where both neonatal nurses and midwives would work together. Midwives would provide care for mothers and their infants in the NICU. The physical proximity of the prenatal maternity ward to the labor and delivery room and the NICU aimed to enhance synergy, cooperation, and communication between the staff of these units.

A parent representative was invited to take part in The Beginning of Life Group so that patient and parent perspectives were taken into account. The representative held discussions with a larger group of parents in a peer-support group in order to bring their views into the planning process.

Information gathered from the staff and secretaries regarding supportive functions proved useful to the design group.

The planning group assessed patient and information flows in order to avoid unnecessary traffic within the hospital and to increase the efficiency of the units. Tools such as value stream mapping were utilized for a patient flow analysis, starting from pregnant women and caesarean sections through to neonatal intensive care and transitions to home. Bottlenecks, functional problems, other forms of waste in the process, and potentials for synergy were identified using root cause analysis. Comments and problems were marked with yellow and red tags, respectively. Furthermore, simulations using a stopwatch were carried out to assess throughput times of critical connections between operating units. After the analysis, the planning group redesigned the whole process according to the four defined key fundamentals.

The key values in the beginning of life process, especially family-centered care, were not up for compromise. These values were subsequently adopted by each of the six functional design groups planning the new Women's and Children's Hospital. The project coordinator and a Lean consultant worked with each of the groups to ensure the desired design methods and values were comprehended.

Functional planning was followed by layout planning alongside the architects. It was seen as favorable that the design team had the chance to alter the hospital layout. The whole staff was involved in commenting on the layout draft based on their experience with clinical processes.

*3.4. Final Outcome of the Beginning of Life Process.* One of the most beneficial structural changes in the developed functional model was the placement of the prenatal maternity ward, the labor and delivery room, and the NICU on the same floor and in immediate proximity to each other. This was done to enable synergies leading to decreased patient traffic and transfers. This would lead to better collaboration between the staff of different units and more continuity in care.

To ensure efficient use of space, functional triage models were suggested for both obstetric and neonatal admissions. When there is a triage space that allows staff to observe the mother on entering the hospital or the newborn after birth, it is more likely that they will be admitted to the most suitable ward.

The goal of the obstetric triage model was to combine pregnant women's emergency care process with delivery room admissions. It was planned for the triage to be located in immediate proximity to the prenatal maternity ward, but for either prenatal maternity ward or labor ward midwives to function as triage nurses. The elective maternity outpatient clinic was to be separate from the emergency care. All acute care was to proceed through a single pathway, in which a midwife was to admit the new patient. All telephone consultations from outside the hospital were to be taken in a centralized call center in the triage space, allowing mothers to be monitored from home before arriving at the hospital (e.g., in the latency phase). Mothers were to be assessed for care or follow-up needs and then either transferred from the triage to the labor and delivery room, to the prenatal maternity ward, or back home if labor was not in progress. Separating the emergency process was expected to decrease traffic in both the maternity outpatient clinic and the labor and delivery room. The labor and delivery room could therefore focus on mothers in active labor and delivery as the prenatal maternity ward would admit emergency patients. The rooms in the prenatal maternity ward were planned for one patient, but with an additional bed for the spouse according to the philosophy of family-centered care.

The inclusion of triage for newborns means that they can be monitored and treated in an adequately sized and equipped stabilization room located in the labor and delivery unit until the need for more extensive intensive care is identified or ruled out. Newborn infants may therefore avoid NICU admission if the symptoms resolve spontaneously and the initial laboratory tests or X-rays rule out the need for longer or more intensive monitoring or treatment. This saves staff costs as well as reserving space for specialized functions. The stabilization room was to have space for a mother's bed next to the newborn.

The integration of obstetric operating rooms for caesarean sections in the labor and delivery room makes the transfer to operation quicker, improves the safety of the mother and the newborn, and improves the efficient use of space as one stabilization room can be used for all newborns whether they are born vaginally or by caesarean section.

In the NICU, single family rooms were designed to accommodate the immediate family of an infant. Modifiable rooms in the NICU enable the care of both mother and infant in one room from admission until transition to home. Importantly, this decreases parent-infant separation for this vulnerable infant population and for parents who are developing an attachment relationship with their child. Parents and family members expressed their appreciation for a feeling of individuality (individual/customized welcome signs and guides), peacefulness (no other patients in the room), and protection of privacy (possibility of blocking visual contact to the room).

The innovations in hospital structures set new demands for the HC personnel, which need to be acknowledged for the benefits of the new structure to be realized. Parents and family members expressed their sensitivity to and the importance of staff attitudes and explained how the feeling of being welcomed affects their willingness to utilize hospital space and to participate in the care of their infant in the hospital. The staff needed to acquire new skills as the new process was different to the old practice, which comprised separate staff for mothers and infants and less parental involvement in the hospital care of their infant. In 2009 the H1 NICU developed and initiated a goal-oriented training program for the entire staff about delivering care in partnership with parents (Close Collaboration with Parents Training Program™) [16] to prepare staff for the new architecture.

The family rooms were to be located as close as possible to the central monitoring stations to minimize the distance between the staff and their patients. The central monitoring stations were seen as valuable for maintaining good teamwork between staff members. A curve-shaped layout was seen as functional for this purpose.

The functional model for the beginning of life process can be seen in Figure 2.

The new model incorporated several desired benefits for patients, parents, and the hospital. The functional model for the beginning of life process simplified and streamlined patient flows and made them more flexible. The new model is believed to create a positive effect on infants' recovery and growth, as well as lowering patient and parent stress level due to increased physical and emotional closeness. Increased feelings of security and decreased levels of stress for the mother may also result from enabling the father's presence. If parents or support persons can be present within the hospital, the workload of hospital personnel might reduce in the long run:

(i) Parents are able to participate in the care of their infants.

(ii) The spouse is able to participate in the care of the mother.

(iii) The patient discharge process may become quicker.

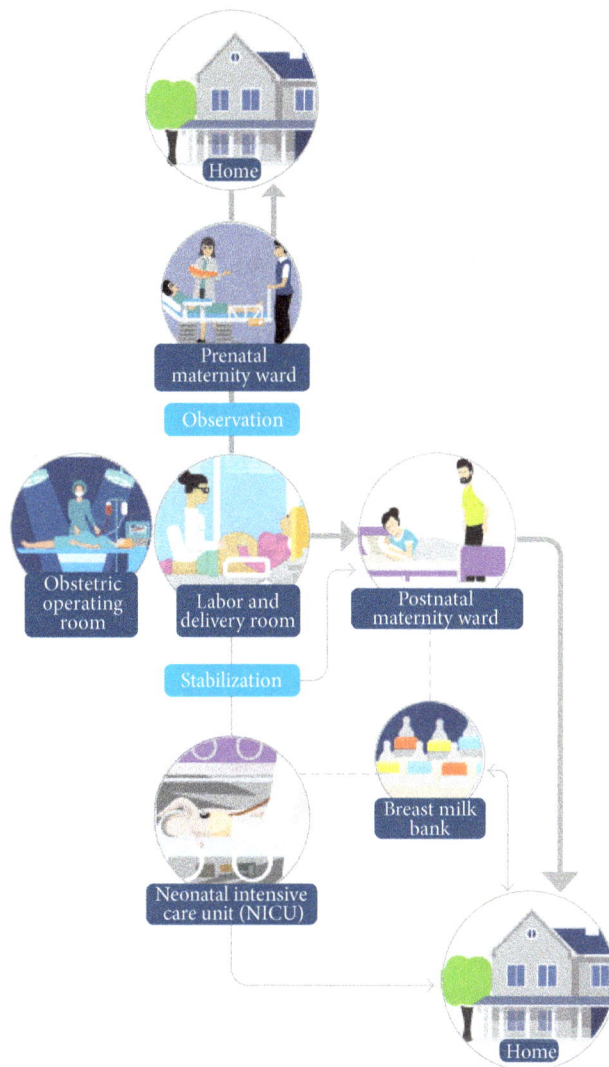

FIGURE 2: The newly developed H1 patient flow process model for the care of pregnant women and newborns. The new process minimizes parent-infant separation by, for example, locating more extensive stabilization for a sick newborn in the delivery room and by designing single family rooms with privacy and facilities for parents to stay overnight alongside their infant. Waste decreases and patient safety improves by, for example, decreasing the need for transitions between hospital wards and by preventing hospital infections with single family rooms. The delivery room and the NICU being in close proximity of each other and on the same floor increases synergy, especially in emergency situations.

3.5. *Challenges Encountered.* The original plans of The Beginning of Life Group were significantly altered during subsequent phases of the building project because the original budget estimate was reduced from €207 million to €158 million. This meant that major spatial reductions had to be made, which in turn decreased the functionality of the space. The required compromises impacted work processes due to heightened competition for space between the units in the hospital.

The design group wished they had been able to engage in earlier and closer contact and communication with the project architects. H1 cooperated with an architect company along the way but committed to them relatively late in the planning process, after funding for the architects had already been agreed upon. Optimally, the architects would have been included in the functional planning group. The functionality had to be explained and demonstrated separately to the architects, which significantly delayed the completion of sketches and also wasted time and effort in the planning process. Several FD group members were not satisfied with the initial sketches by the architects. Thus, the group decided to design the initial sketch of the new hospital independently, without the guidance of architects. After H1 committed to the architecture company, the exchange of information and the relationship gradually improved.

## 4. Discussion

*4.1. What Has Been Learned?* Many functional weaknesses of the old hospital were identified by the leaders and the experienced staff, who were active in initiating preparation for the FD several years before the official mandate was given to prepare a functional plan for a new hospital. The process of learning about different solutions and their strengths, weaknesses, and relevance to the local project was time consuming. It was able to be done cost-effectively when combined with other professional travel during the early stages of the process.

When the official FD phase finally began, a large amount of documentation had been studied and several international visits and work periods in modern design settings had been carried out. The information had been discussed and reflected on in staff meetings. This facilitated the FD process and improved the design quality.

The planning group represented a wide range of professionals who had extensive experience in their roles and many international experiences to draw on for comparison. The inclusion of a patient representative in the planning group was seen as beneficial as her presence and active participation emphasized the patient perspective. Moreover, her contacts with key stakeholders were believed to facilitate the design process. It was seen as a significant weakness that the architects responsible for the layout were not chosen early on in the process, and thereby not included in the group. A real-time link with an architect company might have created solutions to problems which remained unseen in this process.

While clinicians' responsibilities can limit their participation in FD work groups [17], H1 allocated protected FD time for key persons, which proved to be a practical solution. Management needed to carefully weigh their options, such as which clinicians should be assigned to FD work and how intensely they should participate. Even though assigning an experienced HC professional to actively participate in an FD project may at first seem expensive, the investment is likely to benefit the design of the new building and lead to an increased capability of the clinicians to develop work processes suited to the new work environment.

When the total budget was decided, significant compromises had to be made. At this stage, the clearly determined

key values and core goals were critical to keep in mind as priorities. In the planning phase, the priority level of each key value was carefully considered and established. Thus, H1 was able to develop structures for providing family-centered care, for supporting patient safety, and for implementing Lean principles and cooperation.

In Finland, HC is largely provided by the public sector. Thus, competition between hospitals differs from countries in which local, privately funded hospitals compete against each other. Lack of financial competition supports open knowledge sharing between hospitals both within and between countries. Humbleness and open-mindedness in sharing knowledge, FD information, and learning from and collaborating should be prioritized in areas where human lives are at stake [18]. In addition to better functional outcomes, information sharing is cost-efficient as it has the potential to prevent nonfunctional solutions and costly design mistakes. New forums and tools for learning and spreading vital FD information among HC practitioners are required [19].

The main focus for healthcare technology assessment (HTA) frameworks is to evaluate the properties and effects of a certain health technology, addressing the direct and intended effects and consequences of the technology. This helps in informed decision-making regarding health technologies. The HTA Core model is a methodological framework for production and sharing of HTA information [20]. It consists of a standardized set of HTA questions, recommends use of already existing guidance and guidelines, and includes a common reporting structure for presenting findings in a standardized format. Although it might have been useful to provide a proven international bridge between the state-of-the-art evidence-based research and the world of decision-making, it was not implemented due to the designers not being aware of the HTA Core model.

*4.2. Family-Centered Care.* As the top priority for the beginning of life process, family-centered care is likely to provide several benefits. First of all, single family rooms bring family members together and provide privacy, individuality, a sense of closeness, peacefulness, and protection, which have been shown to benefit all family members [21]. There is large, untapped potential for family members to improve the quality of care in both adult and neonatal care. Although the benefits may generate some economic savings for the hospital, the greatest advantages are likely to be seen in the improved wellbeing and satisfaction of the patients and their family members. In the case of newborn care, the benefits for the developing parent-infant relationship and for parents' psychological wellbeing are likely to improve the long-term outcomes of the infants.

Modifiable single family rooms in neonatal intensive care units support three of the key values of the planning: family-centered care, patient safety, and waste minimization. This model increases time efficiency as patients stay in one room for the duration of their hospital stay. The same care team also works with families for the entire time, which is favorable because lack of continuity is one of the most common complaints from parents [22]. This model also prevents hospital-acquired infections and thereby patient and staff safety [23]. Hospital-acquired infections prolong the hospital stay [24] and increase later developmental problems [25]. Therefore, the prevention of infection decreases both short- and long-term costs.

In order to successfully integrate parents in the care team it is advisable to prepare staff with training and practice in advance. In traditional intensive care units, parents have commonly had a passive role, primarily being recipients of information. To make the parents' role meaningful, they need to become information providers and active decision makers alongside staff [16]. Hospital design can emphasize the role of the family: parents need to have facilities that allow them to stay in the unit for several weeks, including overnight sleeping facilities, sanitary facilities, facilities for preparing meals and washing laundry, and rooms for socializing with other families in the unit. In addition, siblings need a play space separate to patient's room. The family rooms should be comfortable and let in daylight so that a long-term stay will be tolerable. Many hospitals have made the move to single family room units without an increase in staffing. Even if greater distances between patient beds and increased parental support requires more time input from staff, the investment is paid back when the parents become more independent in the care routines of their infant. In some hospitals, a move to the single family room model has led to shorter hospital stays [26] but this phenomenon has not been seen in all hospitals [27].

*4.3. Patient Safety.* A complex care process for mothers and infants includes many challenges. It is not necessarily known beforehand who requires more medical attention. Close collaboration and information sharing between staff that specializes in obstetrical and newborn care is crucial for success. The physical closeness of the maternal prenatal ward, the labor and delivery room, and the NICU is especially vital in emergency situations.

*4.4. Lean Thinking.* H1 utilized a unique method of conveying information to the functional work groups in the FD project: a project coordinator from the beginning of life process joined all of the other planning groups and divulged information and working methods. The working methods included value stream mapping, the Lean framework, and brainstorming sessions using extreme models as the starting point [12, 13]. Thus, utilizing this experienced specialist, who participated in each functional work group, proved crucial because the FD groups saved time in their working processes. This arrangement also enabled a standardized protocol to be carried out. The goal for each functional group was to set their own, customized FD priorities and incorporate their specialized needs into the building layout. The Lean ideology of streamlining patient care processes was taught to the user group representatives. Based on work flow processes, layouts for the new building were designed.

As the budget unexpectedly decreased during the project, significant spatial reductions had to be undertaken. Attempting to find answers, H1 FD personnel resorted to Lean hospital design, which suggested the centralization of HC work processes in order to utilize the space efficiently, with a focus on critical connections for patient flow [3]. H1

embraced these proposals and was successful in managing the reductions.

The triage model aimed to organize HC personnel among the care pathways in a way that would, ideally, suit the patient flow. By utilizing value stream maps, each step among the patient care pathway was optimized and the bottlenecks that were hindering the provision of efficient patient care were eliminated [28]. The key innovation was in combining care processes so that the route traveled by the patient was as quick and effortless as possible. A wide array of research supports centralizing and streamlining acute care processes to emphasize fluent patient flow [29, 30]. Multiprofessional assessment of the patient, with the possibility of observation time in an early phase, saves patient transfers as well as time later in the care process. Furthermore, home monitoring before delivery and early discharge lowers patient care expenses.

*4.5. Future Challenges.* Despite the vast majority of scientific evidence pointing to the benefits of family-centered care [31, 32], mixed opinions and uncertainty have prevailed in some HC institutions [33]. Thus, gaining management approval to adopt and implement solutions such as single family rooms may prove difficult. H1's Beginning of Life Group made calculations to convince the management of the benefits of initial investment for larger single family rooms. This was cumbersome as there is a lack of cost-benefit analyses related to single family room design.

## 5. Conclusions

In the wake of stifling pressure to create enhanced facilities for providing efficient HC, H1 FD personnel have demonstrated self-initiative and creativity in laying the groundwork for the FD process. Rigorous preparation has paid dividends and facilitated the FD process. Family-centered care, patient safety, Lean thinking, and cooperation were chosen by The Beginning of Life Group as the key values needed to achieve the core goals for the new hospital. This strategy was successful, as the four fundamentals have made a strong imprint on the FD process and have visibly guided it.

The FD based on functional planning is a good start. The ultimate quest lies in implementing the new functional schemes into the new facilities. Thus, the employees hold the keys to making the changes enabled by the new design. Implementing the functional principles among the staff is an ongoing process. Strong, determined, and insightful leadership should provide a solid foundation.

## Competing Interests

The authors declare that there is no conflict of interests regarding the publication of this paper.

## Acknowledgments

The authors are grateful to the Finnish Work Environment Fund and the Finnish Institute of Occupational Health for funding the research. They would also like to thank the following colleagues for their generous information sharing:

Dr. Michelle Walsh and Dr. Jonathan Fanaroff from Rainbow Babies and Children's Hospital, Cleveland, Ohio; Elizabeth MacMillan, RN, from Sunnybrook Hospital, Toronto; and Dr. Uwe Ewald from Uppsala University Hospital.

# References

[1] J. Reijula, N. Nevala, M. Lahtinen, V. Ruohomäki, and K. Reijula, "Lean design improves both health-care facilities and processes: a literature review," *Intelligent Buildings International*, vol. 6, no. 3, pp. 170–185, 2014.

[2] J. Reijula, J. Kouri, L. Aalto, R. Miettunen, and K. Reijula, "Healthcare facility design development in Kuopio University Hospital," *Intelligent Buildings International*, 2015.

[3] N. Grunden and C. Hagood, *Lean-Led Hospital Design: Creating the Efficient Hospital of the Future*, Productivity Press, Boca Raton, Fla, USA, 2012.

[4] P. P. Sun, "An integrated project delivery process: providing information, sustainability, and humanization for the last independent hospital in San Francisco," in *Proceedings of the 28th International Public Health Seminar*, Firenze, Alinea, 2009.

[5] B. L. Sadler, L. L. Berry, R. Guenther et al., "Fable hospital 2.0: the business case for building better health care facilities," *Hastings Center Report*, vol. 41, no. 1, pp. 13–23, 2011.

[6] E. Schreuder, L. van Heel, R. Goedhart, E. Dusseldorp, J. M. Schraagen, and A. Burdorf, "Effects of newly designed hospital buildings on staff perceptions: a pre-post study to validate design decisions," *Health Environments Research and Design Journal*, vol. 8, no. 4, pp. 77–97, 2015.

[7] J. Reijula, R. Holopainen, E. Kähkönen, K. Reijula, and I. D. Tommelein, "Intelligent HVAC systems in hospitals," *Intelligent Buildings International*, vol. 5, no. 2, pp. 101–119, 2013.

[8] J. Reijula, E. Reijula, and K. Reijula, "Insight into healthcare design: lessons learned in two university hospitals," *Journal of Facilities Management*, vol. 14, no. 3, 2016.

[9] J. S. Toussaint and L. L. Berry, "The promise of lean in health care," *Mayo Clinic Proceedings*, vol. 88, no. 1, pp. 74–82, 2013.

[10] J. P. Womack and D. Miller, *Going Lean in Health Care*, Institute for Healthcare Improvement, Cambridge, Mass, USA, 2005.

[11] M. Graban, *Lean Hospitals—Improving Quality, Patient Safety and Employee Engagement*, CRC Press, Boca Raton, Fla, USA, 2012.

[12] S. Karvonen, H. Korvenranta, M. Paatela, and T. Seppälä, "Production flow analysis: a tool for designing a lean hospital," *World Hospitals and Health Services*, vol. 43, no. 1, pp. 28–31, 2007.

[13] S. Karvonen, M. Lehto, and J. Elo, "Patient flow analysis: planning a new surgery unit," *British Journal of Health Care Management*, vol. 18, no. 2, pp. 96–102, 2012.

[14] J. K. Liker, *The Toyota Way: 14 Management Principles from the World's Greatest Manufacturer*, McGraw-Hill Press, New York, NY, USA, 2004.

[15] S. Karvonen, *U2 Patient Flow Analysis*, Turku University Hospital, Turku, Finland, 2012.

[16] S. Ahlqvist-Björkroth, Z. Boukydis, A. M. Axelin, and L. Lehtonen, "Close Collaboration with Parents™ Intervention to Improve Parents' Psychological well-being and child development: description of the Intervention and Study Protocol," *Behavioural Brain Research*, 2016.

[17] A. J. Ramirez, J. Graham, M. A. Richards et al., "Burnout and psychiatric disorder among cancer clinicians," *British Journal of Cancer*, vol. 71, no. 6, pp. 1263–1269, 1995.

[18] S. Ryu, S. H. Ho, and I. Han, "Knowledge sharing behavior of physicians in hospitals," *Expert Systems with Applications*, vol. 25, no. 1, pp. 113–122, 2003.

[19] M. N. K. Boulos, I. Maramba, and S. Wheeler, "Wikis, blogs and podcasts: a new generation of Web-based tools for virtual collaborative clinical practice and education," *BMC Medical Education*, vol. 6, article 41, 2006.

[20] K. Lampe, M. Mäkelä, M. V. Garrido et al., "The HTA core model: a novel method for producing and reporting health technology assessments," *International Journal of Technology Assessment in Health Care*, vol. 25, no. 2, pp. 9–20, 2009.

[21] H. Chaudhury, A. Mahmood, and M. Valente, "Advantages and disadvantages of single-versus multiple-occupancy rooms in acute care environments: a review and analysis of the literature," *Environment & Behavior*, vol. 37, no. 6, pp. 760–786, 2005.

[22] K. Finlayson, A. Dixon, C. Smith, F. Dykes, and R. Flacking, "Mothers' perceptions of family centred care in neonatal intensive care units," *Sexual and Reproductive Healthcare*, vol. 5, no. 3, pp. 119–124, 2014.

[23] M. E. Detsky and E. Etchells, "Single-patient rooms for safe patient-centered hospitals," *The Journal of the American Medical Association*, vol. 300, no. 8, pp. 954–956, 2008.

[24] A. Ohlin, L. Björkman, F. Serenius, J. Schollin, and K. Källen, "Sepsis as a risk factor for neonatal morbidity in extremely preterm infants," *Acta Paediatrica*, vol. 104, no. 11, pp. 1070–1076, 2015.

[25] A. Mitha, L. Foix-L'Hélias, C. Arnaud et al., "Neonatal infection and 5-year neurodevelopmental outcome of very preterm infants," *Pediatrics*, vol. 132, no. 2, pp. e372–e380, 2013.

[26] A. Örtenstrand, B. Westrup, E. B. Broström et al., "The Stockholm neonatal family centered care study: effects on length of stay and infant morbidity," *Pediatrics*, vol. 125, no. 2, pp. e278–e285, 2010.

[27] B. M. Lester, K. Hawes, B. Abar et al., "Single-family room care and neurobehavioral and medical outcomes in preterm infants," *Pediatrics*, vol. 134, no. 4, pp. 754–760, 2014.

[28] J. Reijula and I. D. Tommelein, "Lean hospitals: a new challenge for facility designers," *Intelligent Buildings International*, vol. 4, no. 2, pp. 126–143, 2012.

[29] L. D. Martin, S. E. Rampersad, D. K. W. Low, and M. A. Reed, "Process improvement in the operating room using Toyota (Lean) methods," *Revista Colombiana de Anestesiologia*, vol. 42, no. 3, pp. 220–228, 2014.

[30] E. W. Dickson, S. Singh, D. S. Cheung, C. C. Wyatt, and A. S. Nugent, "Application of lean manufacturing techniques in the emergency department," *The Journal of Emergency Medicine*, vol. 37, no. 2, pp. 177–182, 2009.

[31] M. F. Petersen, J. Cohen, and V. Parsons, "Family-centered care: do we practice what we preach?" *Journal of Obstetric, Gynecologic, & Neonatal Nursing*, vol. 33, no. 4, pp. 421–427, 2004.

[32] A. Maria and R. Dasgupta, "Family-centered care for sick newborns: a thumbnail view," *Indian Journal of Community Medicine*, vol. 41, no. 1, pp. 11–15, 2016.

[33] I. Van De Glind, S. De Roode, and A. Goossensen, "Do patients in hospitals benefit from single rooms? A literature review," *Health Policy*, vol. 84, no. 2-3, pp. 153–161, 2007.

# 3

# Stress Detection Using Low Cost Heart Rate Sensors

**Mario Salai, István Vassányi, and István Kósa**

*Medical Informatics R&D Centre, University of Pannonia, Egyetem Utca 10, Veszprém 8200, Hungary*

Correspondence should be addressed to István Vassányi; vassanyi@almos.vein.hu

Academic Editor: Valentina Camomilla

The automated detection of stress is a central problem for ambient assisted living solutions. The paper presents the concepts and results of two studies targeted at stress detection with a low cost heart rate sensor, a chest belt. In the device validation study ($n = 5$), we compared heart rate data and other features from the belt to those measured by a gold standard device to assess the reliability of the sensor. With simple synchronization and data cleaning algorithm, we were able to select highly (>97%) correlated, low average error (2.2%) data segments of considerable length from the chest data for further processing. The protocol for the clinical study ($n = 46$) included a relax phase followed by a phase with provoked mental stress, 10 minutes each. We developed a simple method for the detection of the stress using only three time-domain features of the heart rate signal. The method produced accuracy of 74.6%, sensitivity of 75.0%, and specificity of 74.2%, which is impressive compared to the performance of two state-of-the-art methods run on the same data. Since the proposed method uses only time-domain features, it can be efficiently implemented on mobile devices.

## 1. Introduction

Stress is commonly defined as a feeling of strain and pressure [1]. There is evidence that stress is linked with many diseases, playing a crucial role in the development of cardiovascular diseases [2], diabetes [3], or asthma [4], and it also significantly influences the later course of these diseases. Stress is related to life style; therefore, especially for mobile automated lifestyle counseling and analysis services, the need arises to identify stress automatically during daytime, using physiological data from various sensors. If stress could be reliably and automatically identified, this could directly help users manage stress situations, and it could also be used in medical intelligence applications, for example, in refining blood glucose predictions for diabetics during daytime under influence of stress. However, the available methods for automated stress detection based on low price, ubiquitous sensors, are yet immature. Telemonitoring and self-management systems [5–9] extend the horizons of traditional health care using only point of care measurement data, but the proper interpretation and reliability of the results depend on the reliability of the measured data and the sensor itself.

The two crucial questions related to this problem are as follows:

(i) Whether low price physiological sensors are reliable enough compared to "gold standard" devices accepted by and used in clinical practice.

(ii) Which sensors and algorithms can provide a reliable method for stress detection, at an affordable price and minimal user interaction.

This paper describes our efforts and results in answering these questions. The rest of this paper is organized as follows. Section 1 gives an overview on applicable technologies and related research. In Section 2, we describe our methods for a small scale device validation and the methods used in the main clinical study that compared heart rate variability (HRV) features between relaxation and mental stress periods. We also present here a simple stress detection algorithm. Section 3 presents the measurement results of the two studies, with the latter compared with two state-of-the-art algorithms. We conclude the strengths and weaknesses of this study and the newly designed stress detection algorithm in Section 4.

The most commonly used physiological markers of stress are as follows:

(i) Galvanic skin response (GSR): using changes in skin conductivity. During stress, resistance of skin drops due to increased secretion in sweating glands [10].

(ii) Electromyogram (EMG): measuring electrical activity of the muscles. Stress causes differences in the contraction of the muscles which can be used to identify stress [11, 12].

(iii) Skin temperature: changes in temperature of the skin are related to the stress level [13].

(iv) Electrical activity of the heart: the most commonly used stress marker parameters derived from the electrocardiograph (ECG) are the heart rate (HR) and the heart rate variability (HRV) [14].

Stress can also be detected using other, less common markers like accelerometer [15], key stroke dynamics [16], or blinking [17]. It is also common to use a combination of several markers at the expense of an increased system cost and user involvement. Fernandes et al. used GSR and blood pressure (BP) markers [18] for determining stress. Sun et al. describe mental stress detection using combined data from ECG, GSR, and accelerometer [19]. De Santos Sierra et al. in [20] used GSR and HR. Rigas et al. used ECG, GSR, and respiration for detecting stress while driving [21]. Wijsman et al. used ECG, respiration, GSR, and EMG of trapezius muscles for mental stress detection [22]. Riera et al. combined EEG and EMG markers [23]. Singh and Queyam used GSR, EMG, respiration, and HR [24] for detecting stress during driving. Pupil diameter, ECG, and photoplethysmogram were used as markers by Mokhayeri et al [25]. Baltaci and Gokcay used pupil diameter and temperature features in stress detection [26], while Choi used HRV, respiration, GSR, EMG, acceleration, and geographical location [27].

New noncontact methods have also been developed recently to measure stress states. Some of them are hyperspectral imaging technique [28], human voice [29, 30], pupil diameter [31], visible spectrum camera [32], or using stereo thermal and visible sensors [33].

However, observing several markers for identifying stress requires an increasing number of input sensors which in turn increases the overall price and lowers applicability. Prices for heart rate meters range from $70 to $500 USD; GSR devices range from $100 to $500 USD, while EMG devices have price ranges from $450 USD up to $1750 USD. Systems combining multiple sensors are priced much higher. For such systems prices fall between $550 USD and $5700 USD, which already can be considered excessive for a mass telemedical lifestyle counseling application. Therefore, in an ambient assisted living (AAL) system, the number of input sensors should be kept minimal. In the rest of the paper, we focus on the simplest and most researched sensor input, that is, the electrical activity of the heart.

As for the reliability of HRV sensors, there are still surprisingly few reviews reported in the literature to date on the validation of the information content of low cost sensors compared to a clinically accepted "gold standard" device. Some devices that were tested for validity are the SenseWear HR Armband [34], the Smart Health Watch [35], the Actiheart [36, 37], the Equivital LifeMonitor [38], and the PulseOn [39]; and also the Bioharness multivariable monitoring device from Zephyr has been tested for validity [40, 41] and reliability [41, 42]. In all cases, a gold standard

device was used simultaneously with the device under test as a method for validating data. However, the validated devices above are high-end devices with a considerable price which present an obstacle for the penetration of telemedicine. For example, the Bioharness device has a price around $550 USD, whereas the price of low cost heart rate meters varies from $70 USD to $100 USD. The lack of reliability tests of low cost devices was our motivation for our device validation study.

For automated stress detection, several methods have been published which use only HRV. In 2008, Kim et al. collected HRV data from sixty-eight subjects [43]. HRV data were collected during three different time periods. High stress decreased HRV features. A maximum classification accuracy of 66.1% was achieved. Melillo et al. in 2011 used nonlinear features of HRV for real-life stress detection [44]. HRV data were collected two times, during university examination and after holidays, on 42 students. Most of HRV features significantly decreased during stress period. Stress detection with classification accuracy of 90% was reported using two *Poincaré* plot features and Approximate Entropy. One year later, using the same data, they designed a classification tree for automatic stress detection based on LF and pNN50 HRV features with sensitivity of 83.33% [45]. In 2013, Karthikeyan et al. created stress detection classifiers from ECG signal and HRV features [46]. Vanitha and Suresh used a hierarchical classifier to classify stress into four levels with a classification efficiency of 92% [47] in 2014. In 2015 Munla et al. used an SVM-RBF classifier to predict driver stress with an accuracy of 83% [48].

## 2. Methods

The main goal of this study is the development of a reliable, robust, low price stress detection method suitable for mobile health applications. The study included two distinct phases. In the first phase (device validation study) we tested the reliability of a low cost telemedical heart rate sensor against an accepted medical device. In the second phase we performed and evaluated a clinical study, using the validated telemedical sensor.

### 2.1. Device Validation Study

*2.1.1. Sensor Selection and Measurement Protocol.* Among many low cost devices, we have chosen and analyzed CardioSport TP3 Heart Rate Transmitter device, a simple commercial chest belt, as a source of heart rate data, because this is one of the few devices that can measure both heart rate and millisecond accurate RR time interval data. Since this device does not have its own memory for storing data, we used a Nexus 7 tablet with Android version 4.4.2 to connect to the device with the bluetooth 4.0 protocol and store the measured data on the tablet. The reference "gold standard" device was a Schiller MT-101/MT-200 Holter device which was designed for clinical use (see Figure 1).

Five healthy male volunteers used the two devices simultaneously during a 24-hour long period in order to make the measurements (see Figure 1). For chest belt sensors, the temporary detachment or dislocation of the sensor during

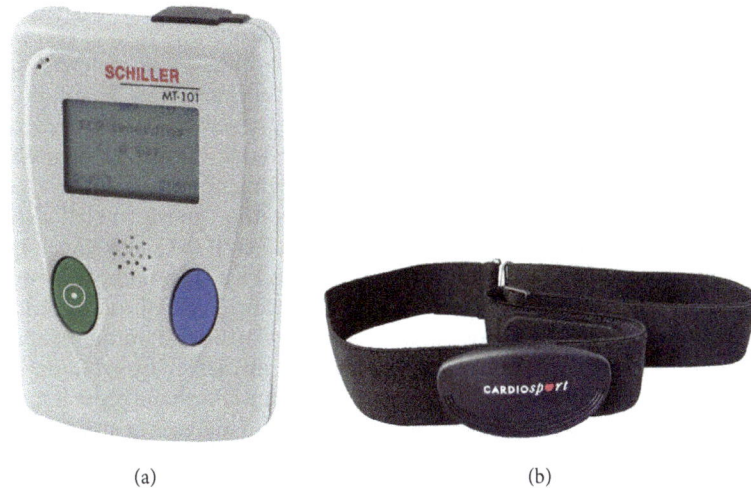

(a) (b)

FIGURE 1: The Schiller MT-101/MT-200 device (a) and the CardioSport TP3 Heart Rate Transmitter device (b).

physical activity or sleep is a common source of errors according to our experiences. Though this problem could be mitigated by using tapes for fixing the device firmly to the body, we felt that such discomfort would not be tolerated in a real AAL situation, so we did not use tapes and used only the daytime 12 hours of the overall signal for analysis. After the monitoring period, we collected the devices and stored the measured data in a unified database.

The protocol was reviewed and approved by the institutional ethics review board in January 2014. The volunteers expressed their informed consent to participate and expressed that they understand the goals of the study before the experiment.

The comparison of the measured data was a hard task due to the different designs of the gold standard and the telemedical device. However, we wanted to compare signals directly in the time domain and also to develop a data cleaning algorithm for the removal of the noisy parts of the CardioSport device measurements, without using the gold standard data. As the chest belt is not firmly attached to the body, even a slight movement of the device could sometimes cause signal loss (especially during sleep). Therefore, we created a software module for synchronization and data cleaning before any further analysis. Data cleaning meant to remove obviously bad data (artifacts) and to keep only "good" data segments of sufficient length, because, as a rule of thumb, both HRV and *Poincaré* plot computation require data chunks of at least 5 minutes. Even though the data cleaning algorithm removes lots of data from the original signal, such a procedure poses no great obstacles for further calculations since we still have enough "good" data during daytime.

*2.1.2. Synchronization Procedure.* Since the time stamps of the measured records can shift due to device buffering, we used a simple procedure to synchronize the data measured by the CardioSport device with those measured by the gold standard device in order to facilitate their comparison. The algorithm uses a sliding window that passes from the beginning of the chest belt signal to the end and calculates the absolute error between the two signals. When sliding is over, the location of the sliding window with the minimum absolute error is considered as the point where the two signals should be synchronized. This applies only if the correlation of the data in the sliding window and the same amount of data from the gold standard are higher than a minimum set by the user. If these conditions are met, the algorithm copies data from the sliding window into a newly generated third signal which represents the chest belt signal fully synchronized with the gold standard signal. If conditions are not met, the third signal is filled with zeros. At the end, the algorithm extracts all the highly correlated segments from the third signal skipping zero values. Also, a file with all the merged segments is generated for general analysis. The algorithm uses the following 5 main parameters, with their values determined empirically in parentheses:

(i) Window size: how much data is copied from the signal into the sliding window (default: 200).

(ii) Window shift step: number of samples by which we shift the sliding window in each iteration (default: 50).

(iii) Absolute error window: how much data will be used to calculate the minimum absolute error (default: 200).

(iv) Maximum error distance: number of samples by which we shift the absolute error window in order to find the minimum absolute error (default: 1000).

(v) Minimum correlation: minimum correlation, expressed as a percentage, required for the two signals to consider data in the chest belt signal accurate (default: 97%).

*2.1.3. Statistical Analysis and Data Processing.* We performed time- and frequency-domain analysis and computed the correlation and mean absolute percentage error of the two measurements. We also compared the slope of the scatter plot diagrams of the two measurements.

The time- and frequency-domain analysis for HRV was performed in Kubios HRV analysis software, while the rest of the analysis was performed in Microsoft Excel.

We developed a simple *data cleaning algorithm* to be used in a real telemedical scenario, for automatically finding good parts of the signal, even without gold standard data. This means finding gaps and abnormal values and skipping them. First, we compare the timestamp of each data item with the timestamp of the previous one. If the difference between the timestamps is bigger than 3 seconds, we mark this data as a gap. Three seconds is used for gap detection because the chest belt has a buffering system that can tolerate short detachments of the device from the body. If more than 3 seconds is used, some data could be missing which could cause errors in further data analysis. In the second step we identify abnormal values in the signal. It is important to emphasize that we do not modify the data in any way as this could potentially result in false results in the subsequent analysis. Instead, abnormal values are treated the same way as gaps. The abnormal values are identified by observing the mean value of 20 contiguous samples (10 previous and 10 following ones). If this mean value differs from the value of the current sample by more than 300, we consider it invalid and mark as gap/error in the signal. Finally, we extract the good segments from the signal with a length of more than 5 minutes.

### 2.2. Clinical Study

#### 2.2.1. Measurement Protocol.
46 healthy volunteers, mostly university and high school students (27 men and 19 women; average age: 24.6 years), participated in the experiment. The experiment was divided into two parts with a duration of 10 minutes each, so the whole procedure lasted for 20 minutes. In the first part, the participants were asked to try to relax in upright sitting position while listening to relaxation music. The second part of the experiment was a mental task designed to serve as a source of mental stress. We used the Stroop color test smartphone game [49] which is commonly applied to induce mental stress in similar studies. In this game, the user must connect colors to labels at an ever increasing pace. Since controlled breathing and posture have been reported before influencing HRV features, we asked the participants not to control their breathing and to sit still in the same position during the whole experiment. This was also necessary to prevent the detachment of the chest belt from the body. RR intervals were recorded using the CardioSport TP3 Heart Rate Transmitter. The participant was asked about her/his subjective stress levels on a relative scale three times, that is, before the experiment, after the relaxation part, and after the game playing part. The answers along with her/his age and gender were recorded in a simple questionnaire (see Appendices A-B). The reason for such questions was that, though less expected, game playing may be more relaxing for some people than music, and only if we actually succeeded in raising the stress level in the second part compared to the first part, can we expect any algorithm or method to detect the

stress. After the recording, the device was unmounted from the participant.

The protocol was reviewed and approved by the institutional ethics review board in January 2014. The volunteers expressed their informed consent to participate and expressed that they understand the goals of the study before the experiment.

After the experiment all data was stored in a unified database, and the data cleaning algorithm described in Section 2.1 was run on both 10-minute parts of each record. Those participants whose records contained no "clean" segments of at least 5 minutes in both parts were excluded from the further analysis. Similarly, we excluded those who—despite our efforts for provoking stress in the experiment—reported no increase of stress level due to game playing.

#### 2.2.2. Statistical Analysis.
We used the Kubios software package for getting HRV features and later we analyzed and compared data using the MedCalc software and Microsoft Excel. Wilcoxon paired-samples test was used as a tool for determining significant changes between the two parts of the experiment for the measured values of the HRV features and a $p$ value of $< 0.05$ was considered as significant. Correlation, percentage differences, average percentage differences, and minimum percentage differences were also calculated for all the observed HRV features.

#### 2.2.3. Stress Detection Algorithm.
We developed a simple algorithm to detect stress that uses only time-domain HRV features. The reason for excluding frequency-domain features is that they require much more computing power to calculate than time-domain features, an argument that we should consider in a solution designed for mobile devices. We used a combination of the mean HR, pNN50, and RMSSD features to identify stress. A sliding window over the HR signal was divided into four equal parts. We tested various lengths of the sliding window and the shortest width of the window that achieved good result was 560 RR intervals with shift of 20 RR intervals in each step. We used brute force technique to find best threshold values for each HRV feature. As a result, stress is detected by the algorithm if the mean heart rate in the fourth part compared to the first part increases by more than 5%, and RMSSD and pNN50 values decrease by more than 9% in the fourth part compared to the third part. We must emphasize here that this algorithm does not detect rest state. So for the sake of calculating accuracy, specificity, and sensitivity, rest state is considered if stress was not detected. The state of the subject after stressor is also not recognized. Therefore, instead of detecting the subject's physiological state of stress, the purpose of our algorithm is to detect those stressful events which have negative impact on the subject's current state but which may or may not lead the subject into a stressful state. A series of stressful events instead of a single major event can also gradually put the subject into a stressful condition. In a binary classification model this could lead to the false conclusion that only the last event was the one which caused stress, while all the previous events are not taken into consideration and remain hidden.

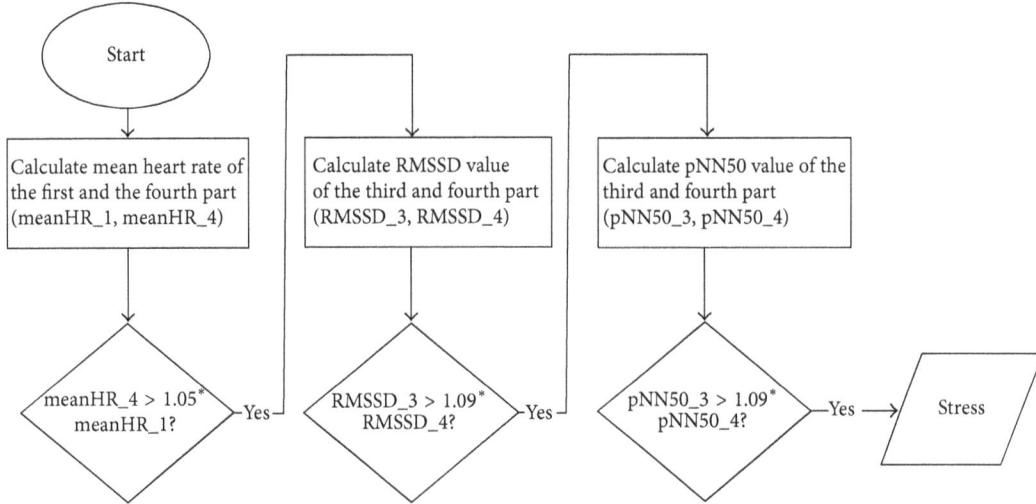

FIGURE 2: Flow chart of stress detection algorithm.

We note that though it is true that the HRV features may be due to other factors such as depression and mood, we postulate that these factors do not change during the experiment. In contrast, the proposed method uses a well-defined *change* in the HRV features to detect the beginning of the (induced) stressful state; therefore we expect no false positive stress detections due to such factors.

Figure 2 shows a summary flow chart of the proposed stress detection algorithm which implements the above procedure.

In order to test the power of this algorithm, we compared its performance to two state-of-the-art algorithms from the same author, Melillo et al. [31, 32], on the same dataset.

*2.2.4. Performance Comparison to a Linear HRV Algorithm.* The algorithm described in [45] uses the pNN50 feature from the time domain and the LF feature from the frequency domain to create a simple classification tree. Stress is detected if LF < 899.58 and pNN50 > 0.9873 or if LF > 277.28 and pNN50 < 0.9873. Restful state is detected if LF > 899.59 or if LF > 277.28 and pNN50 < 0.9783.

For extracting the LF and pNN50 features, we used the same software as the authors of this algorithm, Kubios. Our experiment consisted of two 10 minutes long periods so we extracted two 5 minutes long segments from relaxation part and two 5-minute segments from game playing part. If stress was detected in any one of them, we marked the whole 10-minute part as STRESS. If both parts were detected as REST, then whole 10-minute part was marked as REST.

*2.2.5. Performance Comparison to a Nonlinear HRV Algorithm.* A stress detection method based on nonlinear analysis [44] was the next algorithm we used. This algorithm uses three nonlinear features: Poincaré plot SD1, Poincaré plot SD2, and Approximate Entropy (En). According to the method, stress is found if

$$10.64 + 203.99 \cdot SD1 - 108.74 \cdot SD2 - 8.26 \cdot En\,(0.2) \tag{1}$$
$$> 0.$$

TABLE 1: Signal durations after the synchronization process.

| Subject number | #1 | #2 | #3 | #4 | #5 |
|---|---|---|---|---|---|
| Duration (hh:mm:ss) | 2:06:18 | 10:53:28 | 8:45:40 | 10:30:17 | 7:46:56 |

To reconstruct this algorithm we used Microsoft Visual C# to calculate Approximate Entropy based on formula described by authors. A sliding window was used to scan the whole relaxation part as well as the game playing part. If stress was found in any step, we marked the whole 10-minute period as STRESS and, similarly, if rest was detected on all steps of whole part, we marked that part as REST.

In order to compare the performances of the three methods, we computed the accuracy, specificity, and sensitivity for each of them. For this, we registered a true positive result if the method marked the game playing part as STRESS, a true negative result if the relax music part was marked as REST, a false positive result if the relax music part was marked as STRESS, and a false negative result if the game playing part was marked as REST.

## 3. Results

*3.1. Device Validation Study: Comparison with the Gold Standard.* After running the synchronization process, we got segments of highly correlated data. Figure 1 shows how the lengths of signal segments are distributed. We can see that most segments are 3–18 minutes long. The longest segment that is highly correlated with the gold standard data is 110 minutes long. The default parameter settings minimize the number of overly short (<5 min) segments. Most of the bad segments (Figure 3) are shorter than one minute, and only one bad segment was 60 minutes long.

The synchronization procedure resulted in highly (>97%) correlated synchronized data segments with various durations. Table 1 shows the overall duration of signals. Subject #1

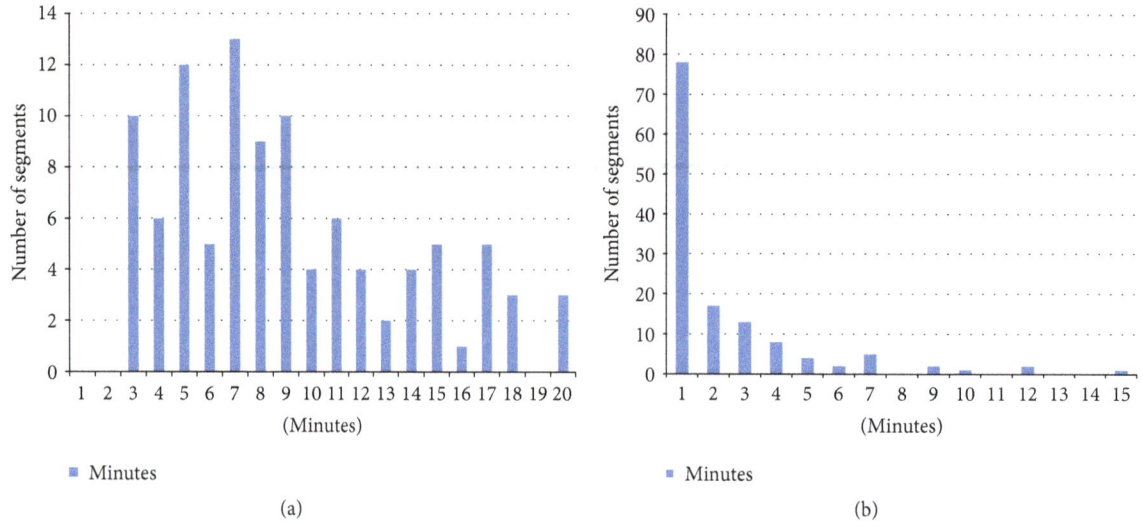

FIGURE 3: Distribution of highly (a) and low correlated (b) segment lengths for all subjects after synchronization procedure.

TABLE 2: Time-domain results after the synchronization process.

| Subject number | Mean RR (ms) | | | STD RR (ms) | | |
|---|---|---|---|---|---|---|
| | Schiller | CardioSport | Error | Schiller | CardioSport | Error |
| #1 | 738.27 | 755.47 | 2.28% | 123.34 | 125.09 | 1.40% |
| #2 | 704.04 | 720.42 | 2.27% | 91.35 | 93.47 | 2.27% |
| #3 | 907.63 | 928.88 | 2.29% | 90.40 | 92.83 | 2.62% |
| #4 | 854.53 | 874.50 | 2.28% | 144.74 | 148.00 | 2.20% |
| #5 | 937.01 | 958.97 | 2.29% | 107.18 | 109.41 | 2.04% |
| Average | 850.80 | 870.69 | 2.28% | 108.42 | 110.93 | 2.11% |

had the lowest usable time with only 2 hours and 6 minutes. The most probable reason for such a low time is the chest hair which reduced the contact between electrodes and the skin. For this reason, this subject was excluded from calculation of average results.

Table 2 shows results in time domain for the Schiller and the CardioSport devices after using our algorithm for the synchronization of signals. The time-domain analysis shows pretty close values for both mean RR values and standard deviation. The formula used for computing the standard deviation of RR intervals is as follows:

$$\text{STD RR} = \sqrt{\frac{1}{N-1}\sum_{j=1}^{N}\left(\text{RR}_j - \overline{\text{RR}}\right)^2}. \quad (2)$$

Average mean RR values for Schiller and CardioSport devices are 850.80 and 870.69, respectively. Average STD RR for the Schiller device is 108.42 and it is 110.93 for the CardioSport device.

The frequency-domain analysis is presented in Table 3. The absolute power was compared for very low frequency (VLF: 0–0.04 Hz), low frequency (LF: 0.04–0.5 Hz), and high frequency (HF: 0.15–0.4 Hz) and ratio between low frequency and high frequency (LF/HF). The results show no significant difference between Schiller and CardioSport device values.

The average mean absolute percentage error (MAPE) between the two signals is 2.32% with a high average correlation of 99.67%.

*3.2. Device Validation Study: Data Cleaning Method.* We run the data cleaning algorithm described in Section 2 on the data recorded by the chest belt. The duration of the resulting signal is shown in Table 4. Similar to the synchronization process, we got a very short duration for one subject and we excluded this subject from further analysis. It is important to note that, due to the noise on Schiller device records, we had to remove noisy parts from the "gold standard" signal as well. Therefore, even though the signal was recorded for 12 hours continuously, the overall duration is much less. The calculation shows that, in the worst scenario, only 45% of the signal can be used for analysis using this data cleaning method. However, in the best scenario, this number reaches 95%. This leads to a conclusion that results are quite subject dependent.

Table 5 shows the results of data analysis in the time domain after removing bad parts with the data cleaning algorithm. We can see that the mean RR intervals for the Schiller and the CardioSport devices are 851.14 and 871.23 and the standard deviations are 104.61 and 106.35, respectively. In general, the CardioSport device has slightly greater values but they are very close.

TABLE 3: Frequency-domain analysis after the synchronization process.

| Subject number | Schiller Absolute power (ms$^2$) | | | | CardioSport Absolute power (ms$^2$) | | | | Error | | | |
|---|---|---|---|---|---|---|---|---|---|---|---|---|
| | VLF | LF | HF | LF/HF | VLF | LF | HF | LF/HF | % VLF | % LF | % HF | % LF/HF |
| #1 | 7937.6 | 3086 | 1578 | 1.956 | 8444 | 3224 | 1330 | 2.4235 | 6.00 | 4.28 | 18.65 | 19.29 |
| #2 | 5431.5 | 626.6 | 245 | 2.557 | 5723 | 659.3 | 250.9 | 2.6281 | 5.09 | 4.96 | 2.35 | 2.71 |
| #3 | 4251.2 | 1927 | 494.4 | 3.898 | 4543 | 2055 | 538.8 | 3.8146 | 6.42 | 6.23 | 8.24 | 2.19 |
| #4 | 12682 | 1790 | 636.5 | 2.813 | 13514 | 1869 | 621.5 | 3.0077 | 6.16 | 4.23 | 2.41 | 6.47 |
| #5 | 6139.8 | 1212 | 476.7 | 2.542 | 6465 | 1274 | 481.4 | 2.6459 | 5.03 | 4.87 | 0.98 | 3.93 |

TABLE 4: Signal durations after the data cleaning process.

| Subject number | #1 | #2 | #3 | #4 | #5 |
|---|---|---|---|---|---|
| Duration (hh:mm:ss) | 1:28:10 | 11:20:03 | 6:15:38 | 9:27:07 | 4:29:44 |

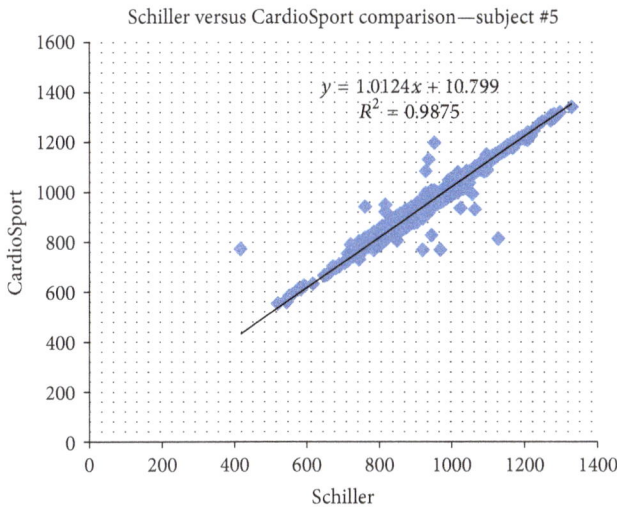

FIGURE 4: Comparison of CardioSport and Schiller device after data cleaning.

The minimum, maximum, and average percentage errors on the whole signal were calculated using a 5 minutes long sliding window with one-minute shift step (Table 6). Only one subject had a very high maximum error value of 33.86%. By visual examination, we determined that the cause of this high error percentage was in fact the presence of artifacts in the "gold standard" Schiller device measurements. Despite that, average error values are at a very low level of 2.20%.

Figure 4 demonstrates the typical relationship between the CardioSport and Schiller measurements using a scatter plot for subject #5. All slope values are close to 1. The lowest slope value is 0.9757, while the highest value is 1.0184. The average mean absolute percentage error (MAPE) between the two signals was 2.62% with a high average correlation of 98.76%.

3.3. Clinical Study. Five subjects were excluded from further analysis because they reported a decrease (instead of the expected increase) of their stress level while playing the Stroop game. As an explanation, some participants reported that playing the game was much more joyful than relaxation music. Others reported that the game kept their mind focused and that the relaxation music brought them back to their problems and duties of the day. Some also reported anxiety about the experiment itself which vanished while playing. After removing these records, we run the data cleaning algorithm which identified 10 noisy records, probably due to too much movement. These were also excluded, so the active dataset decreased to 31 subjects' records (20 men and 11 women; average age = 24.7 years).

Table 7 shows $p$ values of the Wilcoxon paired-samples test, for the relax versus stress parts, for the relevant HRV features ($n = 31$).

We found a statistically significant difference for the following time-domain features: mean RR ($p = 0.0001$), mean HR ($p = 0.0001$), pNN50 ($p = 0.0103$), NN50 ($p = 0.0128$), RMSSD ($p = 0.0255$), and HRV triangular index ($p = 0.0456$). In frequency domain, two features showed statistically significant difference: HF (ms$^2$) with $p = 0.0054$ and LF (ms$^2$) with $p = 0.0128$. The VLF (%) feature was also close but not significantly different ($p = 0.0745$). In nonlinear analysis, the SD1 feature showed a statistically significant difference ($p = 0.0268$). The average percentage differences and the minimum percentage differences are shown in Table 8.

Table 9 shows the correlations between the important features during the relaxation part of experiment. We can see very high positive correlation (higher than 0.9) between the following features: NN50 and RMSSD (0.94818), pNN50 and RMSSD (0.935664), and pNN50 and NN50 (0.98966). Poincaré plot SD1 feature was highly correlated with HF (ms2) feature. Only one very high negative correlation was found between features mean RR and mean HR (−0.99452).

Figure 5 shows, as an example, the values of an observed feature (mean HR) for the relaxation period and the game playing period, respectively.

3.4. Clinical Study: Stress Detection Performance Compared to Other Methods. The accuracy, sensitivity, and specificity values for correctly detecting stress are shown in Table 10 for

TABLE 5: Time-domain analysis after the data cleaning process.

| Subject number | Mean RR (ms) | | | STD RR (ms) | | |
|---|---|---|---|---|---|---|
| | Schiller | CardioSport | Error | Schiller | CardioSport | Error |
| #1 | 707.80 | 724.03 | 2.24% | 136.04 | 138.63 | 1.87% |
| #2 | 700.40 | 716.70 | 2.27% | 91.33 | 93.24 | 2.05% |
| #3 | 899.20 | 920.97 | 2.36% | 99.67 | 99.77 | 0.10% |
| #4 | 846.46 | 866.25 | 2.28% | 139.26 | 142.33 | 2.16% |
| #5 | 958.49 | 981.00 | 2.29% | 88.16 | 90.08 | 2.13% |
| Average | 851.14 | 871.23 | 2.29% | 104.61 | 106.35 | 1.66% |

TABLE 6: Minimum, maximum, and average percentage error.

| Subject number | Minimum error | Maximum error | Average error |
|---|---|---|---|
| #1 | 0.08% | 3.50% | 1.50% |
| #2 | 0.01% | 7.71% | 2.12% |
| #3 | 0.04% | 33.86% | 3.22% |
| #4 | 0.13% | 6.72% | 1.92% |
| #5 | 0.07% | 5.11% | 2.22% |
| Average | 0.06% | 13.35% | 2.37% |

TABLE 7: Statistical significance of the observed features ordered by $p$ value.

| Feature | $p$ value |
|---|---|
| Mean RR | 0.0001 |
| Mean HR | 0.0001 |
| HF ($ms^2$) | 0.0054 |
| pNN50 | 0.0103 |
| NN50 | 0.0128 |
| LF ($ms^2$) | 0.0128 |
| RMSSD | 0.0255 |
| Poincaré plot, SD1 | 0.0268 |
| HRV triangular index | 0.0456 |
| VLF (%) | 0.0745 |
| STD RR | 0.1583 |
| HF (%) | 0.1583 |
| Poincaré plot, SD2 | 0.2725 |
| LF/HF | 0.4565 |
| VLF ($ms^2$) | 0.4565 |
| TINN | 0.5967 |
| Power (n.u.)-HF | 0.7390 |
| Power (n.u.)-LF | 0.7539 |
| STD HR | 0.9687 |

our algorithm, the linear algorithm proposed by Melillo et al., and the nonlinear algorithm proposed by the same authors.

## 4. Discussion

Stress is a very complex subject and measuring stress is not an easy task. There are many markers that could be used, many algorithms that could be applied, and many forms of

TABLE 8: Average percentage difference and minimum percentage difference for the features computed from the HR signal.

| Feature | Average percentage difference | Minimum percentage difference |
|---|---|---|
| Mean HR | 6.88 | 0.94 |
| RMSSD | 27.86 | 3.98 |
| pNN50 | 72.76 | 3.88 |

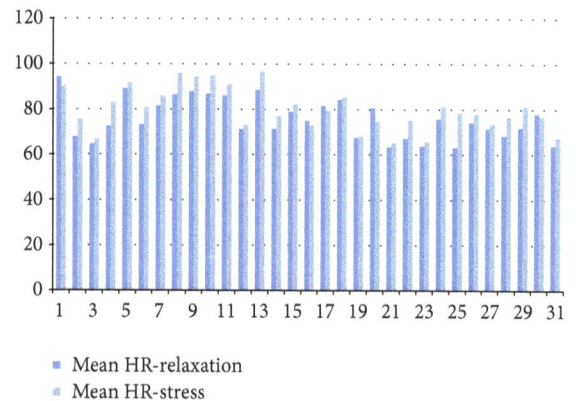

■ Mean HR-relaxation
■ Mean HR-stress

FIGURE 5: Mean HR feature for all subjects during relaxation and while playing game.

stress which could be observed. Heart rate variability, being simple and noninvasive, has recently become one of the most popular methods for detecting stress. Still, this is not an easy task, since HRV is not a single value; rather, it consists of many features that can be observed in time domain and frequency domain or using nonlinear analysis. The literature generally reports that, under mental stress, the mean RR, pNN50, STD RR, and RMSSD features decrease, while the mean HR and LF features increase significantly. However, significant differences for the same features and sometimes even opposite results (e.g., LF feature) are also reported. One probable cause for this inconsistency in literature could be the fact that stress is not the only condition that influences changes in HRV. Physical activity, body posture, breathing, age, gender, and illnesses all have a great influence on HRV. In this paper, we analyzed various HRV features in order to find those that change significantly under mental stress and proposed a simple stress detection algorithm.

TABLE 9: Correlation of observed features during relaxation part.

|  | Mean RR | Mean HR | RMSSD | NN50 | pNN50 | HRV t.i. | LF (ms$^2$) | HF (ms$^2$) | P.P., SD1 |
|---|---|---|---|---|---|---|---|---|---|
| Mean RR | 1.00 | | | | | | | | |
| Mean HR | −0.99 | 1.00 | | | | | | | |
| RMSSD | 0.29 | −0.28 | 1.00 | | | | | | |
| NN50 | 0.38 | −0.37 | 0.95 | 1.00 | | | | | |
| pNN50 | 0.48 | −0.47 | 0.94 | 0.99 | 1.00 | | | | |
| HRV t.i. | 0.25 | −0.25 | 0.78 | 0.77 | 0.75 | 1.00 | | | |
| LF (ms$^2$) | 0.08 | −0.09 | 0.15 | 0.17 | 0.16 | 0.28 | 1.00 | | |
| HF (ms$^2$) | 0.20 | −0.20 | −0.09 | −0.03 | 0.00 | −0.21 | 0.33 | 1.00 | |
| P.P., SD1 | 0.12 | −0.13 | −0.01 | 0.01 | 0.03 | −0.15 | 0.51 | 0.89 | 1.00 |

TABLE 10: Performance comparison of the three stress detection methods.

| Feature | Melillo linear | Melillo nonlinear | Our method |
|---|---|---|---|
| Accuracy | 61.29% | 50.00% | 74.60% |
| Sensitivity | 61.29% | 29.03% | 75.00% |
| Specificity | 61.29% | 70.97% | 74.19% |

In the device validation study, we tested the reliability of a low cost heart rate meter. The CardioSport TP3 heart rate meter device was used simultaneously with a professional ECG recorder (Holter) device. We compared the results using standard deviation, correlation, and scatter plot diagram with slope of the regression line which are commonly used in literature [36, 40, 50]. However, before we analyzed the results, we used a simple data cleaning algorithm to eliminate noisy parts without using any data correction. The data cleaning process reduces the overall duration of the signal but it increases its quality. After data cleaning, all results of the CardioSport device were very close to the Schiller device with an average correlation of 98.73%. The downside of the data cleaning algorithm is that it will delete sections of the signal even with the slightest detachment. Hopefully, with advance in wearable sensors, new forms of heart rate monitors like rings or bracelets with firmer attachment to body will be available.

In the next step, we demonstrated how a simple mental stressor can influence HRV features significantly. Our findings are not very different from previous research, showing that HRV can indeed be used as an indicator of mental stress. We found that, under the influence of mental stress, mean HR increased, while mean RR, pNN50, RMSSD, and HRV triangular index decreased. Contrary to the results from literature, we did not find a statistically significant difference in STD RR feature ($p = 0.1583$). This could be explained by the fact that we analyzed only 10 minutes in each part of the experiment, while STD RR feature describes long-term variability. A limitation of our study is that we only analyzed the influence of mental stress. Physical or emotional stress could influence observed features in a completely different way.

For some subjects, the experiment failed to provoke mental stress which is of course a shortcoming of the experiment setup; however, it would be very hard to design a method that is successful in all cases. The Stroop test was chosen because it is easy to implement and is generally accepted in the literature for such purposes. Since it increases the speed of the game proportionally with the user's results, it should increase the stress level regardless of the subjects' cognitive level. We believe that other factors, such as the subject's prior experience and motivation for playing computer games, are harder to control.

As a conclusion of this study we created a robust stress detection algorithm. Unlike other stress detection algorithms which use several stress markers [51, 52], we used only HRV features for stress detection but with relatively high stress identification ratio. We were able to get an accuracy rate of 74.60%, somewhat below the 85% reported by the algorithm in [53]; however, the latter uses the full electrocardiogram (ECG) measurement compared to using only RR intervals in our case.

If we compare our algorithm with other algorithms for stress detection using only HR and HRV parameters, we can say that we achieved higher identification rate than the algorithm in [43] and a worse result than [48] or [45] and around 15% worse compared to [44, 47] but we used only time-domain features for stress identification instead of frequency-domain features or using nonlinear analysis which are much more expensive to calculate.

Since performance of particular algorithm depends on multiple parameters like type of stressor, number of subjects, methods used, and so forth, we compared the performance of our algorithm with two state-of-the-art algorithms. Although our algorithm showed lower declared accuracy, the comparison of its performance on the same dataset showed much better results than the algorithm that uses nonlinear HRV features [44] and slightly better performance than the algorithm that uses linear HRV [45] features for stress detection. We think that the poor performance of the two tested methods could partly be due to the fact that our stressor, the Stroop game, was not as strong as the university exam stressor used for the development of the Melillo algorithms or driving [48]. Such results show that the same algorithm can give very different results on different dataset meaning that comparing strictly by accuracy values is not good indicator if comparison is not performed on the same dataset.

A weakness of the proposed algorithm is that it only detects events that provoke stress for a particular subject. It cannot classify the current state of a subject in given moment. However, this was not the intention of our algorithm from the beginning and we propose using combination of our algorithm with typical classification algorithms for achieving greater insight into stressful events and a subject's current state.

A strength of our algorithm is that an event or a series of stressful events could be detected before entering into a stressful state defined by classification algorithms. The user could be informed by sound, vibration, or other kinds of alert when stressful event happens, leading to greater awareness about daily stressors. Also, this algorithm is very simple and easy to implement in mobile environments due to the fact that all HRV features are chosen only from time domain.

## 5. Conclusions

From this research we can conclude that even a simple low cost heart rate monitor device can detect features that change significantly under the influence of mental stress. Using these results we created a simple stress detection algorithm that is being integrated in the Lavinia lifestyle counseling mobile application [54] for further testing and refinement in real-life stress situations. If stress detection proves to be reliable for larger samples, it will be used in the blood glucose prediction models developed for diabetics.

## Appendix

## A. The Instructions for the Clinical Study

*Experiment: Measuring Physiological Effects of Heart Rate Parameters during Various Situations*

*Instructions to Participants.* During this experiment we will measure physiological parameters of various situations. First, we will measure parameters during listening to relaxation music and then we will measure the same parameters during playing simple Android based game using mobile phone. You will need to fill data in the questionnaires three times: before experiment starts, after the relaxation music stops, and at the end of experiment. If you feel any discomfort during this experiment, you can stop at any time:

*Personal Data*

> Name or code: —
>
> Age: —
>
> Gender: M/F

*How to Play.* In this game screen is divided in four parts. In each part word is shown with different color. Words are color names like red, blue, purple, black, green,…. You need to touch the word which is colored in the color of the word. For example, if word red is colored with black, then you skip

it, but if the word red is colored in red color, then you need to press that word. If you make a mistake, game ends. You need to get as high score as possible. For every choice, you have only a limited amount of time. If time runs out, game is over. You can play as many games as you can during 10 minutes:

*Example*

| Red | Blue |
|-----|------|
| Green | Black |

Correct                                                   Incorrect

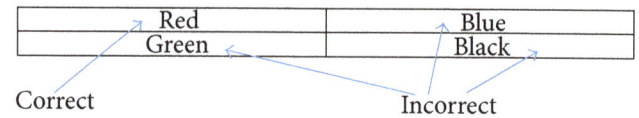

Word red is colored red so this is *correct* choice.

Word green is colored with black color so this is *incorrect* choice.

Word blue is colored with orange color so this is *incorrect* choice.

Word black is colored with blue color so this is *incorrect* choice.

## B. Experiment Data and Questionnaire

*Experiment Data*

> Date: —
>
> Protocol

> > Give person the paper with experiment description. Let him/her read whole description (including "how to play" section). Ask if they understand the experiment. Tell the person that in this experiment they will first listen one relaxation song and then they will play simple game. Show the person how to play game shortly if necessary. Explain to person that during whole experiment he/she will need to wear chest belt for collecting heart rate data.
> >
> > Ask the person to put chest belt. Ensure privacy for person to put chest belt on.

> > > Time (hh:mm): —

> > Establish bluetooth connection between chest belt and Android device. Write down time when this occurs.

> > > Time (hh:mm): —

> > Ask the person about current perceived stress level from 1 to 10 where 1 is no stress and 10 is maximum stress level and write down perceived stress level

> > > Time (hh:mm): —
> > > Perceived stress level: —

> > Tell the person to relax while listening relaxation music. Start playing relaxation music and write the exact start time (when you hit the play button)

> > > Time (hh:mm): —

When music stops, write down the time of the event. Ask the person about perceived stress level after listening the song from 1 to 10 where 1 is no stress and 10 is maximum stress level. Write down perceived stress level

Time (hh:mm): —
Perceived stress level: —

Ask person to play Android based game for the next 10 minutes. Write the start time and set countdown timer to at least 10 minutes.

Time (hh:mm): —

At the end of 10 minutes, tell person to stop playing and write down the time. Ask person about perceived stress level after playing game from 1 to 10 where 1 is no stress and 10 is maximum stress level. Write down perceived stress level

Time (hh:mm): —
Perceived stress level: —

## Abbreviations

| | |
|---|---|
| AAL: | Ambient assisted living |
| BP: | Blood pressure |
| ECG: | Electrocardiograph |
| EMG: | Electromyogram |
| GSR: | Galvanic skin response |
| HF: | High frequency |
| HR: | Heart rate |
| HRV: | Heart rate variability |
| LF: | Low frequency |
| MAPE: | Average mean absolute percentage |
| NN50: | The number of pairs of successive beat-to-beat or NN intervals that differ by more than 50 ms |
| pNN50: | The proportion of NN50 divided by total number of NNs |
| RMSSD: | The square root of the mean of the squares of the successive differences between adjacent intervals |
| RR (interval): | R wave to R wave interval |
| VLF: | Very low frequency. |

## Competing Interests

The authors declare that there are no competing interests regarding the publication of this paper.

## References

[1] A. Mitra, "Diabetes and stress: a review," *Ethnomedicine*, vol. 2, no. 2, pp. 131–135, 2008.

[2] A. Steptoe and M. Kivimäki, "Stress and cardiovascular disease: an update on current knowledge," *Annual Review of Public Health*, vol. 34, no. 1, pp. 337–354, 2013.

[3] A. M. Heraclides, T. Chandola, D. R. Witte, and E. J. Brunner, "Work stress, obesity and the risk of type 2 diabetes: gender-specific bidirectional effect in the whitehall II study," *Obesity*, vol. 20, no. 2, pp. 428–433, 2012.

[4] Y.-M. Oh, Y. S. Kim, S. H. Yoo, S. K. Kim, and D. S. Kim, "Association between stress and asthma symptoms: a population-based study," *Respirology*, vol. 9, no. 3, pp. 363–368, 2004.

[5] S. Patel, H. Park, P. Bonato, L. Chan, and M. Rodgers, "A review of wearable sensors and systems with application in rehabilitation," *Journal of NeuroEngineering and Rehabilitation*, vol. 9, no. 1, article 21, 2012.

[6] A. Pantelopoulos and N. G. Bourbakis, "A survey on wearable sensor-based systems for health monitoring and prognosis," *IEEE Transactions on Systems, Man and Cybernetics Part C: Applications and Reviews*, vol. 40, no. 1, pp. 1–12, 2010.

[7] A. Pantelopoulos and N. Bourbakis, "A survey on wearable biosensor systems for health monitoring," in *Proceedings of the 30th Annual International Conference of the IEEE Engineering in Medicine and Biology Society (EMBS '08)*, pp. 4887–4890, Vancouver, Canada, August 2008.

[8] S. Ortmann, P. Langendorfer, and C. S. Lanyi, "Telemedical assistance for ambulant rehabilitation of stroke patients," *Brain Injury*, vol. 26, Meeting Abstract 0650, no. 4-5, pp. 644–645, 2012.

[9] Y. Zhang, H. Liu, X. Su, P. Jiang, and D. Wei, "Remote mobile health monitoring system based on smart phone and browser/server structure," *Journal of Healthcare Engineering*, vol. 6, no. 4, pp. 717–738, 2015.

[10] Y. Shi, N. Ruiz, R. Taib, E. Choi, and F. Chen, "Galvanic skin response (GSR) as an index of cognitive load," in *Proceedings of the Extended Abstracts on Human Factors in Computing Systems (CHI EA '07)*, San Jose, Calif, USA, 2007.

[11] U. Lundberg, R. Kadefors, B. Melin et al., "Psychophysiological stress and emg activity of the trapezius muscle," *International Journal of Behavioral Medicine*, vol. 1, no. 4, pp. 354–370, 1994.

[12] J. Wijsman, B. Grundlehner, J. Penders, and H. Hermens, "Trapezius muscle EMG as predictor of mental stress," in *Proceedings of the 1st Wireless Health Conference (WH '10)*, pp. 155–163, ACM, October 2010.

[13] T. Yamakoshi, K. Yamakoshi, S. Tanaka et al., "Feasibility study on driver's stress detection from differential skin temperature measurement," in *Proceedings of the 30th Annual International Conference of the IEEE Engineering in Medicine and Biology Society (EMBS '08)*, pp. 1076–1079, Vancouver, Canada, August 2008.

[14] J. Taelman, S. Vandeput, A. Spaepen, and S. V. Huffel, "Influence of mental stress on heart rate and heart rate variability," in *Proceedings 4th European Conference of the International Federation for Medical and Biological Engineering (IFMBE '09)*, pp. 1366–1369, 2009.

[15] E. Ceja, V. Osmani, and O. Mayora, "Automatic stress detection in working environments from smartphones' accelerometer data: a first step," *IEEE Journal of Biomedical and Health Informatics*, 2015.

[16] S. D. W. Gunawardhane, P. M. D. Silva, D. S. B. Kulathunga, and S. M. K. D. Arunatileka, "Non invasive human stress detection using key stroke dynamics and pattern variations," in *Proceedings of the International Conference on Advances in ICT for Emerging Regions (ICTer '13)*, pp. 240–247, Colombo, Sri Lanka, December 2013.

[17] A. Marcos-Ramiro, D. Pizarro-Perez, M. Marron-Romera, and D. Gatica-Perez, "Automatic blinking detection towards stress

discovery," in *Proceedings of the 16th International Conference on Multimodal Interaction (ICMI '14)*, pp. 307–310, Istanbul, Turkey, November 2014.

[18] A. Fernandes, R. Helawar, R. Lokesh, T. Tari, and A. V. Shahapurkar, "Determination of stress using blood pressure and galvanic skin response," in *Proceedings of the International Conference on Communication and Network Technologies (ICCNT '14)*, pp. 165–168, Sivakasi, India, December 2014.

[19] F.-T. Sun, C. Kuo, H.-T. Cheng, S. Buthpitiya, P. Collins, and M. Griss, "Activity-aware mental stress detection using physiological sensors," in *Mobile Computing, Applications, and Services*, M. Gris and G. Yang, Eds., vol. 76 of *Lecture Notes of the Institute for Computer Sciences, Social Informatics and Telecommunications Engineering*, pp. 211–230, Springer, New York, NY, USA, 2012.

[20] A. De Santos Sierra, C. S. Ávila, J. Guerra Casanova, and G. B. Del Pozo, "A stress-detection system based on physiological signals and fuzzy logic," *IEEE Transactions on Industrial Electronics*, vol. 58, no. 10, pp. 4857–4865, 2011.

[21] G. Rigas, Y. Goletsis, and D. I. Fotiadis, "Real-time driver's stress event detection," *IEEE Transactions on Intelligent Transportation Systems*, vol. 13, no. 1, pp. 221–234, 2012.

[22] J. Wijsman, B. Grundlehner, H. Liu, H. Hermens, and J. Penders, "Towards mental stress detection using wearable physiological sensors," in *Proceedings of the Annual International Conference of the IEEE Engineering in Medicine and Biology Society*, Boston, Mass, USA, August-September 2011.

[23] A. Riera, A. Soria-Frisch, A. Albajes-Eizagirre et al., "Electrophysiological data fusion for stress detection," *Studies in Health Technology and Informatics*, vol. 181, pp. 228–232, 2012.

[24] M. Singh and A. B. Queyam, "A novel method of stress detection using physiological measurements of automobile drivers," *International Journal of Electronics Engineering*, vol. 5, no. 2, pp. 13–20, 2013.

[25] F. Mokhayeri, M.-R. Akbarzadeh-T, and S. Toosizadeh, "Mental stress detection using physiological signals based on soft computing techniques," in *Proceedings of the 18th Iranian Conference of Biomedical Engineering (ICBME '11)*, pp. 232–237, Tehran, Iran, December 2011.

[26] S. Baltaci and D. Gokcay, "Role of pupil dilation and facial temperature features in stress detection," in *Proceedings of the 22nd Signal Processing and Communications Applications Conference (SIU '14)*, pp. 1259–1262, Trabzon, Turkey, April 2014.

[27] J. Choi, *Minimally-invasive wearable sensors and data processing methods for mental stress detection [Ph.D. dissertation]*, Texas A&M University, 2011, http://hdl.handle.net/1969.1/ETD-TAMU-2011-12-10674.

[28] T. Chen, P. Yuen, M. Richardson, G. Liu, and Z. She, "Detection of psychological stress using a hyperspectral imaging technique," *IEEE Transactions on Affective Computing*, vol. 5, no. 4, pp. 391–405, 2014.

[29] H. Lu, D. Frauendorfer, M. Rabbi et al., "StressSense: detecting stress in unconstrained acoustic environments using smartphones," in *Proceedings of the 14th International Conference on Ubiquitous Computing (UbiComp '12)*, pp. 351–360, ACM, Pittsburgh, Pa, USA, September 2012.

[30] A. K. Mishra and O. S. Vaidya, "Attributes detection for allocation of resources with stress detection from speech," *International Journal of Electronics, Electrical and Computational System*, vol. 3, no. 4, pp. 61–66, 2014.

[31] P. Ren, A. Barreto, J. Huang, Y. Gao, F. R. Ortega, and M. Adjouadi, "Off-line and on-line stress detection through processing of the pupil diameter signal," *Annals of Biomedical Engineering*, vol. 42, no. 1, pp. 162–176, 2014.

[32] B. Kaur, S. Moses, M. Luthra, and V. N. Ikonomidou, "Remote stress detection using a visible spectrum camera," in *Independent Component Analyses, Compressive Sampling, Large Data Analyses (LDA), Neural Networks, Biosystems, and Nanoengineering XIII*, vol. 9496 of *Proceedings of SPIE*, May 2015.

[33] M. N. Haji Mohd, M. Kashima, K. Sato, and M. Watanabe, "Mental stress recognition based on non-invasive and non-contact measurement from stereo thermal and visible sensors," *International Journal of Affective Engineering*, vol. 14, no. 1, pp. 9–17, 2015.

[34] M. B. Crawley, *Validation of the Sensewear Hr Armband for Measuring Heart Rate and Energy Expenditure*, The Pennsylvania State University, 2003.

[35] C. M. Lee and M. Gorelick, "Validity of the smarthealth watch to measure heart rate during rest and exercise," *Measurement in Physical Education and Exercise Science*, vol. 15, no. 1, pp. 18–25, 2011.

[36] J. Kristiansen, M. Korshøj, J. H. Skotte et al., "Comparison of two systems for long-term heart rate variability monitoring in free-living conditions—a pilot study," *BioMedical Engineering OnLine*, vol. 10, article 27, 2011.

[37] S. Brage, N. Brage, P. W. Franks, U. Ekelund, and N. J. Wareham, "Reliability and validity of the combined heart rate and movement sensor actiheart," *European Journal of Clinical Nutrition*, vol. 59, no. 4, pp. 561–570, 2005.

[38] Y. Liu, S. H. Zhu, G. H. Wang, F. Ye, and P. Z. Li, "Validity and reliability of multiparameter physiological measurements recorded by the equivital lifemonitor during activities of various intensities," *Journal of Occupational and Environmental Hygiene*, vol. 10, no. 2, pp. 78–85, 2013.

[39] J. Parak, A. Tarniceriu, P. Renevey, M. Bertschi, R. Delgado-Gonzalo, and I. Korhonen, "Evaluation of the beat-to-beat detection accuracy of PulseOn wearable optical heart rate monitor," in *Proceedings of the 37th Annual International Conference of the IEEE Engineering in Medicine and Biology Society (EMBC '15)*, pp. 8099–8102, Milan, Italy, August 2015.

[40] J. A. Johnstone, P. A. Ford, G. Hughes, T. Watson, and A. T. Garrett, "Bioharness™ multivariable monitoring device. Part I: validity," *Journal of Sports Science and Medicine*, vol. 11, no. 3, pp. 400–408, 2012.

[41] J. A. Johnstone, P. A. Ford, G. Hughes, T. Watson, A. C. S. Mitchell, and A. T. Garrett, "Field based reliability and validity of the bioharness multivariable monitoring device," *Journal of Sports Science and Medicine*, vol. 11, no. 4, pp. 643–652, 2012.

[42] J. A. Johnstone, P. A. Ford, G. Hughes, T. Watson, and A. T. Garrett, "Bioharness™ multivariable monitoring device: part. II: reliability," *Journal of Sports Science and Medicine*, vol. 11, no. 3, pp. 409–417, 2012.

[43] D. Kim, Y. Seo, J. Cho, and C.-H. Cho, "Detection of subjects with higher self-reporting stress scores using heart rate variability patterns during the day," in *Proceedings of the 30th Annual International Conference of the IEEE Engineering in Medicine and Biology Society (EMBS '08)*, pp. 682–685, August 2008.

[44] P. Melillo, M. Bracale, and L. Pecchia, "Nonlinear Heart Rate Variability features for real-life stress detection. Case study: students under stress due to university examination," *BioMedical Engineering Online*, vol. 10, no. 1, article 96, 2011.

[45] P. Melillo, C. Formisano, U. Bracale, and L. Pecchia, "Classification tree for real-life stress detection using linear heart rate variability analysis. Case study: students under stress due to university examination," in *Proceedings of the IFMBE World Congress on Medical Physics and Biomedical Engineering*, pp. 477–480, Beijing, China, May 2012.

[46] P. Karthikeyan, M. Murugappan, and S. Yaacob, "Analysis of stroop colorword test-based human stress detection using electrocardiography and heart rate variability signals," *Arabian Journal for Science and Engineering*, vol. 39, no. 3, pp. 1835–1847, 2014.

[47] L. Vanitha and G. R. Suresh, "Hierarchical SVM to detect mental stress in human beings using Heart Rate Variability," in *Proceedings of the 2nd International Conference on Devices, Circuits and Systems (ICDCS '14)*, pp. 1–5, Combiatore, India, March 2014.

[48] N. Munla, M. Khalil, A. Shahin, and A. Mourad, "Driver stress level detection using HRV analysis," in *Proceedings of the International Conference on Advances in Biomedical Engineering (ICABME '15)*, pp. 61–64, Beirut, Lebanon, September 2015.

[49] Color Stroop game, February 2016, https://play.google.com/store/apps/details?id=com.citroon.colortest.

[50] A. A. Flatt and M. R. Esco, "Validity of the ithletetm smart phone application for determining ultra-short-term heart rate variability," *Journal of Human Kinetics*, vol. 39, no. 1, pp. 85–92, 2013.

[51] J. A. Healey and R. W. Picard, "Detecting stress during real-world driving tasks using physiological sensors," *IEEE Transactions on Intelligent Transportation Systems*, vol. 6, no. 2, pp. 156–166, 2005.

[52] A. De Santos Sierra, C. S. Ávila, G. B. Del Pozo, and J. Guerra Casanova, "Stress detection by means of stress physiological template," in *Proceedings of the 3rd World Congress on Nature and Biologically Inspired Computing (NaBIC '11)*, pp. 131–136, Salamanca, Spain, October 2011.

[53] Listen to Your Heart: Stress Prediction Using Consumer Heart Rate Sensors, February 2016, http://cs229.stanford.edu/proj2013/LiuUlrich-ListenToYourHeart-StressPredictionUsing-ConsumerHeartRateSensors.pdf.

[54] Lavinia—lifestyle mirror application, http://lavinia.hu/introduction-and-publications/.

# 4

# A Quantitative Analysis of Cold Water for Human Consumption in Hospitals in Spain

**A. G. González,[1] J. García-Sanz-Calcedo,[2] D. R. Salgado,[3] and A. Mena[4]**

[1]School of Design Engineering, Department of Mechanical, Energy, and Materials Engineering, University of Extremadura, 06800 Mérida, Spain

[2]Department of Projects, University of Extremadura, 06007 Badajoz, Spain

[3]School of Industrial Engineering, Department of Mechanical, Energy, and Materials Engineering, University of Extremadura, 06007 Badajoz, Spain

[4]School of Industrial Engineering, Department of Engineering Design and Projects, University of Huelva, 21003 Huelva, Spain

Correspondence should be addressed to J. García-Sanz-Calcedo; jgsanz@unex.es

Academic Editor: John S. Katsanis

An estimation of the water used for human consumption in hospitals is essential to determine possible savings and to fix criteria to improve the design of new water consumption models. The present work reports on cold water for human consumption (CWHC) in hospitals in Spain and determines the possible savings. In the period of 2005–2012, 80 Eco-Management and Audit Schemes (EMAS) from 20 hospitals were analysed. The results conclude that the average annual consumption of CWHC is $1.59\,\mathrm{m^3/m^2}$ (with a standard deviation of $0.48\,\mathrm{m^3/m^2}$), $195.85\,\mathrm{m^3/bed}$ (standard deviation $70.07\,\mathrm{m^3/bed}$), or $53.69\,\mathrm{m^3/worker}$ (standard deviation $16.64\,\mathrm{m^3/worker}$). The results demonstrate the possibility of saving $5{,}600{,}000\,\mathrm{m^3}$ of water per year. Assuming the cost of water as approximately $1.22\,\text{€}/\mathrm{m^3}$, annual savings are estimated as $6{,}832{,}000\,\text{€}$. Furthermore, $2{,}912\,\mathrm{MWh}$ of energy could be saved, and the emission of $22{,}400$ annual tonnes of $CO_2$ into the atmosphere could be avoided.

## 1. Introduction

The hospital is a tertiary sector building in which, due to the nature of its usage, a large number of human resources are needed. The objectives outlined by the European Council in March 2007 were initially to reduce the total energy consumption by 20% (based on the 2005 consumption) and to cut greenhouse emissions by 20% to below the emissions recorded in 1990. These objectives were designed to reduce the use of resources [1].

Although the quantity of water available on Earth today is sufficient to cover the needs of the population, continual inappropriate and excessive usage could lead to a lack of resources within a few years. To overcome this situation, a change in current consumption rates is crucial. This would focus on (i) the preservation of water and an improvement in water management, (ii) encouragement of a greater respect and sensitivity towards the usage of water, and (iii) a more balanced distribution and emphasis on its ecological and social value [2].

In Spain, annual water consumption in cities totals $5{,}000{,}000{,}000\,\mathrm{m^3}$, which is 20% of the country's total consumption. The average daily usage is 171 litres per person, at a cost between $0.91\,\text{€}/\mathrm{m^3}$ and $1.69\,\text{€}/\mathrm{m^3}$ depending on the region [3].

At European Union level, the Water Framework Directive sets objectives to be achieved by all member states, but water quantities are relatively less considered than water quality, and achieving the goals often requires collaboration as water is a shared resource that requires a holistic and integrated approach [4].

The Pacific Institute for Studies in Development, Environment and Security highlights the importance of the hospitals in the construction sector, for its usage of large quantities of water in most procedures [5]. The areas where water consumption in a hospital is high are as follows: patients rooms 20%, domestic hot water (DHW) 15%, laundry areas 15%, maintenance of green areas 10%, therapeutic pools 9%, kitchens 8%, cleaning 5%, refrigeration towers 5%,

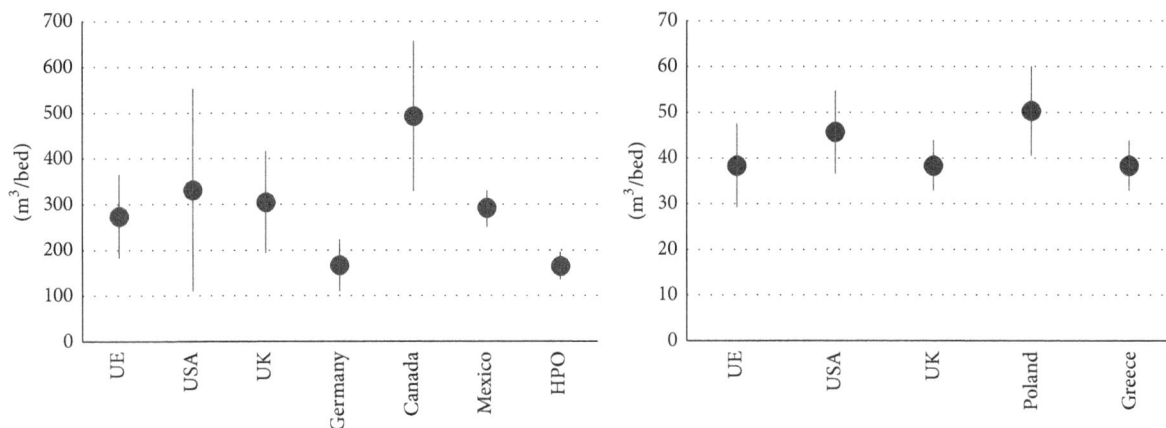

FIGURE 1: Annual average consumption of CWHC and DHW in healthcare centres per hospital bed.

sterilization 5%, heating ventilation and air conditioning (HVAC) 4%, and others 4% [6].

The typical ratios of usage across European hospitals indicate an average annual consumption between 182.5 and 365 m³ per bed [7]. However, these indicators fluctuate greatly depending on the locations under study, the type of establishment, the date of construction, the number of users, the number of workers, and the possible green areas it may have. In the USA this consumption ranges from 109.5 to 552.61 m³/bed [8–10] and in the UK from 193.45 to 415.37 m³/bed [11] and in Germany, as reported in some studies, it lies in the range 109.5–223.02 m³/bed [12], reaching a maximum of 247.84 m³/bed [13]. Canadian studies reveal even higher ratios between 328.5 and 657 m³/bed [14]. Other examples of these figures come from the Mexican Institute of Water Technology, which reports annual consumption as 292 m³/bed [15], whereas the Pan-American Health Organization (PAHO) indicates 164.25 m³/bed [16].

To assess hot water consumption, a series of studies was carried out. These studies show that the annual average per hospital bed varies between 29.2 m³/bed and 47.45 m³/bed in Europe [17] and between 36.5 and 54.75 m³/bed in the USA [18]. In Greece, this figure ranges between 32.85 and 43.8 m³/bed [19, 20]. Bujak [21] estimated that the average annual consumption of hot water in a hospital lies between 40.52 and 60.05 m³/bed. Figure 1 shows the values of annual average consumption ratios of CWHC and DHW per hospital bed.

Though some studies related to the management of water consumption in Spain have been undertaken [22], methods for saving water have not yet been studied in a systematic form, even though expectations of saving water are high. This information is based on studies of 903 hospitals, which were operative in 2013, and extends to a total of 163,585 beds. However, the potential energy saving in hospitals has elsewhere been studied [23].

The small amount of research, which has been done up until now, has only been carried out on a small number of sample buildings and therefore has little statistical relevance. The purpose of the present work is to analyse and assess the consumption of CWHC in hospitals in Spain, depending on different variables, and to estimate the possibilities of savings.

## 2. Methodology

To obtain valuable data with high statistical significance in the results, an analytical study was performed between 2005 and 2012 in 20 Spanish hospitals, which had been built between 1980 and 2005.

Data was collected and analysed according to the regulations of EMAS [24], a voluntary environmental management instrument which recognises those organizations which not only have set up an environmental management system [25] but also have reached an agreement of continual improvement, which is verified through independent audits [26, 27]. EMAS is a management tool developed for companies and other organizations, to evaluate, inform, and improve their environmental achievements. 80 EMAS statements have been analysed in hospitals [28].

The consumption of CWHC in 20 hospitals was examined between 2005 and 2012. Table 1 shows the list of particular hospitals under study. A reduction factor for the consumption of CWHC has been applied in the case of hospitals with gardening areas (reduction factor 10%) or laundry facilities (reduction factor 15%) [29, 30].

The figures for the number of beds and the number of workers analysed by the EMAS were obtained from annual data published by the Ministry of Health [31]. In both cases the figures were acquired by calculating the average in relation to the range of years. In order to calculate the area of the hospital, only the built surface area (m²) of the facilities has been taken into consideration.

In the present study, two different analyses were conducted. Firstly, an analysis of three water consumption indicators was carried out, namely, the average annual water consumption in relation to built surface area (floor area), the number of workers, and the number of beds. The second analysis was conducted in order to obtain more detailed results from the statistical data used in this research, for which analysis of variance (ANOVA) tests were carried out using the factors presented in Table 2. In this sense, it is important to note that an ANOVA test requires all samples to

TABLE 1: List of hospitals under study.

| Hospital | Management | Area (m²) | Number of workers | Number of beds | CWHC (m³/year) | Province |
|---|---|---|---|---|---|---|
| Hospital Asepeyo de Coslada | Private | 22,000 | 389 | 200 | 31,536 | Madrid |
| HM Universitario de Madrid | Private | 7,717 | 257 | 110 | 10,074 | Madrid |
| HM Universitario Montepríncipe | Private | 19,521 | 503 | 197 | 40,147 | Madrid |
| HM Universitario Torrelodones | Private | 10,808 | 291 | 136 | 12,928 | Madrid |
| HM Universitario Sanchinarro | Private | 33,989 | 520 | 190 | 24,692 | Madrid |
| Hospital Clínico San Carlos | Public | 175,000 | 5,811 | 996 | 271,270 | Madrid |
| Hospital Juan Ramón Jiménez | Public | 126,241 | 2,685 | 725 | 215,232 | Huelva |
| Hospital Costa del Sol | Public | 24,408 | 1,271 | 366 | 71,690 | Málaga |
| HAR de Benalmádena | Public | 7,077 | 300 | 48 | 8,184 | Málaga |
| Hospital Virgen de las Nieves | Public | 42,734 | 4,977 | 1,075 | 266,767 | Granada |
| Hospital Victoria Eugenia | Private | 7,330 | 372 | 39 | 9,889 | Sevilla |
| Hospital General de Valencia | Public | 18,209 | 2,184 | 550 | 145,773 | Valencia |
| Fundación Hospital Calahorra | Public | 6,683 | 382 | 91 | 36,195 | La Rioja |
| Hospital Galdakao-Usansolo | Public | 72,000 | 1,599 | 383 | 131,730 | Vizcaya |
| Hospital de Zumárraga | Public | 14,125 | 470 | 130 | 23,801 | Guipúzcoa |
| Hospital Asepeyo Sant Cugat | Private | 15,000 | 350 | 120 | 23,194 | Barcelona |
| Hospital de Figueres | Private | 18,186 | 643 | 168 | 36,857 | Gerona |
| Hospital de Manacor | Public | 28,333 | 1,076 | 226 | 62,330 | Baleares |
| Hospital de Palamós | Private | 21,151 | 643 | 136 | 30,455 | Gerona |
| Hospital Perpetuo Socorro | Private | 10,409 | 237 | 195 | 12,568 | Las Palmas |

TABLE 2: Classification of the factors considered in the statistical analysis of the collected data.

| Factors | Distribution regarding factors |
|---|---|
| Type of management (TM) | Public |
|  | Private |
| Gross Domestic Product (GDP) | GDP 1: <20,000 € |
|  | GDP 2: 20,000 €–25,000 € |
|  | GDP 3: 25,000 €–30,000 € |
|  | GDP 4: >30,000 € |
| Heating degrees-day year (HDDY) | HDDY 1: 0° to 250°C |
|  | HDDY 2: 250° to 500°C |
|  | HDDY 3: 500° to 750°C |
|  | HDDY 4: 750° to 1000°C |
|  | HDDY 5: 1,000° to 1,250°C |
|  | HDDY 6: 1,250° to 1,500°C |
|  | HDDY 7: >1,500°C |
| Hospital category depending on the number of beds (HCNB) | HCNB 1: <200 beds |
|  | HCNB 2: 200 to 500 beds |
|  | HCNB 3: 500 to 1,000 beds |
|  | HCNB 4: >1,000 beds |
| Geographic location (GL) | Madrid |
|  | Andalucía |
|  | Valencia |
|  | Rioja |
|  | País Vasco |
|  | Cataluña |
|  | Canarias |
| Range of years | 2005–2007 |
|  | 2008–2012 |

follow a normal distribution and to have the same variance. To prove that these indicators verify a normal distribution, the Levene test (an inferential statistic used to assess the equality of variances for a variable calculated for two or more groups) [32] was used. ANOVA is a statistical tool used to determine whether there are any significant differences between the means of three or more unrelated groups of data. In particular, ANOVA compares the means between the groups and determines whether any of those means are significantly different from each other.

The Gross Domestic Product (GDP) is the monetary value of all finished goods and services produced within a country's borders during a specific period of time, and it is considered a representative indicator that measures the growth or decrease of goods and services production. GDP is one of the primary measures used by decision-makers and financial and other institutions to evaluate the health of the economy. An increase in real GDP is interpreted as a sign that the economy is doing well, while a decrease indicates that the economy is not working at its full capacity. Real GDP is linked to other macro-economic variables such as employment, economic cycles, productivity, and long-term economic growth. In this sense, it is reasonable to consider that the GDP can be related to the services offered by hospitals and that such services could directly be related to the water consumption. The GDP has been divided into four ranges in this study (Table 2).

Heating degrees-day year (HDDY) is defined as the sum of the difference between a reference temperature and the average temperature of the day (taking into account all the days in a period) when such a temperature is lower than 15°C:

$$\text{HDDY (°C)} = \sum_{i=1}^{n} \left(15 - \frac{T_{\max} + T_{\min}}{2}\right) \cdot X_c, \quad (1)$$

where $T_{\max}$ and $T_{\min}$ represent the maximum and the minimum daily temperature, respectively, and $X_c$ is a logical coefficient that will equal unity when the average daily temperature is lower than 15°C and zero for values exceeding 15°C.

## 3. Results

In this section, firstly, the analysis of the correlation between the average annual consumption of water and the three indicators considered (built surface area, number of workers, and number of beds) is presented. Secondly, the ANOVA tests according to the factors listed in Table 2 are presented. The following results are obtained from the water consumption data given in Table 1.

*3.1. Correlations between Average Annual Consumption of CWHC and Built Surface Area, Number of Workers, and Number of Beds.* All possible correlations were accounted for to further conclude that a linear dependence is that which best describes the sample behaviour. This is in good agreement with some studies on hospital management elsewhere reported [33], which modelled the correlation among built surface area, number of workers, and number of beds.

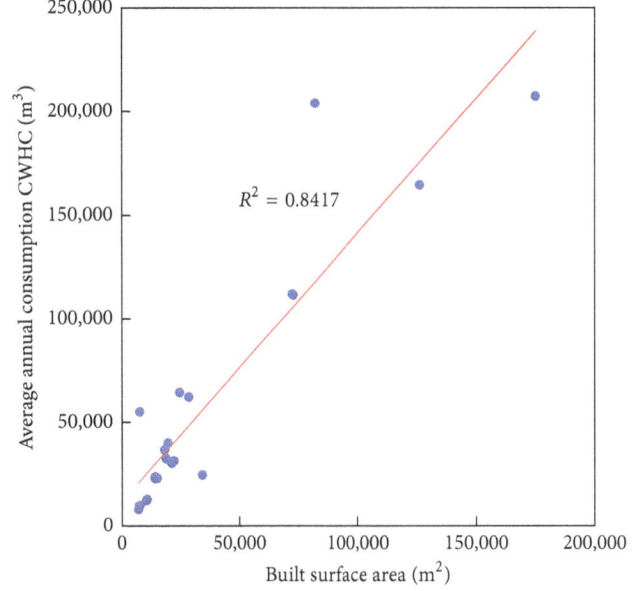

FIGURE 2: Relation between the average annual consumption of CWHC and the built surface area in a hospital.

*3.1.1. Relation between Average Annual Consumption of CWHC and the Built Surface Area (A).* The relation between consumption of CWHC and the built surface area of a hospital is shown in Figure 2, which indicates a good correlation factor ($R^2 = 0.8417$).

Equation (2) shows the mathematical expression for the linear fit in Figure 1:

$$\text{WC} = 1.30A + 11{,}791, \quad (2)$$

where WC represents the average annual consumption of CWHC in m³ and $A$ the built surface area in m² of a hospital, respectively.

*3.1.2. Relation between the Average Annual Consumption of CWHC and the Number of Workers (NW).* In this case, the correlation factor ($R^2 = 0.9046$) shows a higher relation than in the above case. Figure 3 shows the correlation between the average annual consumption of CWHC and the number of workers in a hospital, and (3) sets the mathematical expression for the corresponding linear fit:

$$\text{WC} = 38.26\text{NW} + 15{,}221, \quad (3)$$

where WC represents the average annual consumption of CWHC in m³ and NW the number of workers in a hospital, respectively.

*3.1.3. Relation between the Annual Average Consumption of CWHC and the Number of Beds (NB).* Finally, the plot and the regression expression for the relation between the average annual consumption of CWHC (in m³) and the number of beds (NB) are indicated in Figure 4 and in (4), respectively. Note the correlation coefficient ($R^2 = 0.9172$) is

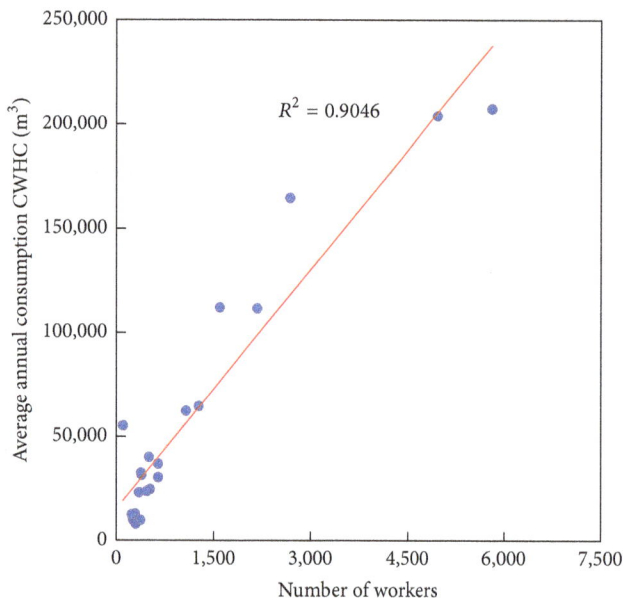

FIGURE 3: Relation between the average annual consumption of CWHC and the number of workers in a hospital.

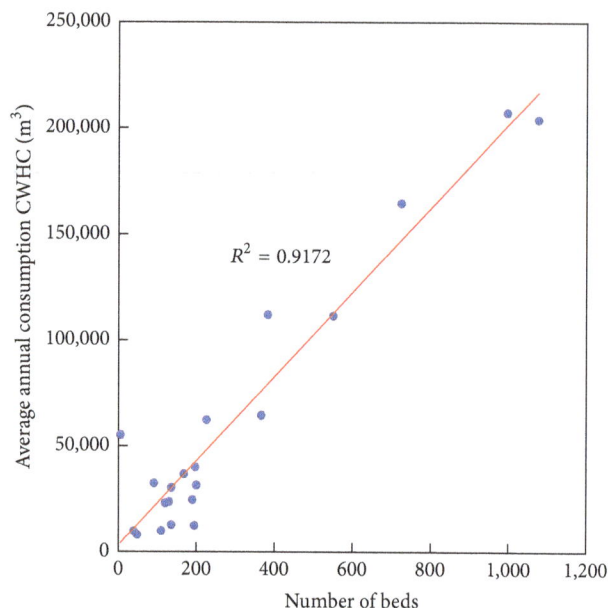

FIGURE 4: Relation between the average annual consumption of CWHC and the number of beds in a hospital.

the highest for the three analysed indicators to estimate water consumption in a hospital:

$$WC = 198.77NB + 3,284, \qquad (4)$$

where WC represents the average annual consumption of CWHC in m$^3$ and NB the number of beds in a hospital.

*3.2. ANOVA Results.* In this subsection, the results obtained from the statistical analysis of variance (ANOVA) are presented. The factors listed in Table 2 as well as the ratios between the average annual consumption of CWHC in a Spanish hospital and the three abovementioned water consumption indicators (built surface area, number of workers, and number of beds in a hospital, resp.) are next analysed. Table 3 lists the obtained $p$ values in the analysis of variance. The null hypothesis in ANOVA test states that the population means for all conditions are the same. In order to determine whether any of the differences between the means are statistically significant, the $p$ value should be compared to the significance level to assess the null hypothesis. A significance level of 0.05 (denoted by $\alpha$) is assumed for the present study, provided such value is regarded to perform appropriately. If the $p$ value is less than or equal to the significance level, that is, $p$ value $\leq 0.05$, the null hypothesis can be rejected and it could be concluded that not all of population means are equal. Otherwise, if the $p$ value is greater than the significance level, there is not enough evidence to reject the null hypothesis that the population means are all equal.

*3.2.1. Water Consumption as Related to the Type of Management (TM).* Considering the type of management in a hospital as a factor, the results of ANOVA test present significant differences ($p < 0.05$) between the average annual water consumption in a hospital and one of three indicators

used, namely, the indicator related to the number of beds, where great differences ($p = 0.03$) have been observed, as shown in Table 3. The $p$ value is widely used in statistical hypothesis testing, specifically in null hypothesis significance testing. In statistical studies, one first chooses a model (the null hypothesis) and a threshold value for $p$, called the significance level of the test, traditionally 1% or 5%, and denoted as $\alpha$. If the $p$ value is less than or equal to the chosen significance level ($\alpha$), the test suggests that the observed data is inconsistent with the null hypothesis, and so the null hypothesis must be rejected. For typical analysis, using the standard $\alpha = 0.05$ cutoff, a widely used interpretation is that a small $p$ value ($\leq 0.05$) indicates strong evidence against the null hypothesis, so it is rejected; and a large $p$ value ($> 0.05$) indicates weak evidence against the null hypothesis (fail to reject). For the particular case of type of management (TM), Table 3 shows that $p < 0.05$ only for the indicator accounting for the number of beds, which means that there is a strong evidence against the null hypothesis.

*3.2.2. Water Consumption as Related to Gross Domestic Product (GDP).* The results from the ANOVA test considering the GDP as a factor show great differences in the three statistical indicators as can be observed in Table 3. In other words, it can be concluded that there is no direct GDP link with the consumption of water according to the area, the number of workers, nor the number of beds.

*3.2.3. Water Consumption as Related to Heating Degrees-Day Year (HDDY).* Taking into account the HDDY factor, the outcome of the test shows differences in one of the three indicators, namely, the indicator of the number of beds ($p = 0.03$). However, there is no evidence of variance for the indicator of the area ($p = 0.39$) and for that of the number

TABLE 3: Analyses of variance.

| Test factors | Consumption ratios | | |
| --- | --- | --- | --- |
| | $\dfrac{\text{m}^3 \text{ average water consumption}}{\text{m}^2 \text{ built surface area}}$ | $\dfrac{\text{m}^3 \text{ average water consumption}}{\text{Number of workers}}$ | $\dfrac{\text{m}^3 \text{ average water consumption}}{\text{Number of beds}}$ |
| Type of management (TM) | $p = 0.14$ | $p = 0.88$ | $p = 0.03^*$ |
| Gross Domestic Prod. (GDP) | $p = 0.52$ | $p = 0.27$ | $p = 0.23$ |
| Heating degrees-day year (HDDY) | $p = 0.39$ | $p = 0.27$ | $p = 0.03^*$ |
| Hospital categories (HCNB) | $p = 0.01^*$ | $p = 0.79$ | $p = 0.51$ |
| Geographical location (GL) | $p = 0.71$ | $p = 0.36$ | $p = 0.01^*$ |
| Range of years (2005–2007 and 2008–2012) | $p = 0.03^*$ | $p = 0.12$ | $p = 0.23$ |

*At the 0.05 level, the population means are significantly different.

TABLE 4: Fischer test for means comparison with 0.05 of significance level.

| HCNB | Mean diff. | SEM | $t$-value | Prob. | Sig. | LCL | UCL |
| --- | --- | --- | --- | --- | --- | --- | --- |
| 3-1 | −0.11 | 0.24 | −0.45 | 0.66 | 0 | −0.62 | 0.40 |
| 2-1 | 0.68 | 0.24 | 2.83 | 0.01 | 1 | 0.17 | 1.19 |
| 2-3 | 0.79 | 0.31 | 2.57 | 0.02 | 1 | 0.14 | 1.44 |
| 4-1 | 1.05 | 0.39 | 2.68 | 0.02 | 1 | 0.22 | 1.88 |
| 4-3 | 1.16 | 0.43 | 2.66 | 0.02 | 1 | 0.23 | 2.08 |
| 4-2 | 0.37 | 0.43 | 0.84 | 0.41 | 0 | 0.56 | 1.29 |

of workers ($p = 0.27$). Thus, there is no direct relationship between HDDY and the water consumption in hospitals in Spain according to the area and number of workers. There is however a link between HDDY and the number of beds.

### 3.2.4. Water Consumption as Related to the Hospital Categorization in terms of the Number of Beds (HCNB).
The analysis of variance considering the category of the hospital as a factor (Table 2) shows great differences among the three statistical indicators, specifically that related to the built surface area of the hospital (Table 3).

Due to the existence of these substantial differences, the Fisher test was carried out in order to thoroughly examine these differences, and it proves that there is no direct link between the category of a hospital (HCNB) and the water consumption in relation to the number of workers or beds (Table 4). There is, however, a link between the HCBN and the built surface area of the hospital. The Fisher test is a statistical significance test used to compare sample means and is proved to be valid for any sample size.

Table 4 lists data corresponding to the analysis of the sample means of various hospital types, according to their HCNB factor. In particular, mean diff. stands for the difference between the means of the two compared samples in each row. The standard error of the mean (SEM) is a measure of how far a particular sample mean is likely to be from the true population mean and is always smaller than the

standard deviation (SD). All other terms ($t$-value, prob., and Sig.) allow evaluation of the degree of similarity between the means of the samples compared. Finally, the lower and upper confidence limits (LCL and UCL) define the 95% confidence interval for the true mean difference between the means.

### 3.2.5. Water Consumption as Related to Geographic Location (GL).
The results collected when considering location as a factor show significant differences in the average annual water consumption of CWHC in a hospital in relation to the number of beds ($p = 0.01$) and no statistical significance according to the built area of the hospital ($p = 0.71$) nor the number of workers ($p = 0.36$). Therefore, it can be concluded that there is a direct relationship between the water consumption based on its location and the number of beds in a hospital.

### 3.2.6. Water Consumption as Related to the Range of Years.
According to the results, the consumption of water according to the number of beds and workers and built area of the hospitals, one of the main explanations of such a significant reduction in CWHC between 2005 and 2007 is the impact of the sensitization and awareness campaigns about water savings. ANOVA test was carried out in order to show the influence of this campaign by using the average consumption of water as a main factor between the abovementioned years and then again from 2007 until 2012. Substantial differences

TABLE 5: Classification according to percentiles and type of statistic indicator.

| Indicator | Average annual consumption in $m^3$ of CWHC | | | | | |
| | Percentiles | | | | | |
| | 10% | 25% | 50% | 75% | 90% | Average |
|---|---|---|---|---|---|---|
| $\dfrac{\text{Average water consumption } (m^3)}{\text{Built surface area } (m^2)}$ | 1.18 | 1.28 | 1.49 | 1.80 | 2.23 | 1.59 |
| $\dfrac{\text{Average water consumption } (m^3)}{\text{Number of workers}}$ | 34.87 | 43.63 | 50.92 | 62.56 | 79.90 | 53.69 |
| $\dfrac{\text{Average water consumption } (m^3)}{\text{Number of beds}}$ | 94.71 | 167.29 | 198.02 | 224.73 | 277.72 | 195.85 |

TABLE 6: Annual average consumption of water given by EMAS.

| | | |
|---|---|---|
| | HCNB 1 | 194 |
| $\dfrac{\text{Average water consumption } (m^3)}{\text{Number of beds}}$ | HCNB 2 | 197 |
| | HCNB 3 | 200 |
| | HCNB 4 | 203 |

were noted in one of the three indicators, namely, the statistical significance (Table 3) in the indicator related to the built surface area ($p = 0.03$), though there is no such a link for the number of workers ($p = 0.12$) nor for the number of beds ($p = 0.23$). Therefore, taking into account the water consumption, there is no direct link with the number of workers nor with the number of beds. There is, however, a direct relation to the built surface area of the hospital.

The final ratio of this study is 195.85 $m^3$/year/bed. Significant consumption averages are shown in Figure 5 according to the statistical indicators. Table 5 shows the classification according to percentiles and type of statistic indicator.

If 34.24 $m^3$ water per hospital bed is assumed as average saving and 163,585 beds are taken to be available nationwide by the time the present study was carried out, the above results yield a potential annual water saving in Spanish hospitals of 5,600,000 $m^3$. This implies an annual saving of 6,832,000 € if the cost of water is assumed as 1.22 €/$m^3$. Additionally it is possible to achieve an energy saving of 2,912 MWh, which would avoid the emission of 22,400 tonnes of $CO_2$ into the atmosphere every year. To work out this saving, an atmospheric emission of 4 kg of $CO_2$ for every $m^3$ of water has been calculated, which accounts for the emissions due to impulsion, purification, and depuration and for an energetic intensity of 0.52 kWh/$m^3$ [34].

The indicators listed in Table 6 have been acquired through the investigation of the averages of different analysed EMAS.

## 4. Discussion

Any action to improve the efficiency of a hospital ought to account for both the climatic and working conditions in this kind of building. It must not disregard other requirements, for instance, the accessibility, safety, and reliability of its facilities.

Another factor that has to be analysed is the presence of *Legionella*, which is usually present in cooling towers and hydrological networks and in the production equipment of domestic hot water, mainly in accumulation stores where the stratification conditions boost its proliferation [35]. Interruptions in the water supply may create, in any section of the hydrological network, the conditions required for the bacteria to thrive and thus pollute the water once the supply is restored. In addition to this, sand and dust contain inactive forms of *Legionella*, which can move through the air and then plant themselves, thus polluting the cooling tower collectors. On one hand, purges in the facilities contribute to a reduction in the risk of this bacteria spreading but on the other hand, the water consumption level greatly increases.

An important element of the saving of water has been seen to be directly linked to the daily management of a hospital [36], in which it is possible to directly control the water consumption associated with both workers and users. Therefore it is suggested that workers increase their awareness of the importance of saving water through additional training and campaigns to optimise the sensitivity surrounding water saving and the rational use of water. The rain must also be used advantageously; it can be collected from the roof and used to irrigate green areas. This is an option, which would reduce the consumption of CWHC and consequently its environmental impact. The storage of this water, however, is not recommended. Another advisable strategy is to use specially constructed wells for the watering of green areas. Greywater, which comes from showers and sinks, must not be reused under any circumstances in this kind of building, as aseptic conditions take priority.

Measures for energy saving in hospital management should mainly focus on both domestic hot water savings and the increase of energy efficiency in production installations, given that such facilities are typically linked to high rates of energy consumption. However, efforts should also be made to account for the exploitation, channelling, and recovery of water from cooling/condensation towers and for the installation of electronic counters to monitor consumption rates and potential leaks.

The installation of atomizers, specific saving devices to be screwed in taps and showers, is also recommended. Air is injected to the water flow so that the speed of the flow stream is increased and the flow rate is thus reduced. Even though atomizers apparently increase the flow rate, water savings

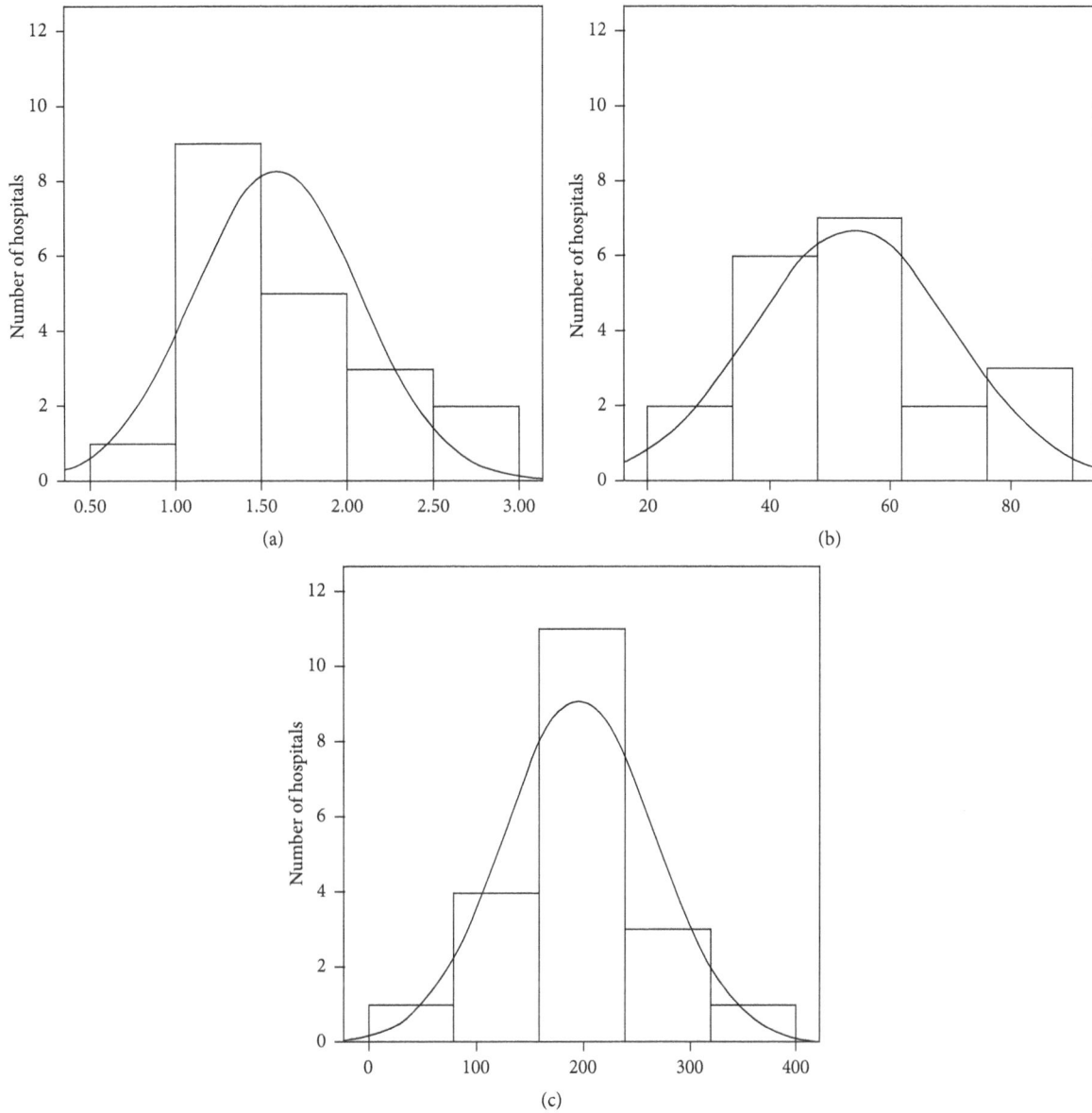

FIGURE 5: Average consumption in m$^3$ of CWHC for each indicator: (a) built surface area, (b) number of workers, and (c) number of beds.

associated with their use are reported to range between 30% and 50%.

With regard to gardening, savings of around 25–30% can be achieved by landscape adaptation of the surroundings through xeriscape techniques, by the selection of native species, and by the use of efficient and programmable irrigation systems.

The use of floor cleaning devices based on microfiber fabric in hospitals is proved to reduce water consumption as well as decrease the needs for chemicals.

In all cases ISO-14000 and EMAS certifications are suggested procedures for improved management of hospital infrastructures, as can be seen from different ISO-14000 studies [37] and EMAS studies [38]. Being in possession of such certificates implies a greater ability to implement the improvement of the hospital image and environmental

surroundings. At the same time, environmentally speaking, wastage and how it is discharged cannot be overlooked nor omitted.

The information related to the environmental efficiency of Spanish hospitals registered in EMAS is sufficient but there are certain deficiencies in the indicators (surface built area, number of beds, and number of workers) that make it difficult to make a comparative evaluation. This is because the chosen indicators are not always used with the same criteria, and consequently they do not quantify the analysed parameter appropriately. In turn, this is likely to be because of a wrongly chosen indicator. There are studies which indicate such deficiencies according to the used indicators, like the EVER study [39].

The results of this research can be useful to quantify the exact cost of water consumption. It could be interesting to repeat the same study in different organizations and hospitals in other countries, in order to establish some comparisons.

The results are extrapolated to similar buildings with limitations due to the wide variety of healthcare building designs mainly based on architectural conception, climate conditions, interior facilities, and building locations.

## 5. Conclusion

It can be concluded that there is a link between the cold water for human consumption (CWHC) in hospitals and the built surface area of the hospital ($A$) and the number of beds (NB). However, the number of workers (NW) has no significant statistical relation to such consumption.

Furthermore, it has been proved that the factors based on the hospital category depending on number of beds (HCNB), type of management (TM), heating degrees-day year (HDDY), and geographic location (GL) have a direct relationship with water consumption. There is no such link regarding the GDP.

The statistical indicator of the number of workers (NW) is not considered appropriate to be used as a ratio to quantify the consumption of water. This indicator is the most used in EMAS and it has been proved throughout this study that it is not consistent enough and it is not adequately quantified.

## Nomenclature

$A$: Value of the built area in a hospital, $m^2$
HDDY: Heating degrees-day year, °C
NB: Total number of beds in a hospital
NW: Number of workers in a hospital
$T_{max}$: Maximum daily temperature, °C
$T_{min}$: Minimum daily temperature, °C
WC: Average annual consumption of CWHC, $m^3$
$X_c$: Logical coefficient.

## Competing Interests

The authors declare no potential competing interests.

## Acknowledgments

The authors wish to express their gratitude to the EU Eco-Management and Audit Scheme for the resources provided throughout the development of the present work. This study has been carried out through the Research Project GR-15057 linked to the IV Regional Plan of Research and Investigation from the General Government of Extremadura 2015–2017.

## References

[1] Fundación de la Energía de la Comunidad de Madrid, *Guía de Ahorro y Eficiencia Energética en Hospitales*, 2010.

[2] Ambientum, *El Portal Profesional del Medio Ambiente*, El Consumo de Agua en Porcentajes, 2005.

[3] Ministry of Agriculture, *Food and Environment*, Ministry of Agriculture, Madrid, Spain, 1998.

[4] European Union, "Water performance of buildings," Final Report, European Commission, DG Environment, 2012.

[5] P. H. Gleick, D. Haasz, C. Henges-Jeck et al., *Waste Not, Want Not: The Potential for Urban Water Conservation in California*, Alonzo Printing, Hayward, Calif, USA, 2003.

[6] Best Environmental Practices in the Healthcare Sector, *A Guide to Improve your Environmental Performance*, Institute for Ecopreneurship (IEC), University of Applied Sciences Northwester Switzerland (FHNW), School of Life Sciences (HLS), Sustainable Business Associate (SBA), Royal Scientific Society (RSS), 2006.

[7] F. Daschner, "Substance flow water management-substance flow related water/sewage wastewater management in European hospitals. Water saving- strategies and strategies for reducing wastewater pollution for water saving potentials and pollution control of sewage," Project LIFE99 ENV/D/000455, 1999–2012.

[8] FEMP-Federal Energy Management Program, http://energy.gov/eere/femp/federal-energy-management-program.

[9] The Office of the Reviser of Statutes, State of Minnesota, 2013, https://www.revisor.mn.gov/rules/?id=4715.3600.

[10] Washington State Department of Health, *Water System Design Manual*, Office of Drinking Water Constituent Services Section, 2009.

[11] The Audit Commission for local authorities and the National Health Service in England and Wales, *Untapped Savings: Water Services in the NHS*, NHS Occasional Paper no. 5, Audit Commission, 1993.

[12] A. Reller, *Greener Hospitals. Improving Environmental Performance*, Environment Science Center, University Augsburg, Augsburg, Germany, 2003.

[13] M. Dettenkofer, K. Kuemmerer, A. Schuster et al., "Environmental auditing in hospitals: First results in a University Hospital," *Environmental Management*, vol. 25, no. 1, pp. 105–113, 2000.

[14] New Found Labrador and Department of Environment and Conservation of Canada, *Study on Water Quality and Demand on Public Water Supplies with Variable Flow Regimes and Water Demand*, CBLC Limited, Halifax, UK, 2011.

[15] Comisión Nacional del Agua, *Manual de Agua Potable, Alcantarillado y Saneamiento. Datos Básicos*, 2007, ftp://ftp.cna.gob.mx/Mapas/libros%20pdf%202007/Alcantarillado%20Pluvial.pdf.

[16] Organización Panamericana de la Salud et al., 1999, http://www.paho.org.

[17] K. S. Werner-Verlag, *GmbH*, Sanitäre Haustechnik, Düsseldorf, Germany, 1981.

[18] P. D. Bourkas, *Applications of Installations in Hospitals*, National Technical University of Athens, Athens, Greece, 1999.

[19] J. S. Katsanis, P. G. Halaris, G. N. Malahias, and P. D. Bourkas, "Estimation of energy consumption in hospitals," in *Proceedings of the 5th IASTED International Conference 'Power and Energy Systems'*, June 2005.

[20] J. S. Katsanis, P. G. Halaris, P. T. Tsarabaris, G. N. Malahias, and P. D. Bourkas, *Estimation of Energy Consumption for Domestic Hot Water in Hospitals*, Series on Energy and Power Systems, 2006.

[21] J. Bujak, "Heat consumption for preparing domestic hot water in hospitals," *Energy and Buildings*, vol. 42, no. 7, pp. 1047–1055, 2010.

[22] J. García Sanz-Calcedo, S. Garrido, and F. Fernández Tardío, "Se puede ahorrar energía en la gestión del agua en un hospital," in

*XXVII Congreso Nacional de Ingeniería Hospitalaria*, Asociación Española de Ingeniería Hospitalaria, Santiago de Compostela, Spain, 2009.

[23] J. García-Sanz-Calcedo, "Analysis on energy efficiency in healthcare buildings," *Journal of Healthcare Engineering*, vol. 5, no. 3, pp. 361–374, 2014.

[24] European Communities, "Regulation (EC) No 1221/2009 of the European Parliament and of the Council of 25 November 2009 on the voluntary participation by organizations in a Community eco-management and audit scheme (EMAS), repealing Regulation (EC) No 761/2001 and Commission Decision 2001/681/EC and 2006/193/EC," *Official Journal of European Communities, Brussels*, 2009.

[25] F. Iraldo, F. Testa, and M. Frey, "Is an environmental management system able to influence environmental and competitive performance? The case of the eco-management and audit scheme (EMAS) in the European union," *Journal of Cleaner Production*, vol. 17, no. 16, pp. 1444–1452, 2009.

[26] UK Department of Health, *Environment and Sustainability Health Technical Memorandum 07-04: Water Management and Water Efficiency—Best Practice Advice for the Healthcare Sector*, UK Department of Health, London, UK, 2013.

[27] Water Transformed Sustainable Water Solutions for Climate Change Adaptation, *Identifying & Implementing Water Efficiency & Recycling Opportunities by Service Sector Lecture 4.2*, chapter 4, The Health Sector-Water Savings in Hospitals, Sydney, Australia, 2009.

[28] European Commission, Environment EMAS, http://ec.europa.eu/environment/emas/index_en.htm.

[29] J. S. Katsanis, P. T. Tsarabaris, P. D. Bourkas, P. G. Halaris, and G. N. Malahias, "Estimating water and energy consumption of hospital laundries," *AATCC Review*, vol. 8, no. 7, pp. 32–36, 2008.

[30] Ministerio de Sanidad, Servicios Sociales e Igualdad de España, http://www.msssi.gob.es/estadisticas/microdatos.do.

[31] Schneider Electrics, "Leading techniques for energy savings in healthcare facilities," White Paper on Healthcare, 2006, http://static.schneider-electric.us/assets/pdf/healthcare/whitepapers/Leading Techniques WP.pdf.

[32] N. R. Farnumy and J. L. Devore, *Applied Statistics for Engineers and Scientists*, Duxbury Press, New York, NY, USA, 2nd edition, 2004.

[33] J. García-Sanz-Calcedo, F. López-Rodríguez, and F. Cuadros, "Quantitative analysis on energy efficiency of health centers according to their size," *Energy and Buildings*, vol. 73, pp. 7–12, 2014.

[34] L. Hardy and A. Garrido, Papeles de Agua Virtual no. 6: Análisis y Evaluación de las relaciones entre el agua y la energía en España: Fundación Botín, 2010.

[35] J. G. Sanz-Calcedo and P. Monzón-González, "Analysis of the economic impact of environmental biosafety works projects in healthcare centres in Extremadura (Spain)," *DYNA*, vol. 81, no. 188, pp. 100–105, 2014.

[36] J. García Sanz-Calcedo, F. Cuadros Blázquez, F. López Rodríguez, and A. Ruiz-Celma, "Influence of the number of users on the energy efficiency of health centres," *Energy and Buildings*, vol. 43, no. 7, pp. 1544–1548, 2011.

[37] S. X. Zeng, C. M. Tam, V. W. Y. Tam, and Z. M. Deng, "Towards implementation of ISO 14001 environmental management systems in selected industries in China," *Journal of Cleaner Production*, vol. 13, no. 7, pp. 645–656, 2005.

[38] K. Rennings, A. Ziegler, K. Ankele, S. Hoffman, and J. Nill, "The influence of the EU environmental management and audit scheme on environmental innovations and competitiveness in Germany: an analysis on the basis of case studies and a large-scale survey," ZEW Discussion Papers 03-14, 2003, http://ideas.repec.org/s/zbw/zewdip.html.

[39] EVER Team, EVER: Evaluation of EMAS and Eco-label for their Revision. IEFE, Bocconi University IT, Adelphi Consult—DE, IOEW, Office Heidelberg—DE, SPRU, Sussex University-UK, Valor & Tinge A/S—DK. European Commission, DG, Environment, Brussels, 2005.

# 5

# Length of Hospital Stay Prediction at the Admission Stage for Cardiology Patients Using Artificial Neural Network

**Pei-Fang (Jennifer) Tsai,**[1] **Po-Chia Chen,**[1] **Yen-You Chen,**[1] **Hao-Yuan Song,**[1] **Hsiu-Mei Lin,**[2] **Fu-Man Lin,**[3] **and Qiou-Pieng Huang**[4]

[1]*Department of Industrial Engineering and Management, National Taipei University of Technology, Taipei 10608, Taiwan*
[2]*Division of Health Insurance, Mackay Memorial Hospital, Taipei 10449, Taiwan*
[3]*Medical Affairs Department, Mackay Memorial Hospital, Taipei 10449, Taiwan*
[4]*Registration and Admitting, Mackay Memorial Hospital, Taipei 10449, Taiwan*

Correspondence should be addressed to Pei-Fang (Jennifer) Tsai; ptsai@ntut.edu.tw

Academic Editor: Hélder A. Santos

For hospitals' admission management, the ability to predict length of stay (LOS) as early as in the preadmission stage might be helpful to monitor the quality of inpatient care. This study is to develop artificial neural network (ANN) models to predict LOS for inpatients with one of the three primary diagnoses: coronary atherosclerosis (CAS), heart failure (HF), and acute myocardial infarction (AMI) in a cardiovascular unit in a Christian hospital in Taipei, Taiwan. A total of 2,377 cardiology patients discharged between October 1, 2010, and December 31, 2011, were analyzed. Using ANN or linear regression model was able to predict correctly for 88.07% to 89.95% CAS patients at the predischarge stage and for 88.31% to 91.53% at the preadmission stage. For AMI or HF patients, the accuracy ranged from 64.12% to 66.78% at the predischarge stage and 63.69% to 67.47% at the preadmission stage when a tolerance of 2 days was allowed.

## 1. Introduction

The demand for health care services continues to grow as the population in most developed countries ages. To make health care more affordable, policy makers and health organizations try to align financial incentives with the implementation of care processes based on best practices and the achievement of better patient outcomes. The length of stay (LOS) in hospitals is often used as an indicator of efficiency of care and hospital performance. It is generally recognized that a shorter stay indicates less resource consumption per discharge and cost-saving while postdischarge care is shifted to less expensive venues [1]. It motivates the endeavor to develop a diagnosis-related group (DRG) for patient classification based on the type of hospital treatments in relation to the costs incurred by the hospital. This quality assurance scheme was then linked to the prospective payment system (PPS) and adopted by the federal government in the United States for the Medicare program in 1983. This payment system was found to moderate

hospital cost inflation due to a significant decline in the average length of stay (ALOS), which refers to the average number of days that patients spend in hospital [2]. Under the assumption that patients sharing common diagnostic and demographic characteristics require similar resource intensity, the aim of DRG is to quantify and standardize hospital resource utilization for patients [3].

Other than diagnostic attributes, most research focuses on two types of factors to explain the variation in LOS: patient characteristics and hospital characteristics. In examining data for the National Health Service (NHS) in the United Kingdom, the variation in LOS for those over age 65 was consistently larger across all regions [4]. It was observed that the variation in LOS between hospitals was larger compared to that between doctors in the same hospital [5]. Hospital policy in treatment management can also determine LOS. It was found that psychiatrists were able to predict LOS with significant accuracy, but only for patients they treated. Moreover, the prediction by a hospital coordinator involved in all patient treatments was significantly more correlated to the true LOS than psychiatrists' predictions [6]. A comparison of data from 24 hospitals in Japan showed that inpatient capacity and the ratio of involuntary admissions correlated positively to longer LOS [7]. A higher level of caregiver interaction among nurses and physicians, such as communication, coordination, and conflict management, was significantly associated with lower LOS [8].

The ability to predict LOS as an initial assessment of patients' risk is critical for better resource planning and allocation [9], especially when the resources are limited, as in ICUs [10, 11]. Yang et al. considered timing for LOS prediction in three clinical stages for burn patients: admission, acute, and posttreatment. Using three different regression models, the best mean absolute error (MAE) in the LOS predictions was around 9 days in both the admission and the acute stage and 6 days in the posttreatment stage. With three more treatment-related variables, the results showed that the prediction accuracy was significantly improved in the post-treatment stage [11]. An accurate prediction of LOS can also facilitate management with higher flexibility in hospital bed use and better assessment in the cost-effectiveness treatment [12, 13].

This prediction can even stratify patients according to their risk for prolonged stays [14, 15]. Spratt et al. used a multivariate logistic regression method to identify factors associated with prolonged stays (>30 days) for patients with acute ischemic stroke. In addition to advanced age (>65), diabetes and in-hospital infection were significantly associated with prolonged LOS [14]. Lee et al. analyzed LOS data on childhood gastroenteritis in Australia and, using either the robust gamma mixed regression or linear mixed regression method, found that both gastrointestinal sugar intolerance and failure to thrive significantly affected prolonged LOS [16]. Schmelzer et al. used the multiple logistic regression method and found that both the American Society of Anesthesiologists (ASA) scores and postoperative complications were significant in the prediction of prolonged LOS after a colectomy [17].

Rosen et al. studied the LOS variation for Medicare patients after coronary artery bypass graft surgery (CABG) in 28 hospitals. They found that including deceased patients did not significantly influence the results. Other than age and gender, the most powerful predictors were history of mitral valve disease or cerebrovascular disease and preoperative placement of an intra-aortic balloon pump. Different hospitals varied significantly in their LOS, and the readmission rate was linearly related to longer LOS [18]. Janssen et al. constructed a logistic regression model to predict the probability for patients requiring 3 or more days in ICU after CABG. Only 60% of the patients predicted to be high risks had a prolonged ICU stay [15]. Chang et al. identified that, among preoperative factors, age of more than 75 years and having chronic obstructive pulmonary disease (COPD) were associated with increased LOS for patients who underwent elective infrarenal aortic surgery [19].

Even though diagnosis had been considered the primary factor affecting hospital stays, patients' clinical conditions, such as the number of diagnoses and the intensity of nursing services required, might be as critical in determining LOS variations within some DRGs [20]. One study showed that only 12% of the variation could be explained by patient characteristics and general hospital characteristics for patients with a primary diagnosis of acute myocardial infarction (AMI) [21]. For heart failure patients, Whellan et al. studied data from 246 hospitals for admission predictors for LOS. Patients with longer LOS had a higher disease severity and more comorbidities, such as hypertension, cardiac dysrhythmias, diabetes mellitus, COPD, and chronic renal insufficiency or failure. However, the overall model based on characteristics at the time of admission explained only a modest amount of LOS variation [22].

The purpose of this study is to develop artificial neural network (ANN) models to predict LOS for inpatients with one of the three primary diagnoses: coronary atherosclerosis (CAS), heart failure (HF), and acute myocardial infarction (AMI) in a cardiovascular unit in a Christian hospital in Taipei, Taiwan. A better recognition in critical factors before admission that determine LOS, or a capacity to predict an individual patient's LOS, could promote the development of efficient admission policy and optimize resource management in hospitals. This study aims to use ANN to predict LOS for patients with three primary diagnoses: coronary atherosclerosis (CAS), heart failure (HF), and acute myocardial infarction (AMI) in a cardiovascular unit. Moreover, two stages in LOS prediction are presented: one uses all clinical factors, designated as the predischarge stage, and the other uses only factors available before admission, designated as the preadmission stage. The prediction results obtained at the predischarge stage are then used to evaluate the relative effectiveness in predicting LOS at the preadmission stage.

The remainder of this paper is organized as follows. In Section 2, the method including steps in data collection and processing and prediction model construction is introduced. Then, the prediction results of various artificial neural network (ANN) models are presented in Section 3. The discussion of the results and the conclusion of the research finding is given in Section 4, with the limitations and future research directions.

## 2. Method

*2.1. Data Sources and Data Preprocessing.* This study was approved by the Mackay Memorial Hospital Institutional Review Board (IRB) for protection of human subjects in research. Clinical and administrative data were obtained for cardiology patients discharged between October 1, 2010, and December 31, 2011, in a Christian hospital with two locations in the metropolitan area of Taipei, Taiwan: Taipei branch and Tamshui branch. A total of 2,424 admission cases were collected for patients with one of three primary diagnoses: CAS, HF, and AMI. Then 47 admissions were identified as outliers, with more than three standard deviations from the mean, when fitting for both forward addition regression and backward elimination regression models. For the remaining 2,377 cases, 933 were coronary atherosclerosis (CAS) patients, 872 heart failure (HF) patients, and 572 acute myocardial

TABLE 1: Inpatient characteristics, occurrence, and the associated LOS data in this study.

| Characteristics | | Quantity ($N$ = 2377) | Occurrence (%) | LOS (days) | | |
|---|---|---|---|---|---|---|
| | | | | Mean | SD | Median |
| Sex | Male | 1501 | 63 | 5.05 | 4.97 | 5 |
| | Female | 876 | 37 | 6.89 | 5.98 | 7 |
| Age | Less than 65 | 1059 | 44 | 4.42 | 4.53 | 3 |
| | 65~74 | 493 | 21 | 5.32 | 5.01 | 4 |
| | 75~84 | 541 | 23 | 7.31 | 5.83 | 6 |
| | 85 and above | 284 | 12 | 8.30 | 6.69 | 6 |
| Location | Tamshui branch | 803 | 34 | 6.21 | 5.39 | 5 |
| | Taipei branch | 1574 | 66 | 5.48 | 5.45 | 4 |
| Main diagnosis | Coronary atherosclerosis (ICD414) | 933 | 39 | 2.63 | 2.25 | 2 |
| | Heart failure (ICD428) | 872 | 37 | 8.24 | 5.87 | 7 |
| | Acute myocardial infarction (ICD410) | 572 | 24 | 6.97 | 5.95 | 5 |
| Comorbidity | Myocardial infarction (ICD410/412) | 134 | 6 | 3.99 | 4.08 | 2 |
| | Diabetes (ICD250) | 954 | 40 | 6.24 | 5.85 | 4 |
| | Cerebrovascular disease (ICD433/434/437/438) | 69 | 3 | 7.61 | 6.14 | 6 |
| | Cardiac dysrhythmias (ICD427) | 447 | 19 | 6.81 | 5.20 | 6 |
| | Heart failure (ICD428) | 394 | 17 | 6.27 | 6.20 | 4 |
| | Chronic airway obstruction (ICD496) | 63 | 3 | 5.00 | 4.21 | 4 |
| | Hypertensive disease (ICD401/402/403/404) | 1218 | 51 | 5.07 | 5.00 | 3 |
| | Coronary atherosclerosis (ICD414) | 909 | 38 | 5.39 | 4.45 | 4 |
| Intervention | Percutaneous transluminal coronary angioplasty (PTCA) | 577 | 24 | 4.68 | 4.71 | 3 |
| | Percutaneous coronary intervention (PCI) | 281 | 12 | 4.48 | 4.61 | 3 |
| | Coronary angiography | 1382 | 58 | 3.86 | 3.78 | 2 |
| | Coronary stenting | 750 | 32 | 4.73 | 4.51 | 3 |
| | Cardiac catheterization | 1297 | 55 | 4.01 | 4.13 | 2 |
| | Left ventricular X-ray | 512 | 22 | 3.66 | 3.98 | 2 |
| TW-DRG pay | Yes | 593 | 25 | 2.94 | 3.09 | 2 |
| | No | 1784 | 75 | 6.66 | 5.73 | 5 |

infarction (AMI) patients, as summarized in Table 1. The LOS of any patient in this cardiology unit was defined as from the time of admission to the time of discharge with range from 1 to 35 days, with an average of 5.73, a standard deviation of 5.44, and a median of 4 days. About 63% were male. The age ranges from 21 to 99 years, with an average of 67.07, a standard deviation of 14.35, and a median of 68; 35% were 75 years or older.

An admission case might have zero to multiple comorbidities and similar medical histories were aggregated into comorbidity factors. For example, the history of hypertensive disease includes four types of diseases as identified by ICD-9 codes 401 (essential hypertension) to 404 (hypertensive heart and chronic kidney disease). Each case might have zero to multiple interventions during the admission. Out of a total of 46 types of intervention or diagnostic ancillary services found in the dataset, only the top 6 interventions with more than 5% occurrence in the entire dataset were adopted in this study. The last characteristic, TW-DRG pay, was regarding whether the admission case had been reimbursed by the pay-per-case (i.e., TW-DRG) system implemented

by the National Health Insurance Administration (NHIA). The NHIA in Taiwan provides a universal health insurance system and covers approximately 99% of the population [23]. Except for using fee-for-service payment system, the NHIA started introducing the first phase of TW-DRG with 164 groups from 2010. Since cases in the same DRG are reimbursed with the same amount, it is to encourage hospitals to improve their financial performance by better utilizing medical resources [24]. Among the data collected, 25% were reimbursed through TW-DRG payment by the NHIA.

*2.2. Statistical Analysis.* Pearson's correlation coefficients were used to study the relationships between LOS and each inpatient's characteristics. As summarized in Table 2, it was observed that all characteristics were significantly correlated with LOS except for the comorbidity of chronic airway obstruction (ICD 496). As for the risk factors, the top three significant positive correlated variables for longer LOS were patients with heart failure (ICD 428) as main diagnosis, who were older and female. It was consistent with

TABLE 2: Pearson's correlation coefficient for each inpatient characteristic to LOS.

| Characteristics | Correlation coefficient ($r$) | $p$ value |
|---|---|---|
| Female sex | 0.163** | 0.000 |
| Age | 0.251** | 0.000 |
| Location | 0.063** | 0.002 |
| Main diagnosis | | |
|   Coronary atherosclerosis (ICD414) | −0.459** | 0.000 |
|   Heart failure (ICD428) | 0.351** | 0.000 |
|   Acute myocardial infarction (ICD410) | 0.128** | 0.000 |
| Comorbidity | | |
|   Myocardial infarction (ICD410/412) | −0.078** | 0.000 |
|   Diabetes (ICD250) | 0.077** | 0.000 |
|   Cerebrovascular disease (ICD433/434/437/438) | 0.060** | 0.004 |
|   Cardiac dysrhythmias (ICD427) | 0.096** | 0.000 |
|   Heart failure (ICD428) | 0.044* | 0.032 |
|   Chronic airway obstruction (ICD496) | −0.022 | 0.280 |
|   Hypertensive disease (ICD401/402/403/404) | −0.125** | 0.000 |
|   Coronary atherosclerosis (ICD414) | −0.050* | 0.015 |
| Intervention | | |
|   PTCA | −0.405** | 0.000 |
|   PCI | −0.346** | 0.000 |
|   Coronary angiography | −0.125** | 0.000 |
|   Coronary stenting | −0.200** | 0.000 |
|   Cardiac catheterization | −0.109** | 0.000 |
|   Left ventricular X-ray | −0.084** | 0.000 |
| TW-DRG pay | −0.295** | 0.000 |

($^{**}$ $p$ value < 0.01; $^{*}$ $p$ value < 0.05).

the findings about factors related to prolonged LOS from literature: female, increasing age, and comorbidities such as cerebrovascular disease and diabetes mellitus [18, 19, 22]. The top three significant negative correlated variables for longer LOS were patients with coronary atherosclerosis (ICD 414) as main diagnosis, who went through either percutaneous transluminal coronary angioplasty (PTCA) or percutaneous coronary intervention (PCI).

As shown in Figure 1, the distribution in LOS data was skewed with few cases staying longer than 14 days. The average and standard deviation of LOS for CAS patients were 2.63 days and 2.25 days, respectively. For AMI and HF patients, the average and standard deviations of LOS were 7.74 days and 5.93 days, respectively. The distribution of LOS for CAS patients was significantly different than that for patients with either AMI or HF (with $p$ value < 0.0001), which suggested different prediction models should be built for CAS patients and for non-CAS patients or referred to as AMI and HF patients.

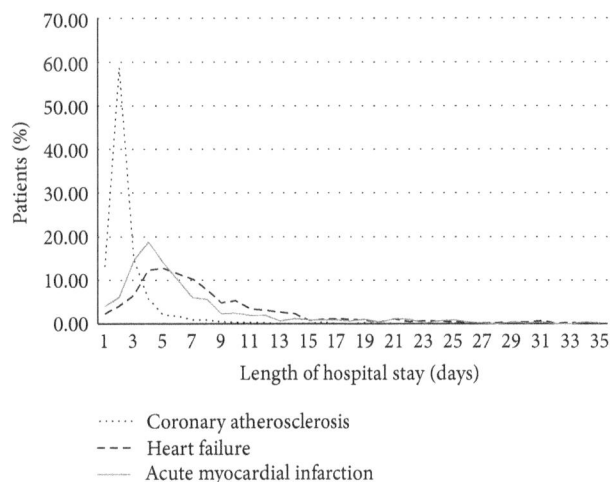

...... Coronary atherosclerosis
--- Heart failure
—— Acute myocardial infarction

FIGURE 1: Distribution of LOS for patients for three major diagnoses: CAS, HF, and AMI.

### 2.3. Structure for Artificial Neural Networks (ANNs).

With the profound growth in clinical knowledge and technology, the development of more sophisticated information systems to support clinical decision making is essential to enhance quality and improve efficiency. Artificial neural networks (ANNs) are useful in modeling complex systems and have been applied in various areas, from accounting to school admission [25]. Walczak and Cerpa proposed four design criteria in artificial neural network (ANN) modeling: the appropriate input variables, the best learning methods, the number of hidden layers, and the quantity of neural nodes per hidden layer [26]. The learning method of ANN can be either supervised or unsupervised, depending on whether the output values should be known before or should be learned directly from the input values. For supervised learning, backpropagation is one of the most commonly used methods due to its robustness and ease of implementation [27].

The clinical benefits of using ANN had been notable in specific areas, such as cervical cytology and early detection of acute myocardial infarction (AMI) [28]. Compared with logistic regression, ANNs were found useful in predicting medical outcomes due to their nature of nonlinear statistical principles and inference [29]. Dybowski et al. adopted an ANN to predict the survival results for patients with systematic inflammatory response syndrome and hemodynamic shock. After improving the performance of ANN iteratively, the predicted outcome was more accurate than using a logistic regression model [30]. Gholipour et al. utilized an ANN model to predict the ICU survival outcome and the LOS for traumatic patients. The results showed that the mean predicted LOS using ANN was not significantly different than the mean of actual LOS [31]. Launay et al. developed ANN models to predict the prolonged LOS (13 days and above) for elder emergency patients (age 80 and over) [32]. Based on the biomedical literature from PUBMED, Dreiseitl and Ohno-Machado showed that the discriminatory performance of ANN models was better or not worse in 93% of the surveyed papers compared to the logistic regression method [33]. Grossi et al. found ANN models outperformed traditional statistic methods in accuracy in various diagnostic and prognostic problems in gastroenterology [34].

The selection of input variables used in an ANN model is critical. Li et al. found that the ANN model using all input variables yielded a slightly higher predictive accuracy than the one using a subset of variables filtered by correlation analysis [35]. Hence, we decided to consider all inpatient characteristics, including gender, age, location, main diagnosis, eight types of comorbidity, six types of intervention, and whether the case met the criteria for TW-DRG reimbursement. These input variables were then categorized into two stages: preadmission stage and predischarge stage, as shown in Table 3. Variables in the preadmission stage included information available prior to hospitalization, such as gender, age, hospital branch (location) to be admitted to, main diagnosis, and comorbidities. In the predischarge stage, additional to variables in the preadmission stage, it includes interventions and whether the case was reimbursed by TW-DRG payment. A case is to be reimbursed by TW-DRG payment, not default pay-per-service, depending on the actual discharge condition such as surgical procedure, treatment, and discharge status according to the NHIA guideline [36].

Separate ANNs were built to predict LOS: one for coronary atherosclerosis (CAS) patients and the other for heart failure or acute myocardial infarction AMI and HF patients. Figure 2 shows the general structure of backpropagation artificial neural networks in this research. The output layer has only one neuron and it generates a number ranged from 0 to 35 to represent the predicted LOS. The size of input layer depends on the number of input variables. Here, the prediction model using input variables in the predischarge stage is referred to as the predischarge model. Likewise, the model using variables in the preadmission stage is referred

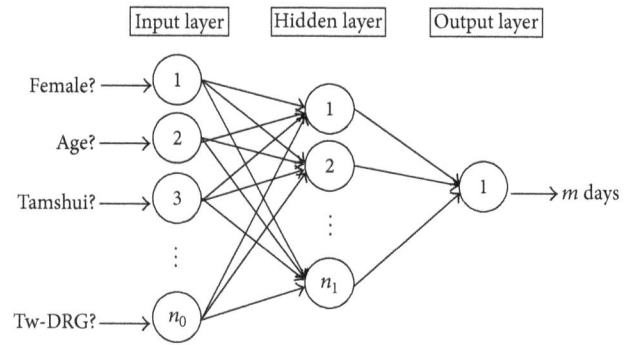

FIGURE 2: General structure of backpropagation artificial neural networks in this study.

to as the preadmission model. For a predischarge model, the input layer in an ANN model has 18 neurons ($n_0$ = 18) for CAS patients. For AMI and HF patients, the value of $n_0$ is 19 with one additional neuron with Boolean value to represent whether the major diagnosis is HF in a predischarge model. In preadmission models, the value of $n_0$ is 11 and 12 for CAS patients and for AMI and HF patients, respectively.

As for the hidden layer, more neurons were found to enable a better closeness-of-fit [37] with lower training errors [38]. However, large ANN size also required more training efforts [39] and could result in overfitting [38]. Some research suggested the number of neural nodes in hidden layers to be between 2/3 to 2 times of the size of the input layer [26, 39, 40].

## 3. Results

In this section, the LOS prediction in predischarge model and preadmission model using ANNs is benchmarked with the results using linear regression (LR) models. All prediction models are implemented using IBM® SPSS® v.21 and IBM SPSS Neural Networks 21. Similar to the preliminary trial run, the original data was separated into training dataset and test dataset. The training dataset included 744 admissions for CAS patients and 1,155 admissions for AMI and HF patients, and the test dataset consisted of 189 admissions for CAS patients and 289 admissions for AMI and HF patients. During training any ANN model, 70% of the training dataset were randomly assigned to the training set and the remaining 30% to the validation set. The training stops when the number of training epochs reaches 2,000 or there is no improvement in validation error for 600 epochs consecutively. For LR models, the entire training dataset was used to generate the linear regression functions.

*3.1. For CAS Patients.* The performance of prediction models is evaluated using the same test dataset. Since the LOS predictions obtained by ANN or LR models are continuous numbers, we further define that a prediction of LOS is considered accurate if the difference is within 1 day from the actual LOS for CAS patients. Moreover, the effectiveness of predictability was measured according to the mean absolute

TABLE 3: Input variables in preadmission and predischarge stages with associated values for ANN models.

| Stage | Variables | Value (Boolean value) | | |
|---|---|---|---|---|
| | | Male (0) | 21~99 | Female (1) |
| Preadmission | Gender | Male (0) | | Female (1) |
| | Age | | 21~99 | |
| | Location | Taipei branch (0) | | Tamshui branch (1) |
| | Main diagnosis (for non-CAS patients) | AMI (0) | | HF (1) |
| | Myocardial infarction (ICD410/412) | Absence (0) | | Presence (1) |
| | Diabetes (ICD250) | Absence (0) | | Presence (1) |
| | Cerebrovascular disease (ICD433/434/437/438) | Absence (0) | | Presence (1) |
| | Cardiac dysrhythmias (ICD427) | Absence (0) | | Presence (1) |
| | Comorbidity — Heart failure (ICD428) | Absence (0) | | Presence (1) |
| | Chronic airway obstruction (ICD496) | Absence (0) | | Presence (1) |
| | Hypertensive disease (ICD401/402/403/404) | Absence (0) | | Presence (1) |
| | Coronary atherosclerosis (ICD414) | Absence (0) | | Presence (1) |
| Predischarge | Percutaneous transluminal coronary angioplasty (PTCA) | No (0) | | Yes (1) |
| | Percutaneous coronary intervention (PCI) | No (0) | | Yes (1) |
| | Coronary angiography | No (0) | | Yes (1) |
| | Intervention — Coronary stenting | No (0) | | Yes (1) |
| | Cardiac catheterization | No (0) | | Yes (1) |
| | Left ventricular X-ray | No (0) | | Yes (1) |
| | Use TW-DRG as payment method | No (0) | | Yes (1) |

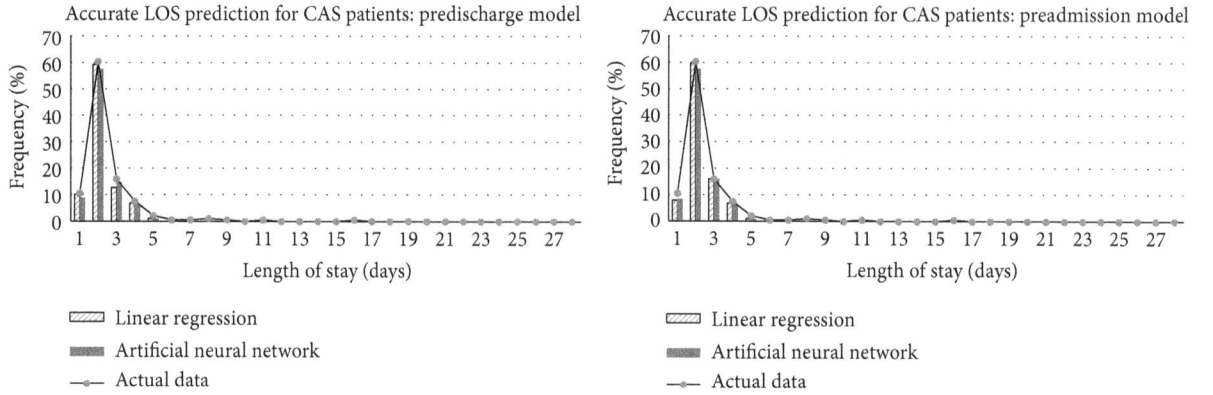

FIGURE 3: Breakdown of accurate LOS predictions using LR and ANN models for CAS patients in the test data.

TABLE 4: Results of predischarge and preadmission models for CAS patients.

| | Predischarge model | | Preadmission model | |
|---|---|---|---|---|
| | LR | ANN | LR | ANN |
| Accuracy (%) | 89.95% | 88.07%~89.64% | 91.53% | 88.31%~89.65% |
| MAE | 1.09 | 1.06~1.11 | 1.00 | 1.03~1.07 |
| MRE | 0.46 | 0.44~0.47 | 0.45 | 0.44~0.47 |

error (MAE) and the mean relative error (MRE), defined as follows:

$$MAE = \frac{\sum_{i=1}^{n} \left| \tilde{Y}_i - Y_i \right|}{n},$$

$$MRE = \frac{\sum_{i=1}^{n} \left( \left| \tilde{Y}_i - Y_i \right| / Y_i \right)}{n},$$

(1)

where $\tilde{Y}_i$ and $Y_i$ are the predicted LOS and actual LOS for the $i$th test data, $i = 1, 2, \ldots, n$, and $n$ is the number of testing instances.

To incorporate the randomness in data selected for training ANN, the results showed in Table 4 are the 95% confidence intervals (95% CI) for accuracy, MAE, and MRE based on 30 runs. All models were quite effective in predicting LOS, with the accuracy rate ranging from 88.07% to 91.53%, the MAE from 1 to 1.11 days, and the MRE from 0.44 to 0.47. Figure 3 shows a detailed look at the distribution in the accurate LOS prediction in the test dataset. It is observed that LR model performed better than ANN model for patients with LOS of 2 days, which was about 60% of the test dataset. However, both LR and ANN models were unable to predict correctly for LOS more than 5 days, which accounted for 3.7% of the test dataset.

*3.2. For AMI and HF Patients.* Same performance indices are used to evaluate the effectiveness of prediction models for AMI and HF patients. Results summarized in Table 5 show that these models are not as effective in predicting LOS as for CAS patients, with the accuracy rate ranging

from 32.99% to 36.33%. The MAE of all models has been quite stable, ranging from 3.76 to 3.97 days and the MRE from 0.69 to 0.77. Further, considering the high degree in the variation of LOS distribution, the definition of accuracy has been extended to include two more scenarios: a tolerance of 1 day is allowed (the difference of LOS prediction to the actual LOS is less than 2 days) or a tolerance of 2 days is allowed (the difference of LOS prediction to the actual LOS is less than 3 days). However, the accuracy rate of these models is increased from 63.69% to 67.47% only even with 2 days of deviation in prediction being allowed as in Table 5.

Figure 4 shows the breakdown in the accurate LOS prediction with no tolerance in the test dataset. It is observed that both LR and ANN models performed better in predicting LOS between 8 and 11 days. In the predischarge model, ANN performs better than LR model for patients with LOS of 3, 5, 6, or 7 days, which is about 60% of the test dataset. Moreover, as shown in the resized charts in Figure 4, ANN models were able to predict correctly for cases with LOS greater than 11 days, which accounts for 14.5% of the test dataset. However, both LR and ANN models were unable to predict correctly for LOS greater than 18 days, which accounts for 5.9% of the test dataset.

*3.3. Validation of ANN Models.* To determine a proper structure for ANN used in this study, a preliminary trial run was first conducted to identify a proper structure for ANN models while assuming that the neuron activation function used for each neuron in the hidden layer was log-sigmoidal function with outputs between 0 and 1 [41]. The original data was separated into two sets: training dataset and test dataset. The training dataset included the first 12-month data, from October 1, 2010, to September 30, 2011, with 744 admissions for CAS patients and 1,155 admissions for AMI and HF patients. The test dataset consisted of the data in the last 3 months, with 189 admissions for CAS patients and 289 admissions for AMI and HF patients.

To avoid overfitting, the training dataset was further separated into two sets: a training set, to update the weights and biases, and a validation set, to stop training when the ANN might be overfitting. In this study, the size of training set and validation set in training all ANN models was assumed

TABLE 5: Results of predischarge and preadmission models for AMI and HF patients.

| | | Predischarge model | | Preadmission model | |
|---|---|---|---|---|---|
| | | LR | ANN | LR | ANN |
| Accuracy (%) | No tolerance | 33.91% | 34.19%~36.24% | 36.33% | 32.99%~35.82% |
| | 1-day tolerance | 55.36% | 50.16%~52.56% | 55.71% | 49.77%~52.82% |
| | 2-day tolerance | 66.78% | 64.12%~66.07% | 67.47% | 63.69%~65.72% |
| MAE | | 3.76 | 3.83~3.91 | 3.76 | 3.87~3.97 |
| MRE | | 0.69 | 0.71~0.74 | 0.72 | 0.73~0.77 |

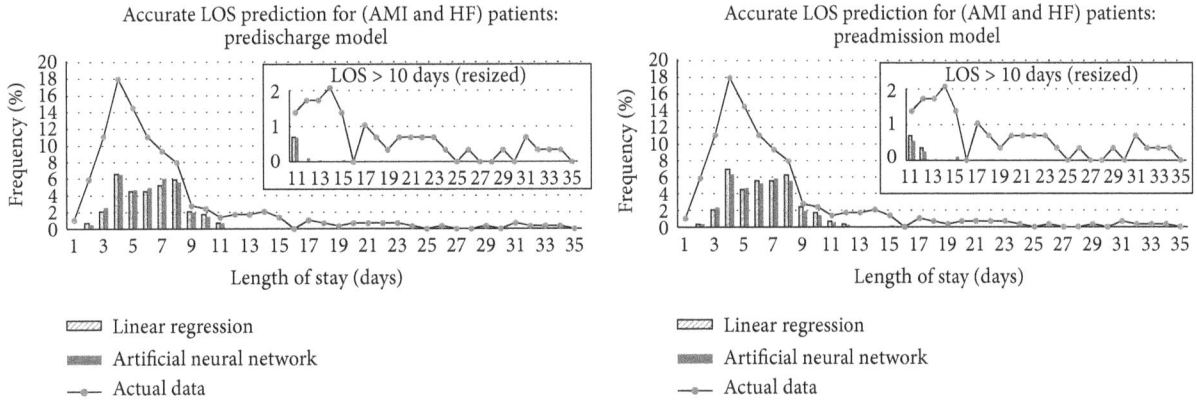

FIGURE 4: Breakdown of accurate LOS predictions (no tolerance) using LR and ANN models for AMI and HF patients in the test data.

to be 70% and 30% of the training dataset. The weights in an ANN were modified using a variable learning rate gradient decent algorithm with momentum [42]. The training stopped when the number of training epochs reached 2,000 or there is no improvement in the validation error for consecutively 600 epochs. After an ANN was trained, the model was then used to obtain the predicted LOS in the test dataset. Furthermore, to avoid the effect of randomness when comparing the results, a fixed training set and validation set were used when training the backpropagation ANNs. Figure 5 shows the root mean squared error (RMSE) for the training set, validation set, and test dataset of trained ANN models with different numbers of neurons in the hidden layer, ranging from 10 to 30. The training errors were found to be slightly decreasing as more neurons were included in the hidden layer. However, no overfitting was observed and the test errors had been quite stable for both models.

To balance between the required training effort and the test errors improvement, the number of neurons in the hidden layer, or the value of $n_1$ in Figure 2, was set to be 13 for all ANN models. Figure 6 shows the weight distribution between input neurons and hidden neurons, as each dot indicates the weight of one of the input neurons to some hidden neuron, and each input neuron has a total of thirteen dots (weights) linked to the hidden layer. It further validates the size of ANN used in this study since the weights had been scattered evenly from −1.5 to 1.5 with only a few dots (weights) close to zero.

## 4. Discussion and Conclusion

This study proposed the use of the neural network techniques to predict LOS for patients in a cardiovascular unit with one of three primary diagnoses: coronary atherosclerosis (CAS), heart failure (HF), and acute myocardial infarction (AMI). The major observation based on the results was that the preadmission models were as effective in predicting LOS as the predischarge models. It was even found that some preadmission models performed slightly better than predischarge models as shown in Tables 4 and 5. This observation indicates that whether a patient might be reimbursed by TW-DRG did not provide additional predictive ability in LOS, and the assumption that a shorter LOS would be preferred in the sake of hospitals' financial performance when DRG was implemented was not applicable in our case hospital.

The benefit of using ANN models was more significant when predicting prolonged LOS for HF and AMI patients. When predicting prolonged LOS, most literature formulated the prediction models to determine whether an admission might belong to a prolonged stay [14, 15, 17] or whether the LOS might be within a fixed range of LOS days [16, 22]. The study by Mobley et al. [43] predicted the exact LOS days for patients in a postcoronary care unit. With 629 and 127 admissions in the training and test file, a total of 74 input variables were used to predict 1 to 20 LOS days in ANNs. The mean LOS was 3.84 days and 3.49 days in the training file and the test file. They showed no significant difference in the distribution from the predicted LOS and from the actual LOS

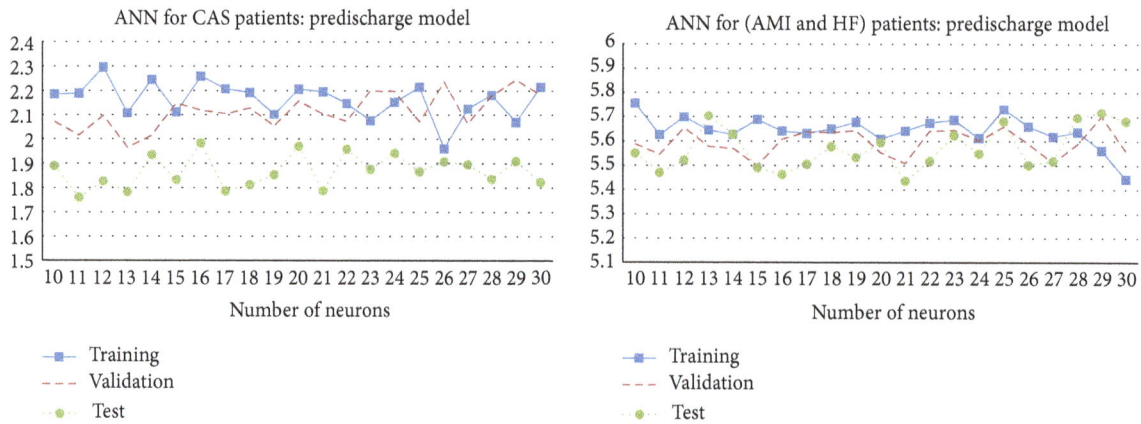

FIGURE 5: The RMSE in training, validation, and test of trained ANN models with 10 to 30 hidden neurons.

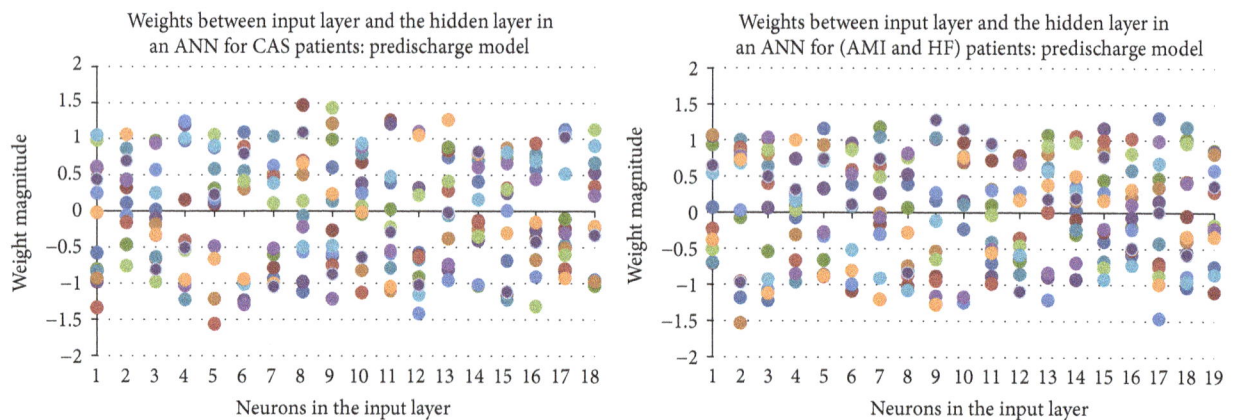

FIGURE 6: Weight distribution of trained ANN in predischarge model with 13 hidden neurons based on one run.

in the test file. However, ANN with two or three hidden layers made no prediction of LOS beyond 5 days [43]. In this study, the mean LOS was 2.65 days and 2.53 days in the training dataset and the test dataset for CAS patients. With only 18 input variables, our models were able to predict correctly for patients with LOS up to 5 days as shown in Figure 3. For AMI and HF patients, the mean LOS was 7.86 days and 7.23 days in the training dataset and the test dataset. Compared with LR method, the ANN model was able to predict patient stays longer than 11 days, as shown in Figure 4.

In general, it is observed that the LR model performed slightly better than ANN models in terms of accuracy as in Tables 4 and 5. It might be due to the reason that each ANN model was built by only 70% of the training dataset, which consisted of the first 12-month data, and the test dataset, which was the remaining 3-month data, had been highly consistent with the previous 12 months. This phenomenon implies that the clinical pathways were well-established in our case hospital.

Limitation of this research is that the major diagnosis and comorbidities for patients are assumed to be well-known in the preadmission stage. Further study is suggested to fully assess the use of ANN models in LOS prediction, especially

for patients who might require longer LOS. Instead of predicting the actual LOS, it might be practical to first categorize LOS into risk groups. More patient characteristics, such as vital signs or lab readings at the time of admission, can be included to improve the performance of LOS predictability.

As the bed supply is limited, the utilization of hospital beds is considered economically critical for most hospitals and any policy related to improving bed utilization has profound impacts on the perception of quality in the provided care and satisfaction of patients and physicians. Currently, hospitalists rely on only aggregated data, such as occupancy rates and average LOS, to access the performance and competitiveness among clinics in the hospital. A reliable LOS prediction in the preadmission stage could further assist in identifying abnormality or potential medical risks to trigger additional attentions for individual cases. It might even allow bed managers to foresee any bottlenecks in bed availability when admitting patients to avoid unnecessary bed transfer between wards.

## Competing Interests

The authors declare that they have no competing interests.

## Acknowledgments

The study has received financial support from the National Taipei University of Technology-Mackay Memorial Hospital Joint Research Program (NTUT-MMH-100-15). The authors would like to thank Cheng-Hsien Mao for insightful inputs and the entire administrative staff from the participating hospital for assistance and support.

## References

[1] OECD, *Average Length of Stay in Hospitals. Health at a Glance 2011*, OECD Indicators, OECD Publishing, 2011.

[2] W. C. Hsiao, H. M. Sapolsky, D. L. Dunn, and S. L. Weiner, "Lessons of the New Jersey DRG payment system," *Health Affairs*, vol. 5, no. 2, pp. 32–45, 1986.

[3] R. B. Fetter, "Diagnosis related groups: understanding hospital performance," *Interfaces*, vol. 21, no. 1, pp. 6–26, 1991.

[4] S. Martin and P. Smith, "Explaining variations in inpatient length of stay in the National Health Service," *Journal of Health Economics*, vol. 15, no. 3, pp. 279–304, 1996.

[5] G. P. Westert, A. P. Nieboer, and P. P. Groenewegen, "Variation in duration of hospital stay between hospitals and between doctors within hospitals," *Social Science and Medicine*, vol. 37, no. 6, pp. 833–839, 1993.

[6] R. D. Serota, A. Lundy, E. Gottheil, S. P. Weinstein, and R. C. Sterling, "Prediction of length of stay in an inpatient dual diagnosis unit," *General Hospital Psychiatry*, vol. 17, no. 3, pp. 181–186, 1995.

[7] H. Imai, J. Hosomi, H. Nakao et al., "Characteristics of psychiatric hospitals associated with length of stay in Japan," *Health Policy*, vol. 74, no. 2, pp. 115–121, 2005.

[8] S. M. Shortell, J. E. Zimmerman, D. M. Rousseau et al., "The performance of intensive care units: does good management make a difference?" *Medical Care*, vol. 32, no. 5, pp. 508–525, 1994.

[9] S. Walczak, W. E. Pofahl, and R. J. Scorpio, "A decision support tool for allocating hospital bed resources and determining required acuity of care," *Decision Support Systems*, vol. 34, no. 4, pp. 445–456, 2002.

[10] M. Verduijn, N. Peek, F. Voorbraak, E. de Jonge, and B. A. J. M. de Mol, "Modeling length of stay as an optimized two-class prediction problem," *Methods of Information in Medicine*, vol. 46, no. 3, pp. 352–359, 2007.

[11] C.-S. Yang, C.-P. Wei, C.-C. Yuan, and J.-Y. Schoung, "Predicting the length of hospital stay of burn patients: comparisons of prediction accuracy among different clinical stages," *Decision Support Systems*, vol. 50, no. 1, pp. 325–335, 2010.

[12] C.-L. Lin, P.-H. Lin, L.-W. Chou et al., "Model-based prediction of length of stay for rehabilitating stroke patients," *Journal of the Formosan Medical Association*, vol. 108, no. 8, pp. 653–662, 2009.

[13] M. Rowan, T. Ryan, F. Hegarty, and N. O'Hare, "The use of artificial neural networks to stratify the length of stay of cardiac patients based on preoperative and initial postoperative factors," *Artificial Intelligence in Medicine*, vol. 40, no. 3, pp. 211–221, 2007.

[14] N. Spratt, Y. Wang, C. Levi, K. Ng, M. Evans, and J. Fisher, "A prospective study of predictors of prolonged hospital stay and disability after stroke," *Journal of Clinical Neuroscience*, vol. 10, no. 6, pp. 665–669, 2003.

[15] D. P. B. Janssen, L. Noyez, C. Wouters, and R. M. H. J. Brouwer, "Preoperative prediction of prolonged stay in the intensive care unit for coronary bypass surgery," *European Journal of Cardio-Thoracic Surgery*, vol. 25, no. 2, pp. 203–207, 2004.

[16] A. H. Lee, M. Gracey, K. Wang, and K. K. W. Yau, "A robustified modeling approach to analyze pediatric length of stay," *Annals of Epidemiology*, vol. 15, no. 9, pp. 673–677, 2005.

[17] T. M. Schmelzer, G. Mostafa, A. E. Lincourt et al., "Factors affecting length of stay following colonic resection," *Journal of Surgical Research*, vol. 146, no. 2, pp. 195–201, 2008.

[18] A. B. Rosen, J. O. Humphries, L. H. Muhlbaier, C. I. Kiefe, T. Kresowik, and E. D. Peterson, "Effect of clinical factors on length of stay after coronary artery bypass surgery: results of the cooperative cardiovascular project," *American Heart Journal*, vol. 138, no. 1, pp. 69–77, 1999.

[19] J. K. Chang, K. D. Calligaro, J. P. Lombardi, and M. J. Dougherty, "Factors that predict prolonged length of stay after aortic surgery," *Journal of Vascular Surgery*, vol. 38, no. 2, pp. 335–339, 2003.

[20] S. E. Berki, M. L. F. Ashcraft, and W. C. Newbrander, "Length-of-stay variations within ICDA-8 diagnosis-related groups," *Medical Care*, vol. 22, no. 2, pp. 126–142, 1984.

[21] E. Chen and C. D. Naylor, "Variation in hospital length of stay for acute myocardial infarction in Ontario, Canada," *Medical Care*, vol. 32, no. 5, pp. 420–435, 1994.

[22] D. J. Whellan, X. Zhao, A. F. Hernandez et al., "Predictors of hospital length of stay in heart failure: findings from get with the guidelines," *Journal of Cardiac Failure*, vol. 17, no. 8, pp. 649–656, 2011.

[23] C. P. Wen, S. P. Tsai, and W.-S. I. Chung, "A 10-year experience with universal health insurance in Taiwan: measuring changes in health and health disparity," *Annals of Internal Medicine*, vol. 148, no. 4, pp. 258–267, 2008.

[24] J.-C. Chen, P.-F. Tsai, and F.-M. Lin, "Simulation study on the effect of diagnosis related group design in length-of-stay and case-mix index for hospitals in Taiwan," in *Proceedings of the IEEE International Conference on Industrial Engineering and Engineering Management*, pp. 1686–1690, Hong Kong, December 2012.

[25] M. Paliwal and U. A. Kumar, "Neural networks and statistical techniques: a review of applications," *Expert Systems with Applications*, vol. 36, no. 1, pp. 2–17, 2009.

[26] S. Walczak and N. Cerpa, "Heuristic principles for the design of artificial neural networks," *Information and Software Technology*, vol. 41, no. 2, pp. 107–117, 1999.

[27] L. R. Medsker and J. Liebowitz, *Design and Development of Expert Systems and Neural Networks*, Prentice Hall, Upper Saddle River, NJ, USA, 1993.

[28] P. J. G. Lisboa, "A review of evidence of health benefit from artificial neural networks in medical intervention," *Neural Networks*, vol. 15, no. 1, pp. 11–39, 2002.

[29] J. V. Tu, "Advantages and disadvantages of using artificial neural networks versus logistic regression for predicting medical outcomes," *Journal of Clinical Epidemiology*, vol. 49, no. 11, pp. 1225–1231, 1996.

[30] R. Dybowski, P. Weller, R. Chang, and V. Gant, "Prediction of outcome in critically ill patients using artificial neural network synthesised by genetic algorithm," *The Lancet*, vol. 347, no. 9009, pp. 1146–1150, 1996.

[31] C. Gholipour, F. Rahim, A. Fakhree, and B. Ziapour, "Using an artificial neural networks (ANNS) model for prediction of intensive care unit (ICU) outcome and length of stay at hospital in traumatic patients," *Journal of Clinical and Diagnostic Research*, vol. 9, no. 4, pp. OC19–OC23, 2015.

[32] C. P. Launay, H. Rivière, A. Kabeshova, and O. Beauchet, "Predicting prolonged length of hospital stay in older emergency department users: use of a novel analysis method, the Artificial Neural Network," *European Journal of Internal Medicine*, vol. 26, no. 7, pp. 478–482, 2015.

[33] S. Dreiseitl and L. Ohno-Machado, "Logistic regression and artificial neural network classification models: a methodology review," *Journal of Biomedical Informatics*, vol. 35, no. 5-6, pp. 352–359, 2002.

[34] E. Grossi, A. Mancini, and M. Buscema, "International experience on the use of artificial neural networks in gastroenterology," *Digestive and Liver Disease*, vol. 39, no. 3, pp. 278–285, 2007.

[35] J.-S. Li, Y. Tian, Y.-F. Liu, T. Shu, and M.-H. Liang, "Applying a BP neural network model to predict the length of hospital stay," in *Health Information Science: Second International Conference, HIS 2013, London, UK, March 25–27, 2013. Proceedings*, vol. 7798 of *Lecture Notes in Computer Science*, pp. 18–29, Springer, Berlin, Germany, 2013.

[36] Bureau of National Health Insurance, *TW-DRGs Improve Healthcare Quality, Efficiency and Fairness*, 2014, http://www.mohw.gov.tw/EN/Ministry/DM1_P.aspx?f_list_no=378&fod_list_no=4999&doc_no=45308.

[37] E. Barnard and L. F. A. Wessels, "Extrapolation and interpolation in neural network classifiers," *IEEE Control Systems*, vol. 12, no. 5, pp. 50–53, 1992.

[38] S. Lawrence, C. L. Giles, and A. Tsoi, "What size neural network gives optimal generalization? Convergence properties of backpropagation," Tech. Rep. UMIACS-TR-96-22 and CS-TR-3617, Institute for Advanced Computer Studies, University of Maryland, College Park, Md, USA, 1996.

[39] Z. Boger and H. Guterman, "Knowledge extraction from artificial neural networks models," in *Proceedings of the IEEE Systems, Man and Cybernetics Conference*, Orlando, Fla, USA, October 1997.

[40] S. Karsoliya, "Approximating number of hidden layer neurons in multiple hidden layer BPNN architecture," *International Journal of Engineering Trends and Technology*, vol. 31, no. 6, pp. 714–717, 2012.

[41] G. Cybenko, "Approximation by superpositions of a sigmoidal function," *Mathematics of Control, Signals, and Systems*, vol. 2, no. 4, pp. 303–314, 1989.

[42] V. N. P. Dao and R. Vemuri, "A performance comparison of different back propagation neural networks methods in computer network intrusion detection," *Differential Equations and Dynamical Systems*, vol. 10, no. 1-2, pp. 201–214, 2002.

[43] B. A. Mobley, R. Leasure, and L. Davidson, "Artificial neural network predictions of lengths of stay on a post-coronary care unit," *Heart & Lung*, vol. 24, no. 3, pp. 251–256, 1995.

# 6

# Quantification of Trunk Postural Stability Using Convex Polyhedron of the Time-Series Accelerometer Data

**Roman Melecky,[1] Vladimir Socha,[1] Patrik Kutilek,[1] Lenka Hanakova,[1] Peter Takac,[2] Jakub Schlenker,[1] and Zdenek Svoboda[3]**

[1]*Faculty of Biomedical Engineering, Czech Technical University in Prague, 272 01 Kladno, Czech Republic*
[2]*Department of Rehabilitation and Spa Medicine, Faculty of Medicine, P. J. Šafárik University in Košice, 040 01 Košice, Slovakia*
[3]*Palacky University of Olomouc, Faculty of Physical Culture, 771 11 Olomouc, Czech Republic*

Correspondence should be addressed to Lenka Hanakova; lenka.hanakova@fbmi.cvut.cz

Academic Editor: Jiann-Shing Shieh

Techniques to quantify postural stability usually rely on the evaluation of only two variables, that is, two coordinates of COP. However, by using three variables, that is, three components of acceleration vector, it is possible to describe human movement more precisely. For this purpose, a single three-axis accelerometer was used, making it possible to evaluate 3D movement by use of a novel method, convex polyhedron (CP), together with a traditional method, based on area of the confidence ellipse (ACE). Ten patients (Pts) with cerebellar ataxia and eleven healthy individuals of control group (CG) participated in the study. The results show a significant increase of volume of the CP (CPV) in Pts or CG standing on foam surface with eyes open (EO) and eyes closed (EC) after the EC phase. Significant difference between Pts and CG was found in all cases as well. Correlation coefficient indicates strong correlation between the CPV and ACE in most cases of patient examinations, thus confirming the possibility of quantification of postural instability by the introduced method of CPV.

## 1. Introduction

Postural stability of the body segments during standing, especially trunk stability, can be negatively influenced by many diseases of the nervous or musculoskeletal system [1]. Patients with these deficits often show instability during stance tasks [2]. Thus, the trunk accelerations during stance can be quantitative indicators of impaired balance control in individuals with neurological disorders [3]. Hence, the evaluation of accelerations suits the needs of clinical practice since they reflect the changes in position as well as the intensity and magnitude of tremor. The biomedical community is currently starting to use the triaxial inertial measurement units (IMU) for high-accuracy measurement of human body segment movements (accelerations and orientations) instead of commonly used force (posturography) platforms used to study the center of pressure (CoP) movements of whole body [4]. Assessment of trunk movements using IMU may yield clearer

insights into balance deficits and provide a considerably cheaper and better diagnostic tool than more traditional, previously documented measures. The IMUs were placed on spinous processes of T1 and/or S1 for measuring the motion of trunk and pelvis during quiet standing. Although the IMU can measure three angles and three accelerations, the techniques to quantify segment movements using only one or two measured quantities were introduced in clinical practice [4]. Thus, in clinical practice, one of the greatest advantages of the IMU compared to traditional posturography platforms, which allow for measuring only the 2D movements in transversal plane, is not used. The reason for this is that the application of the IMU for trunk acceleration measurement during stance is relatively new and the IMU has not been previously used to study the range postural balance problems and patients with specific types of diseases. Thus, the posturography platforms are always the main tool for the study of body movement of the patients, for instance, suffering from cerebellar diseases [5]. Therefore, the first objective of this paper is to test the application of the IMU in an area where IMUs have not been used before and where IMUs will replace conventional posturography platforms.

Since the design is intended to identify connections between trunk movement in space and neurological disorders, it is used to diagnose cerebellar disease characterized by tremor or sway. Cerebellar ataxia can arise as a result of many diseases and present itself with symptoms of coordination, balance, gait, and extremity movements difficulties. Lesions to the cerebellum can cause dyssynergia, dysmetria, dysdiadochokinesia, dysarthria, ataxia of stance and gait, and so forth; see [6, 7]. Deficits can be observed on movements on the same side of the body as the lesion [6]. Clinicians often use motor tasks in order to verify the signs of ataxia [7]. Patients with a cerebellar ataxia diagnosis are interesting not only because of their impaired postural stability but also because there is no effective causal pharmacotherapy. Therefore, it is necessary to look for methods which can enhance the accuracy of evaluation procedures of patients' postural stability during the treatment.

The second objective of the paper is to design and test a new method of quantitative evaluation of 2D data set for the 3D trunk movement measured by IMU. Traditional, more complex methods for processing the measured data and assessing the postural instability, using at least two measured variables, are methods based on the 2D convex hull, 2D confidence ellipse, or length of trajectory obtained by plotting two variables versus each other [8–10]. Usually, these methods are used to evaluate 2D data set from posturography platforms [6]. However, there are limitations of these traditional solutions to quantify postural stability which were originally used to evaluate 2D data set from the posturography platforms and which are now being used to evaluate data from the IMUs. As mentioned before, the limitation is that these methods are based solely on the evaluation of only two variables, each in one of the two human body planes/axes. This can lead to a loss of important information about physical activity, specifically the third physical quantity (i.e., acceleration) of 3D movement. However, we can also model the distribution of the measured 3D data (i.e., three orthogonal accelerations) of human body segment instead of the analysis of 2D data.

Therefore, this study is aimed at introducing a novel method used in the identification of pathological balance control using IMU to measure accelerations as well as the convex polyhedron of plotting three accelerations versus each other (the evaluation of 3D data set of superior-inferior acceleration, mediolateral acceleration, and anterior-posterior acceleration of body segments). It follows practice consisting in the assessment of the convex hull of only two variables (specifically angles) measured by IMU [11]. The convex hull area has already been used in clinical practice to study postural balance problems, but the concept of convex polyhedron volume (CPV) has never been used before in clinical practice to study postural balance problems by three accelerations [8]. The choice for this novel design came from the ability of a single variable which defines the shape of the convex polyhedron used to describe changes in three accelerations, considering wide availability of new cheaper triaxial IMUs

(ordinary cell phones or watches) [12, 13]. The applicability of the convex polyhedron variable describing the body segment movement foreshadows the immense potential of a simple and inexpensive IMU capable of direct evaluation of complex 3D movement (i.e., 3D acceleration) as a whole. Moreover, the combinations of superior-inferior, mediolateral, and anterior-posterior acceleration measurements during specific balance tasks could identify new and specific differences in balance control of patients compared to healthy subjects. The final significant reason for the measurement and evaluation of all three accelerations, instead of only two, is that the calibration of the cheap triaxial IMU may not be accurate, and thus the measurement of all three accelerations minimalizes the loss of information about the 3D movement as a whole. The inclusion of all three accelerations allows us to minimalize the influence of mispositioning the IMU on a body segment. The claim follows the general assumption that acceleration vector in 3D space is defined by the three segments of the vector, while these segments are typically considered in accordance with the Earth's coordinate system axes or anatomical axes of a particular body part. If the sensor is misplaced on the body part or miscalibrated as for the coordinate system, the measured segments of acceleration in their respective axes will be inaccurate. If we choose to examine 3D movement by using only two segments of acceleration, a piece of information may be lost, which is never the case if all three segments are observed. The inclusion of all three accelerations allows us to minimalize the influence of mispositioning of the IMU on a body segment.

The method of recording and processing 3D data thus offers the possibility to measure stability in smaller medical centers or at home by using IMU implemented in, for example, a mobile phone instead of the traditional and spacious posturography platforms. There is also a possibility for patients to perform the therapy, examination, or training at home. The method also eliminates the risk of mispositioning the sensor and loss of vertical movement data and at the same time presents patients and medical staff with an easy-to-interpret 3D data processing method. Therefore, the focus of this work is to identify suitability of the convex polyhedron and IMU data for clinical application.

## 2. Methods and Materials

*2.1. Participants.* In order to test the new methods, it is necessary to compare healthy subjects without any postural balance problems to participants who have postural balance problems. Ten volunteer patients (Pts) (six women and four men; age of 52.2 (SD 11.7) years) with degenerative cerebellar ataxia participated [7]. The patients were recruited from the Faculty Hospital Motol, Prague, Czech Republic. A board-certified neurologist had previously diagnosed progressive cerebellar disease. Diagnostic evaluation included a neurologic examination, laboratory blood tests, and a brain MRI. The patients were measured in the initial phase of the clinic's two-week rehabilitation program. Eleven healthy individuals of control group (CG) (five women and six men; age of 26.0 (SD 6.4) years) were also recruited for comparable analysis. Healthy subjects were recruited from the students/volunteers

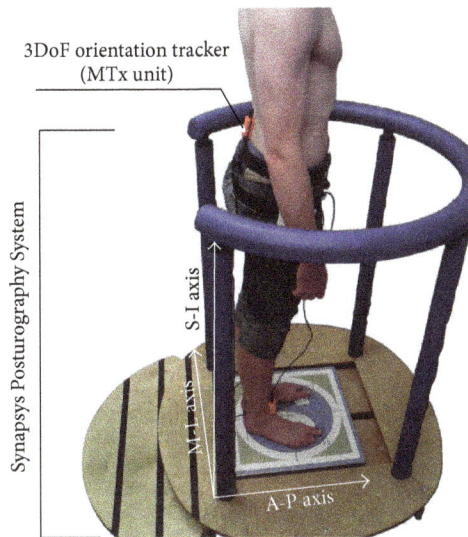

FIGURE 1: The MTx unit used to measure angles and accelerations of the trunk and the Synapsys Posturography System used to measure the COP displacements; S-I: superior-inferior axis, M-L: mediolateral axis, and A-P: anterior-posterior axis.

at Charles University in Prague. In the case of the CG, the diagnostic evaluation included a detailed disease history, a neurological examination, and a routine laboratory testing. The study was performed in accordance with the Helsinki Declaration. The study protocol was approved by the local Ethical Committee and the University Hospital Motol, and an informed consent was obtained from each subject. The subjects were chosen for measurement randomly and on different days.

### 2.2. Measurement Equipment and Test Procedure

*2.2.1. Measurement Equipment.* Xbus Master, a lightweight (330 g) and portable device using Motion Tracker Xsens (product abbreviation: MTx) units for orientation and acceleration measurement of body segments (see Figure 1), was used for measurements of trunk movements. MTx unit with an embedded accelerometer and gyroscope is accurate IMU measuring drift-free 3D orientation and 3D acceleration. The MTx unit was calibrated before each clinical examination by calibration measurement. The MTx unit was set up in a way that the one axis of the coordinate system of the MTx unit was parallel to the anterior-posterior axis, that is, symmetry axis of the fixed stationary platform of the Synapsys Posturography System on which the participants stood, and the other two axes were perpendicular to the anterior-posterior axis (i.e., symmetry axis of the platform) with respect to the direction of Earth's gravity; that is, superior-inferior axis was colinear with the direction of gravity. After calibration, the MTx unit was placed on patient's trunk according to [14, 15], at the level of the lower back (lumbar 2-3); see Figure 1.

The data sets comprised of the three Euler angles (roll ($\Phi$), yaw ($\Psi$), and pitch ($\Theta$)) as well as three orthogonal accelerations ($a_{Sx}$, $a_{Sy}$, $a_{Sz}$) in the accelerometer coordinate system (i.e., three orthogonal components of acceleration

direction corresponding to the three principal axes of the MTx unit accelerometer) were measured using an MTx unit placed on the subjects trunks while Pts and CG were performing a quiet stance on a fixed stationary platform of the Synapsys Posturography System [16, 17]. Conventions of Euler angles are described in [18]. The three accelerations measured by the accelerometer of MTx unit are described in detail in [19].

Also, measurement of the human body center of pressure (COP) displacement (i.e., postural sway) by force platform, Synapsys Posturography System, was performed to compare the data obtained by the traditional method with the data obtained by the IMU. The Synapsys Posturography System provides information about the area of the 95% confidence ellipse of COP excursions [20]. Comparison between COP characteristics and accelerometer data took place due to the fact that COP movement is given by COM (center of mass) movement, position of which follows the position of individual segments. A significant body segment is the trunk on which the accelerometer (i.e., IMU) is placed. Change in the position of the trunk, which is measured as acceleration using IMU, thus directly affects the position of COM and therefore also COP. These data can of course differ with respect to the influence of other segments on the COP position; it is however assumed that the trunk position (or its movement) has the most significant influence on the COP position change. It would be examined and verified whether there is indeed a correlation between the data from the IMU and data from the posturography platform data, which would suggest that the platform is fully replaceable by the IMU.

*2.2.2. Test Procedure.* The body sway of each participant was measured by the Xsens system (Xsens Technologies B.V.) and Synapsys Posturography System (Synapsys Inc.) during quiet stance on a firm surface (FiS) and soft foam surface (FoS) with eyes open (EO) and eyes closed (EC) [21].

The sequence of the four measurement settings for each subject was as follows: EO FiS, EC FiS, EO FoS, and EC FoS. The order of the four settings was set and followed in all participants. The subject's bare feet were positioned next to each other, splayed at the angle of 30°, and arms were always in hanging position. The tasks included standing on both feet for at least 60 seconds [22]. Both systems recorded body activity at the same time; that is, data were recorded simultaneously by both systems. Time synchronization of the measured data (i.e., data from both systems) was achieved by controlling both systems and processing data on the same computer. The measurements usually lasted a few seconds longer, and the initial data have been cut off so that all data sets have a record length of 60 seconds. The data were recorded with a sample frequency of 100 Hz (for both systems). Kalman filter was implemented in the Xbus Kit system and the MT Manager software of the Xbus Kit system was used for data storage.

*2.3. Data Processing Method.* The three Euler angles and three accelerations in the accelerometer coordinate system are used to calculate the accelerations in the global reference system and then in the anatomical coordinate frame. The calculation is based on the rotational matrices. The first rotation matrix

$R_{GS}$ rotates an acceleration vector $\vec{a}_S = \begin{pmatrix} a_{Sx} & a_{Sy} & a_{Sz} \end{pmatrix}^T$ in the sensor coordinate system ($S$) to the global reference system ($G$):

$$\vec{a}_G = R_{GS} \cdot \vec{a}_S, \tag{1}$$

where the matrix $R_{GS}$ is interpreted in terms of Euler angles [23]:

$$R_{GS} = R_\Psi^Z \cdot R_\Theta^Y \cdot R_\Phi^X, \tag{2}$$

where

$$R_\Psi^Z = \begin{bmatrix} \cos\Psi & -\sin\Psi & 0 \\ \sin\Psi & \cos\Psi & 0 \\ 0 & 0 & 1 \end{bmatrix},$$

$$R_\Theta^Y = \begin{bmatrix} \cos\Theta & 0 & \sin\Theta \\ 0 & 1 & 0 \\ -\sin\Theta & 0 & \cos\Theta \end{bmatrix}, \tag{3}$$

$$R_\Phi^X = \begin{bmatrix} 1 & 0 & 0 \\ 0 & \cos\Phi & -\sin\Phi \\ 0 & \sin\Phi & \cos\Phi \end{bmatrix}.$$

The acceleration vector $\vec{a}_G = \begin{pmatrix} a_{Gx} & a_{Gy} & a_{Gz} \end{pmatrix}^T$ in the global reference system is then rotated to the anatomical coordinate frame ($A$):

$$\vec{a}_a = R_{AG} \cdot \vec{a}_G, \tag{4}$$

where second rotation matrix $R_{AG}$ is

$$R_{AG} = R_{\Psi_0}^Z = \begin{bmatrix} \cos\Psi_0 & -\sin\Psi_0 & 0 \\ \sin\Psi_0 & \cos\Psi_0 & 0 \\ 0 & 0 & 1 \end{bmatrix}. \tag{5}$$

The angle $\sin\Psi_0$ is obtained during the calibration process of the MTx unit. The calculated acceleration vector $\vec{a}_A = \begin{pmatrix} a_{AP} & a_{ML} & a_{SI} \end{pmatrix}^T$ represents the superior-inferior acceleration ($a_{SI}$), mediolateral acceleration ($a_{ML}$), and anterior-posterior acceleration ($a_{AP}$). The acceleration vectors, or in other words, time dependent data ($a_{SI}, a_{ML}, a_{AP}$) are plotted as a 3D plot. The set of points is obtained by plotting the accelerations versus each other; see Figure 2. The time of measurement, that is, record length of the data set (60 s), and the sample frequency (100 Hz) affect the number of points in the set. Recording frequency must be sufficiently high to record also a short time and random displacements of the body segment, and no information about the range of motion during maintaining postural stability of stance is lost. Using a greater number of registered points of higher frequency, it is possible to record movement more accurately without losing information on certain phases of rapid movement that is registered through low frequency data collection. For instance, information loss could occur on tremor of segments caused by higher frequencies. Therefore, the data was collected at the frequency of 100 Hz using MT Manager Version 1.7.0,

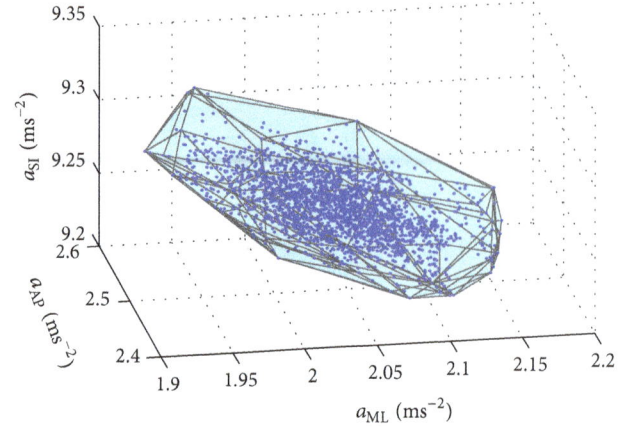

FIGURE 2: Example of a convex polyhedron obtained by plotting superior-inferior (SI), mediolateral (ML), and anterior-posterior (AP) accelerations versus each other.

adjusted for human movements, as recommended by the manufacturer [24]. The choice of the sampling frequency of 100 Hz was made also by following previous studies which used the same system for motion tracking (see [25–29]).

The novel method for identification of pathological balance control is based on mathematical tools for static posturography [20, 30]. We can model the distribution of the measured data by 2D convex hull or 3D convex polyhedron (CP) [31]. A variable which can be used to describe the shape of the 2D convex hull or 3D convex polyhedron can be the area or volume. We used a method based on the description of the distribution of the measured data (i.e., $a_{SI}$, $a_{ML}$, and $a_{AP}$) by CP. In mathematics, the convex hull of a set of points (SP) in the Euclidean space is the smallest convex set that contains SP [32]. The CP may be defined as the intersection of all convex sets containing SP or as the set of all convex combinations of points in SP [33]. The set of points is obtained by plotting three accelerations versus each other; see Figure 2. The CP of a set of points in 3D space is the smallest convex region enclosing all points in the set; see Figure 2. The number of points is determined by the time of measurement (60 s) and the sample frequency (100 Hz). A custom-designed MATLAB program based on the functions of the MATLAB software (MATLAB R2010b, Mathworks, Inc., Natick, MA, USA) was used to calculate the CP of the 3D plot. The convex hull computation in MATLAB uses the Delaunay triangulation [34]. Since there is no known method of calculating the CPV, we can use the equations used to calculate the volume of any polyhedron (PV) [35–37]:

$$PV = \frac{1}{3} \left| \sum_{i=1}^{j} P_{1i} \cdot N_i \cdot A_i \right|, \tag{6}$$

where $A_i$ is the surface area of a planar polygonal face $S_i$:

$$A_i = \frac{1}{2} \left| N_i \cdot \sum_{k=1}^{l} \left( P_{ki} \times P_{(k+1)i} \right) \right|. \tag{7}$$

Thus

$$PV = \frac{1}{6}\left|\sum_{i=1}^{j}\left(P_{1i} \cdot N_i\right) \cdot \left|N_i \cdot \sum_{k=1}^{l}\left(P_{ki} \times P_{(k+1)i}\right)\right|\right|, \quad (8)$$

where $P_{1i}, \ldots, P_{li}$ are the vertices of a planar polygonal face $S_i$ oriented counterclockwise with respect to the outward pointing normal of planar polygonal face and $N_i$ is a unit outward pointing vector normal to specific planar polygonal face $S_i$:

$$N_i = \frac{\left(P_{2i} - P_{1i}\right) \times \left(P_{3i} - P_{1i}\right)}{\left|\left(P_{2i} - P_{1i}\right) \times \left(P_{3i} - P_{1i}\right)\right|}. \quad (9)$$

To calculate the PV, the custom-designed MATLAB program was also used. Because the volume corresponds to the volume of CP of 3D plot obtained by plotting $a_{SI}$, $a_{ML}$, and $a_{AP}$ versus each other, the physical unit of the volume is $m^3 \cdot s^{-6}$. Although the MTx unit also senses the gravitational acceleration, it is not necessary to subtract the gravitational acceleration because the method of calculating the PV uses only changes in the accelerations and the gravitational acceleration is constant and perpendicular to the horizontal plane of the Earth's surface.

The area of the 95% confidence ellipse (ACE) of COP excursions was used to compare the data obtained by the posturography system with data obtained by the IMU. The Synapsys Posturography System directly calculates the areas. Thus, it is not necessary to convert the measured data. The physical unit of the area is $mm^2$.

*2.4. Statistical Analysis.* After calculating the CPV of each patient and healthy subject standing on a FiS and FoS with EO and EC, the Jarque-Bera test was used to test the normal distribution of calculated CPVs. The median (Mdn), minimum (Min), maximum (Max), first quartile (Q1), and third quartile (Q3) of the CPV were then used to compare the results. Also, the Wilcoxon signed rank test and Wilcoxon rank sum test were used to assess the significance of the differences between the measurements results, that is, to compare the different stance conditions and CG with Pts. The significance level was set at $p < 0.05$. Also, Spearman's rank correlation coefficient between the volume of convex polyhedron and the area of the confidence ellipse of COP excursions were calculated to study the differences between the data from IMU and the center of pressure data. The statistical analysis was performed using MATLAB software.

A comparison of the same age groups is not necessary, since studies show that parameters of the body sway of the healthy subjects within the age range between 20 and 60 years vary only slightly [38, 39]. Aoki et al. [38] found that there are insignificant differences in 10–60-year-old subjects in COP sway parameters (i.e., Romberg quotients). Also, a detailed analysis of age-related increase of CoP parameters by the polynomial type of regression showed that the gradual increase of body sway, that is, significant degradation of stability, characterized by increase of CoP oscillations, starts after the age of 60 [39].

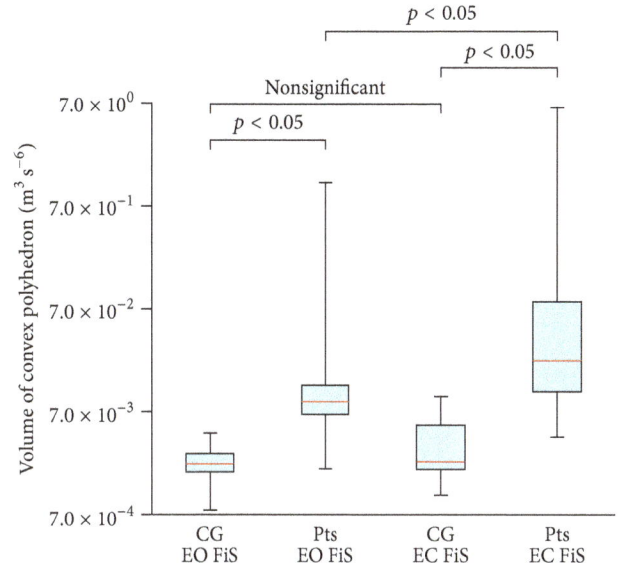

FIGURE 3: Comparison of the volume of convex polyhedron of control group (CG) and patients (Pts) standing on a firm surface (FiS) with eyes open (EO) and eyes closed (EC).

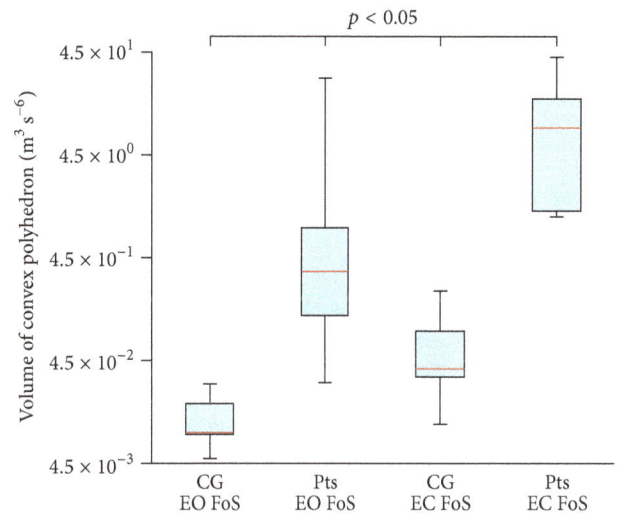

FIGURE 4: Comparison of the volume of convex polyhedron of control group (CG) and patients (Pts) standing on a foam surface (FoS) with eyes open (EO) and eyes closed (EC).

## 3. Results

The statistical data are used to illustrate the differences between the CPVs of Pts and CG; see Figures 3 and 4. Results obtained from the posturography platform are listed as well (see Figures 5 and 6) to provide for the evaluation of the data from IMU by comparing them with the data from the posturography platform. The following plots display the Min, Max, Mdn, Q1, and Q3 for the calculated CPVs and ACEs. Since some calculated values were not distributed normally, the Wilcoxon test was used to compare and analyze the data sets. In all cases of comparisons between the groups of

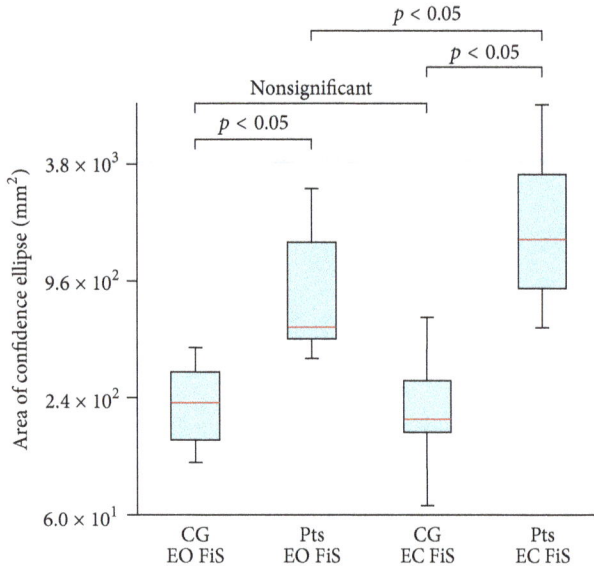

FIGURE 5: Comparison of the area of confidence ellipse of control group (CG) and patients (Pts) standing on a firm surface (FiS) with eyes open (EO) and eyes closed (EC).

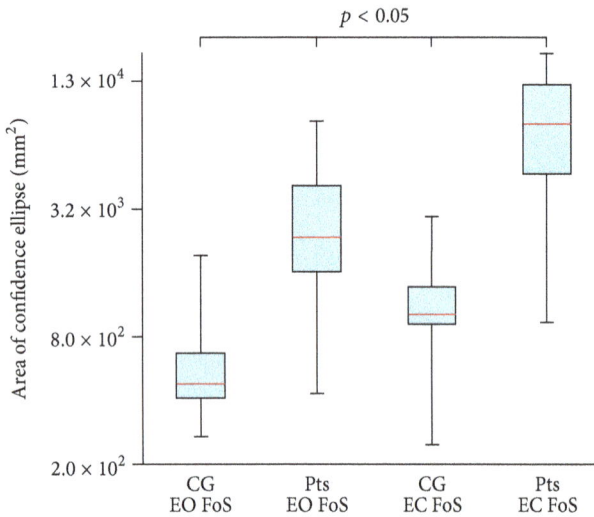

FIGURE 6: Comparison of the area of confidence ellipse of control group (CG) and patients (Pts) standing on a foam surface (FoS) with eyes open (EO) and eyes closed (EC).

data, the effect sizes ranged from moderate to large; that is, calculated values were greater than 0.5. G*Power software (G*Power 3.1.9., Universität Kiel, Germany) was used for the calculations.

*3.1. Comparing Quiet Stance Trials.* The comparison of CG on FiS with EO and CG on FiS with EC ($p = 0.206$) did not show any differences. Differences were found when comparing Pts on FiS with EO and Pts on FiS with EC ($p = 0.014$), CG on FoS with EO and CG on FoS with EC ($p = 0.003$), and Pts on FoS with EO and Pts on FoS with EC ($p = 0.002$). In the case of the CG or Pts with EO and EC standing on the FiS,

TABLE 1: Spearman's rank correlation coefficient between the volume of convex polyhedron and the area of the confidence ellipse of COP excursions of control group (CG) and patients (Pts) standing on a firm surface (FiS) and a foam surface (FoS) with eyes open (EO) and eyes closed (EC).

|  | CG EO | Pts EO | CG EC | Pts EC |
|---|---|---|---|---|
| FiS | 0.03 | 0.53 | 0.37 | 0.93 |
| FoS | 0.03 | 0.83 | 0.18 | 0.70 |

the measured data show the slight increase of the median of the CPVs after the eyes closed phase (Figure 3). In the case of the CG or Pts with EO and EC standing on the FoS, the measured data show a significant increase of the median of the CPVs after the EC phase (Figure 4).

*3.2. Comparing Patients and Healthy Subjects.* Significant differences were found when comparing CG on FiS with EO and Pts on FiS with EO ($p = 0.010$), CG on FiS with EC and Pts on FiS with EC ($p = 0.005$), CG on FoS with EO and Pts on FoS with EO ($p = 0.001$), and CG on FoS with EC and Pts on FoS with EC ($p = 0.001$). In all cases, significant differences between the data for CG and Pts were observed.

The median of the CPVs in Pts standing on the FiS with EO is 4.0 times larger than the median of the CPVs in the CG standing on the FiS with EO. The median of the CPVs in Pts standing on the FiS with EC is 9.7 times larger than the median of the CPVs in the CG standing on the FiS with EC. The median of the CPVs in Pts standing on the FoS with EO is 37.2 times larger than the median of the CPVs in the CG standing on the FoS with EO. The median of the CPVs in Pts standing on the FoS with EC is 222.4 times larger than the median of the CPVs in the CG standing on the FoS with EC.

*3.3. Correlation between the Data from IMU and the Center of Pressure Data.* In the case of the CG with EO standing on the FiS and FoS, the Spearman rank correlation coefficient indicates a negligible correlation between the CPV and ACE. In the case of the CG with EC standing on the FiS and FoS, the correlation between the CPV and ACE is weak. In most cases, the patient examinations show strong correlation between the CPV and ACE; see Table 1. A moderate positive relationship between the data from IMU and the data from force platform was found in all cases.

## 4. Discussion

This study tested and verified a novel method utilizing the volume of convex polyhedron obtained by plotting three accelerations versus each other. It also proved the importance of incorporating the phase of the stance task on a foam surface with EC during the measurement process, since the results between patients with cerebellar ataxia and CG differed the most significantly in the CPVs observed during the FoS stance task, both in the EC and EO phases [40, 41]. This concludes that complicating stance tasks by reducing the mechanoreceptor perception highlights the differences in trunk movements between the CG and Pts. Also, the method identified significant differences between patients and CG in all instances of measurement. The CPV of the CG and Pts differed even in the hundreds of measured units of the CPV.

Although the method yielded results corresponding to those obtained by traditional methods in the case of Pts and CG standing on the FoS with EO and EC, the novel method revealed significant differences in the balance control between Pts and CG [8]. The above findings point to some complexity in the relation between the loss of perception and compensation for this loss by moving the trunk. In the case of the patients, the correlation coefficients indicate moderate and strong positive correlation between the CPV and ACE. The important information for the description of the situation is that very significant changes in the trunk position were seen only in the Pts. The reason for this is that the large movements only in the trunk, which is primarily used to improve the stability of the patient's body, have a great impact on changing the COM of the whole body and which corresponds to the position of the COP [42]. Conversely, in the case of the CG, the correlation coefficients indicate a weak or very weak correlation between the CPV and ACE. The reason for this is that the COP position is a result of a complex kinematic chain. Small movements of the COM of the trunk are overshadowed by movements of other body segments. Thus, in the case of the CG, small changes in trunk position may be different from the changes in position of the center of mass (COM) of the whole body, which differs from the COM of the trunk. Therefore, the lowest correlations correspond to the smallest movements of the torso when CG is standing with eyes open. The final reason why the standard parameter (e.g., ACE) is not correlated to CPV is because the CPV describes the complex 3D trunk accelerations (i.e., 3D movement) and the ACE describes distribution of only 2D data in transversal plane (2D space) and neglects movement in the third direction (i.e., vertical direction) [10]. Even a very small vertical movement which the posturography platform may fail to record can result in a significant change in the CPV. If we assume the area of CPV reflected into the horizontal plane, this may correlate with ACE. However if the reflected CP area is multiplied by a relatively small value of the vertical movement, which might be small compared to the horizontal movement, the volume of the resulting pattern varies according to the number of multiples in the value of vertical movement.

Significant correlations revealed between ACE and CPV during stance on FiS with EC suggest future use of IMU in the evaluation of postural stability in patients with, for example, cerebellar disease at smaller medical centers or even at home. Posturography platforms are spacious and less convenient for use in small medical centers or at home and IMUs might therefore replace the platforms in the therapy process, while enabling the patient to perform postural stability training individually with the IMU implemented in, for example, a mobile phone. Interpretation of the results from the measured data is identical to the interpretation of the results obtained by posturography platforms, and thus their use might be identical as well when it comes to therapy or evaluation of postural stability following surgeries. Based on the above it is clear that the determination and assessment of postural instability may be now additionally carried out

by using the CPV, for example, in the form of examining 3D trunk acceleration. The major difference between utilizing triaxial IMU and the traditional method using 2D trajectory is the ability to describe the trunk movement in all three human body axes/planes. The novel method thus clearly found differences in postural control between Pts and CG and even greater differences in postural stability between Pts and CG. Clinical trials which are generally used to assess an impaired postural stability have large variability (e.g., Clinical Test of Sensory Interaction for Balance and others). This disadvantage could be eliminated using the proposed system and method which can be used to evaluate more subtle changes in postural stability in an individual patient course of treatment. Concluding from what is above mentioned, the potential of CPV may prove instrumental in gaining clearer insight into the postural stability and postural balance problems, which is crucial in medical examination and rehabilitation medicine.

This study also adopted a few limitations. The major one is that the size of the recruited subjects was rather smaller and possibly not fully applicable to the larger scope of population, even though it yielded statistically relevant results and it still might prove the results in a larger study. Another possible limitation is the chance of the existence of difference in comparisons which did not yield a statistically relevant result. However, it is safe to say that the sample of 10 Pts and 11 CG was relevant to design a preliminary study aimed on the study of degenerative cerebellar disorder sufferers using the basic features of the proposed techniques. Moreover, possible limitation might be also the nonhomogenous age groups that were compared. Even though previous works cited that age differences should not pose a significant influence on the presented results [38, 39], it would be interesting to use the presented method to compare age groups and thus verify or refute the influence of age on the relevance of the results.

## 5. Conclusion

All previous applications based on convex hull consider only two variables—two coordinates or two angles—not accelerations [22, 32]. However the three-dimensional version of the convex hull can also be used to study 3D movements of patients measured by triaxial IMU used in clinical practice. There are two main reasons for this design. The first reason is that one variable defining the shape of the 3D convex polyhedron allows us to study the change in the 3D movement as a whole by new and cheaper triaxial IMUs. Moreover, the combinations of the measurement of three accelerations during specific balance tasks could identify new and specific differences in balance control of patients compared to healthy subjects. The second reason for the measurement and evaluation of all three accelerations, instead of only two angles, is that the calibration of the cheap triaxial IMU may not be accurate and thus the measurement of accelerations in all three directions minimalizing the loss of information about the 3D movement as a whole. Particularly cheap IMUs in the contemporary mobile phones or watches, price of which is constantly falling and compared to expensive professional motion capture systems and posturography platforms is already considerably favorable, may find use in smaller medical centers as well as in long distance medicine thanks to the designed method. Also, inclusion of all three accelerations allows for minimalizing the influence of mispositioning of the sensor on a body segment. Thus, with the proposed method, it is capable of providing postural examination in everyday life using a cheap 3D IMU, and it is also possible to use the new method in a wide field of medicine including the rehabilitation with consideration of trunk coordination for physically challenged people.

The designed method and the 3D IMU not only are capable of replacing the expensive posturography platforms, but also they can become their complementary part. Posturography platforms allow for evaluation of body movement as a whole, and the introduced method provides for the evaluation of postural stability of a given segment. The proposed method of the evaluation of IMU data follows the traditional method used with posturography platforms and therefore is already familiar to the medical staff and easily interpreted. The use of parallel measurements of 3D data using IMU and posturography platforms for 2D data would require further research into the applicability of such solution and its contribution for medical examinations, for example, in rehabilitation process. For the future clinical use it would also be appropriate to add dynamic tests of postural stability to the static ones because of the larger complexity of the examination and also because performing the static tests during treatment does not correlate with the improvements of dynamic tests (which are also important for patient life quality).

## Competing Interests

The authors state no conflict of interests.

## Acknowledgments

This work was done in the Joint Department of the Faculty of Biomedical Engineering, CTU, and Charles University in Prague in the framework of Research Program no. VG20102015002 (2010–2015, MV0/VG), sponsored by the Ministry of the Interior of the Czech Republic, and Project SGS16/109/OHK4/1T/17 of Czech Technical University in Prague. The authors would also like to thank Andrej Madoran, BA, for the translation of this paper.

## References

[1] M. Mancini, F. B. Horak, C. Zampieri, P. Carlson-Kuhta, J. G. Nutt, and L. Chiari, "Trunk accelerometry reveals postural instability in untreated Parkinson's disease," *Parkinsonism and Related Disorders*, vol. 17, no. 7, pp. 557–562, 2011.

[2] R. Moe-Nilssen and J. L. Helbostad, "Trunk accelerometry as a measure of balance control during quiet standing," *Gait & Posture*, vol. 16, no. 1, pp. 60–68, 2002.

[3] W. Maetzler, M. Mancini, I. Liepelt-Scarfone et al., "Impaired trunk stability in individuals at high risk for Parkinson's disease," *PLoS ONE*, vol. 7, no. 3, Article ID e32240, 2012.

[4] B. W. Fling, G. G. Dutta, H. Schlueter, M. H. Cameron, and F. B. Horak, "Associations between proprioceptive neural pathway structural connectivity and balance in people with multiple sclerosis," *Frontiers in Human Neuroscience*, vol. 8, article 814, 2014.

[5] S. Kammermeier, J. F. Kleine, T. Eggert, S. Krafczyk, and U. Büttner, "Disturbed vestibular-neck interaction in cerebellar disease," *Journal of Neurology*, vol. 260, no. 3, pp. 794–804, 2013.

[6] M. U. Manto, *Cerebellar, Disorders: A Practical Approach to Diagnosis and Management*, Cambridge University Press, Cambridge, UK, 2010.

[7] O. Čakrt, M. Vyhnálek, K. Slabý et al., "Balance rehabilitation therapy by tongue electrotactile biofeedback in patients with degenerative cerebellar disease," *NeuroRehabilitation*, vol. 31, no. 4, pp. 429–434, 2012.

[8] B. P. C. Van de Warrenburg, M. Bakker, B. P. H. Kremer, B. R. Bloem, and J. H. J. Allum, "Trunk sway in patients with spinocerebellar ataxia," *Movement Disorders*, vol. 20, no. 8, pp. 1006–1013, 2005.

[9] L. F. Oliveira, D. M. Simpson, and J. Nadal, "Calculation of area of stabilometric signals using principal component analysis," *Physiological Measurement*, vol. 17, no. 4, pp. 305–312, 1996.

[10] J. A. Raymakers, M. M. Samson, and H. J. J. Verhaar, "The assessment of body sway and the choice of the stability parameter(s)," *Gait & Posture*, vol. 21, no. 1, pp. 48–58, 2005.

[11] J. Gill, J. H. J. Allum, M. G. Carpenter et al., "Trunk sway measures of postural stability during clinical balance tests: effects of age," *The Journals of Gerontology, Series A: Biological Sciences and Medical Sciences*, vol. 56, no. 7, pp. M438–M447, 2001.

[12] C. U. Manohar, S. K. McCrady, Y. Fujiki, and I. T. Pavlidis, "Evaluation of the accuracy of a triaxial accelerometer embedded into a cell phone platform for measuring physical activity," *Journal of Obesity & Weight loss Therapy*, vol. 1, no. 106, p. 3309, 2011.

[13] V. Socha, P. Kutílek, A. Štefek et al., "Evaluation of relationship between the activity of upper limb and the piloting precision," in *Proceedings of the 16th International Conference on Mechatronics-Mechatronika (ME '14)*, T. Brezina, D. Maga, and A. Stefek, Eds., pp. 405–410, IEEE, Brno, Czech Republic, December 2014.

[14] A. L. Adkin, B. R. Bloem, and J. H. J. Allum, "Trunk sway measurements during stance and gait tasks in Parkinson's disease," *Gait & Posture*, vol. 22, no. 3, pp. 240–249, 2005.

[15] F. Ochi, K. Abe, S. Ishigami, K. Otsu, and H. Tomita, "Trunk motion analysis in walking using gyro sensors," in *Proceedings of the 19th Annual International Conference of the IEEE Engineering in Medicine and Biology Society*, R. J. Jaeger, Ed., pp. 1824–1825, Chicago, Ill, USA, November 1997.

[16] S. T. Aw, G. M. Halmagyi, R. A. Black, I. S. Curthoys, R. A. Yavor, and M. J. Todd, "Head impulses reveal loss of individual semicircular canal function," *Journal of Vestibular Research*, vol. 9, no. 3, pp. 173–180, 1999.

[17] T. J. M. Kennie and G. Petrie, *Engineering Surveying Technology*, Thomson Science and Profesional, Glasgow, UK, 1990.

[18] O. Findling, J. Sellner, N. Meier et al., "Trunk sway in mildly disabled multiple sclerosis patients with and without balance impairment," *Experimental Brain Research*, vol. 213, no. 4, pp. 363–370, 2011.

[19] Á. Gil-Agudo, A. de los Reyes-Guzmán, I. Dimbwadyo-Terrer et al., "A novel motion tracking system for evaluation of functional rehabilitation of the upper limbs," *Neural Regeneration Research*, vol. 8, no. 19, pp. 1773–1782, 2013.

[20] P. Schubert, M. Kirchner, D. Schmidtbleicher, and C. T. Haas, "About the structure of posturography: sampling duration, parametrization, focus of attention (part I)," *Journal of Biomedical Science & Engineering*, vol. 5, no. 9, pp. 496–507, 2012.

[21] F. Honegger, G. J. van Spijker, and J. H. J. Allum, "Coordination of the head with respect to the trunk and pelvis in the roll and pitch planes during quiet stance," *Neuroscience*, vol. 213, pp. 62–71, 2012.

[22] M. Zadnikar and D. Rugelj, "Postural stability after hippotherapy in an adolescent with cerebral palsy," *Journal of Novel Physiotherapies*, vol. 1, no. 1, article 106, 2011.

[23] N. Ying and W. Kim, "Use of dual Euler angles to quantify the three-dimensional joint motion and its application to the ankle joint complex," *Journal of Biomechanics*, vol. 35, no. 12, pp. 1647–1657, 2002.

[24] Xsens, *MTi and MTx User Manual and Technical Documentation 2010*, Xsens Technoloties, Enschede, The Netherlands, 2010.

[25] K. Lebel, P. Boissy, M. Hamel, and C. Duval, "Inertial measures of motion for clinical biomechanics: comparative assessment of accuracy under controlled conditions—effect of velocity," *PLoS ONE*, vol. 8, no. 11, Article ID e79945, 2013.

[26] A. Martínez-Ramírez, P. Lecumberri, M. Gómez, L. Rodriguez-Mañas, F. J. García, and M. Izquierdo, "Frailty assessment based on wavelet analysis during quiet standing balance test," *Journal of Biomechanics*, vol. 44, no. 12, pp. 2213–2220, 2011.

[27] H. M. Schepers, D. Roetenberg, and P. H. Veltink, "Ambulatory human motion tracking by fusion of inertial and magnetic sensing with adaptive actuation," *Medical and Biological Engineering & Computing*, vol. 48, no. 1, pp. 27–37, 2010.

[28] J. Hejda, O. Cakrt, V. Socha, J. Schlenker, and P. Kutilek, "3-D trajectory of body sway angles: a technique for quantifying postural stability," *Biocybernetics and Biomedical Engineering*, vol. 35, no. 3, pp. 185–191, 2015.

[29] H. J. Luinge, *Inertial Sensing of Human Movement*, Twente University Press, Enschede, Nederlands, 2002.

[30] L. Ferrufino, B. Bril, G. Dietrich, T. Nonaka, and O. A. Coubard, "Practice of contemporary dance promotes stochastic postural control in aging," *Frontiers in Human Neuroscience*, vol. 5, article 169, 2011.

[31] M. de Berg, M. van Kreveld, M. Overmars, and O. Schwarz-kopf, *Computational Geometry: Algorithms and Applications*, Springer, Berlin, Germany, 2nd edition, 2000.

[32] B. Chazelle, "An optimal convex hull algorithm in any fixed dimension," *Discrete & Computational Geometry*, vol. 10, no. 1, pp. 377–409, 1993.

[33] D. E. Knuth, *Axioms and Hulls*, Springer, Berlin, Germany, 1992.

[34] F. P. Preparata and S. J. Hong, "Convex hulls of finite sets of points in two and three dimensions," *Communications of the ACM*, vol. 20, no. 2, pp. 87–93, 1977.

[35] B. Grunbaum and V. Klee, "Lectures by Branko Grünbaum and Victor Klee," in *CUPM (Committee on the Undergraduate Program in Mathematics) Geometry Conference Proceedings, Part I: Convexity and Applications*, L. K. Durst, Ed., Mathematical Association of America, 1967.

[36] C. S. Ogilvy, *Excursions in Geometry*, Dover Books on Mathematics, Dover, New York, NY, USA, 1990.

[37] R. Goldman, "Area of planar polygons and volume of polyhedra," in *Graphics Gems II*, J. Arvo, Ed., pp. 170–171, Academic Press, Boston, Mass, USA, 1991.

[38] H. Aoki, S. Demura, H. Kawabata et al., "Evaluating the effects of open/closed eyes and age-related differences on center of foot pressure sway during stepping at a set tempo," *Advances in Aging Research*, vol. 1, no. 3, pp. 72–77, 2012.

[39] D. Abrahamova and F. Hlavacka, "Age-related changes of human balance during quiet stance," *Physiological Research*, vol. 57, no. 6, pp. 1–17, 2008.

[40] J. T. Blackburn, B. L. Riemann, J. B. Myers, and S. M. Lephart, "Kinematic analysis of the hip and trunk during bilateral stance on firm, foam, and multiaxial support surfaces," *Clinical Biomechanics*, vol. 18, no. 7, pp. 655–661, 2003.

[41] M. Patel, P. A. Fransson, D. Lush et al., "The effects of foam surface properties on standing body movement," *Acta Oto-Laryngologica*, vol. 128, no. 9, pp. 952–960, 2008.

[42] T. Teranishi, I. Kondo, S. Sonoda et al., "Validity study of the standing test for imbalance and disequilibrium (SIDE): is the amount of body sway in adopted postures consistent with item order?" *Gait & Posture*, vol. 34, no. 3, pp. 295–299, 2011.

# 7

# Effect of Graded Facetectomy on Lumbar Biomechanics

Zhi-li Zeng,[1] Rui Zhu,[1,2] Yang-chun Wu,[1] Wei Zuo,[1] Yan Yu,[1]
Jian-jie Wang,[1] and Li-ming Cheng[1]

[1]*Spine Division of Orthopaedic Department, Tongji Hospital, Tongji University School of Medicine, 389 Xincun Road, Shanghai
200065, China*
[2]*Department of Histology and Embryology, Tongji University School of Medicine, 1239 Siping Road, Shanghai 200092, China*

Correspondence should be addressed to Rui Zhu; zhurui08@hotmail.com

Academic Editor: Jie Yao

Facetectomy is an important intervention for spinal stenosis but may lead to spinal instability. Biomechanical knowledge for facetectomy can be beneficial when deciding whether fusion is necessary. Therefore, the aim of this study was to investigate the biomechanical effect of different grades of facetectomy. A three-dimensional nonlinear finite element model of L3–L5 was constructed. The mobility of the model and the intradiscal pressure (IDP) of L4-L5 for standing were inside the data from the literature. The effect of graded facetectomy on intervertebral rotation, IDP, facet joint forces, and maximum von Mises equivalent stresses in the annuli was analyzed under flexion, extension, left/right lateral bending, and left/right axial rotation. Compared with the intact model, under extension, unilateral facetectomy increased the range of intervertebral rotation (IVR) by 11.7% and IDP by 10.7%, while the bilateral facetectomy increased IVR by 40.7% and IDP by 23.6%. Under axial rotation, the unilateral facetectomy and the bilateral facetectomy increased the IVR by 101.3% and 354.3%, respectively, when turned to the right and by 1.1% and 265.3%, respectively, when turned to the left. The results conclude that, after unilateral and bilateral facetectomy, care must be taken when placing the spine into extension and axial rotation posture from the biomechanical point of view.

## 1. Introduction

Lumbar stenosis is one of the leading sources of lower back pain worldwide. It is defined as a narrowing of the lumbar spinal canal [1] due to degeneration of the spinal canal and neural foramen. An estimated 73 million people will be over the age of 65 of which 30% are projected to have symptomatic lumbar spinal stenosis in the US by the year 2030 [1]. Surgery is typically required for patients with lumbar stenosis over the age of 65 years [2]. Although nonoperative treatments with accompanying lifestyle modifications and disc microsurgery are becoming more and more popular, the gold standard treatment for lumbar stenosis is still open surgery [2]. The most common surgery for decompression is facetectomy and laminectomy, with the choice of unilateral or bilateral intervention depending on the degree of stenosis. An unfortunate but unavoidable downside to removing anatomical structures of the spine is an altered load-bearing and

motion environment. Greater spinal instability and larger deformation may occur. Knowing the level of instability under physiological loading can help the surgeon to decide whether additional spinal fusion is necessary.

Several groups have reported on the biomechanical behavior of the spine after resecting dorsal lumbar regions using in vitro experimental studies. In 1990, Abumi et al. [3] showed that removing supraspinous/interspinous ligaments did not affect the range of motion but that total facetectomy made the spine unstable. Okawa et al. [4] applied cyclic compressive and bending loads to a cadaveric spinal unit simulating partial facetectomy with intact spinous processes and ligaments. The results showed that facetectomy did not have a significant effect on flexion, but there was a significant effect on compression and extension. Similarly, Zhou et al. [5] performed in vitro unilateral graded facetectomy on 5 cadavers and failed to find any significant negative effects to the range of flexion and extension. However, if the range of graded facetectomy exceeded 50%, spinal stability under lateral bending and axial rotation was greatly impacted. Saying that, the use of cadaveric experiments presents several limitations. The number of the cadaveric specimens is limited and the individual differences in anatomy are not reproducible across multiple experiments. Also, most specimens are from elderly individuals with variations in bone quality [6].

Finite element (FE) analysis is an important method for biomechanical investigations. Material properties can be varied and geometries can be generated and manipulated as desired according to different aims of studies. A number of FE studies around facetectomy have been reported in the literature. In 2003, Zander et al. [7] used a validated FE model to study both facetectomy and laminectomy, recording parameters such as motion, intradiscal pressures (IDP), stress, and facet joint forces. However, only standing and forward bending were investigated. Lee and Teo [8] investigated different spinal motions after laminectomy using a L2-L3 lumbar FE model. The results showed that total laminectomy increased motion and annulus stress, except when under lateral bending. Chen et al. [9] found that posterolateral fusion with hemilaminectomy may relax the stress concentrations on the intervertebral disc above the fusion mass when placed in flexion. Kiapour et al. [10] evaluated the biomechanical mechanism of Dynesys dynamic stabilization which was a semirigid pedicle screw fixation system for graded facetectomy. More recently, Erbulut [11] created an asymmetric FE model of the lumbar spine and subjected it to graded facet injuries in order to study the effect on the range of motion. Total left unilateral medial facetectomy, total bilateral facetectomy, 50% unilateral medial facetectomy, and 75% unilateral medial facetectomy were modeled. However, only the medial section of the segment was involved and only motion parameters were calculated. Involving more parameters, such as pressure and stress, under a range of spinal postures would help to create a more comprehensive biomechanical understanding of the environment in the spine after graded facetectomy.

Therefore, the aim of this study is to construct an FE model of a spinal segment and investigate the biomechanical effect of graded facetectomy on intervertebral rotation (IVR), intradiscal pressure, facet joint forces, and maximum von Mises equivalent stresses for flexion, extension, left/right lateral bending, and left/right axial rotation.

## 2. Materials and Methods

*2.1. Finite Element Model of L3–L5.* A nonlinear finite element model of L3–L5 was constructed from CT image data obtained from a 25-year-old Chinese male without any history of spinal disease. The CT images saved as Digital Imaging and Communications in Medicine format were imported into Simpleware Software (Simpleware Ltd.). After segmentation, feature extraction, smoothing, and mesh processes, the elements and nodes were imported to an FE software for remesh. The vertebrae were meshed using tetrahedral elements, and the intervertebral discs were meshed using hexahedral elements in the ABAQUS software. The FE model consisted of 32,850 nodes and 96,970

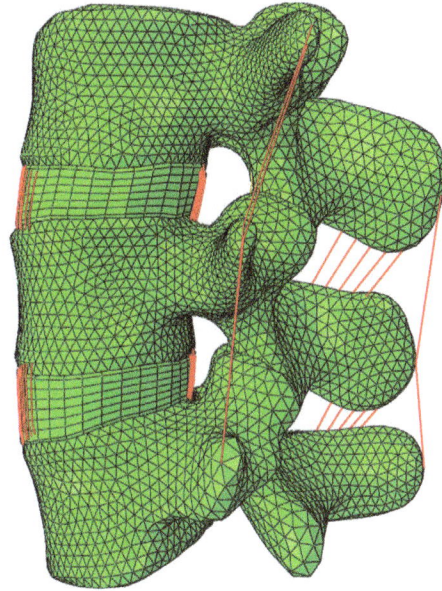

FIGURE 1: Finite element model of L3–L5.

elements. Each vertebra consisted of a cortical shell, a cancellous core, and a posterior bony structure. The 0.5 mm thick cortical shell [12] and the posterior bony structure were modeled as isotropic elastic materials, while the cancellous core was modeled as transverse isotropic. The cartilaginous endplates were 0.8 mm thick [13]. Each intervertebral disc was composed of an incompressible nucleus pulposus and surrounding annulus fibrosus. Rebar elements of two times seven layers were used to represent the fiber and the fiber stiffness decreased from the outside towards the centre [14]. The vertebrae and intervertebral discs were tied together. There was a gap of 0.5 mm [15] between the curved facet joints, and a thin cartilaginous layer of 0.25 mm was created for each facet articular surface. All seven ligaments of the lumbar spine were integrated according to their anatomical positions and were represented by tension-only spring elements with nonlinear material properties [16]. The FE model of L3–L5 is shown in Figure 1, and the material properties are shown in Table 1.

*2.2. Validation.* To validate the model, a moment of 7.5 Nm was applied to the top surface of L3 in the direction of flexion, extension, right lateral bending, and right axial rotation. The inferior endplate of L5 was rigidly fixed. The IVR of L4-L5, the region of concern in this study, was calculated and compared with in vitro data [17]. In addition, the IVR of L3–L5 was compared with in vitro data from whole lumbar specimens [18]. As a whole lumbar spine has five vertebrae and four spinal motion units, a direct comparison is unsuitable. Therefore, a ratio for IVR between L3–L5 and L1–L5 was adopted according to data from Pearcy et al. [19, 20]. This ratio was calculated for flexion-extension, lateral bending, and axial rotation, and the IVR of L3–L5 was justified according to this ratio. A subsequent 500 N axial compressive follower load was also applied and the IDP was estimated and compared with in vivo data [28].

TABLE 1: Material properties used for the different tissues in the finite element model.

| Component | Elastic modulus (MPa) | Poisson ratio | References |
|---|---|---|---|
| Cortical bone | 10,000 | 0.30 | [16] |
| Cancellous bone (transverse isotropic) | 200/140 (axial/radial) | 0.45/0.315 | [21] |
| Posterior bony structures | 3,500 | 0.25 | [14] |
| Ligaments | Nonlinear | | [16] |
| Cartilage of endplate | Hyperelastic, neo-Hookean, $C_{10} = 0.3448$, $D_1 = 0.3$ | | |
| Nucleus pulposus | Incompressible | | [16] |
| Ground substance of annulus fibrosis | Hyperelastic, neo-Hookean, $C_{10} = 0.3448$, $D_1 = 0.3$ | | [22] |
| Fibers of annulus fibrosis | Stiffness decreased from the outer to the centre | | [14] |
| Facet joint | Soft contact | | [15] |

TABLE 2: Loads used to simulate flexion, extension, lateral bending, and axial rotation.

| | Flexion | Extension | Lateral bending | Axial rotation |
|---|---|---|---|---|
| Rohlmann et al. [23, 24] | 1175 N + 7.5 Nm | 500 N + 7.5 Nm | — | — |
| Dreischarf et al. [25, 26] | — | — | 700 N + 7.8 Nm | 720 N + 5.5 Nm |

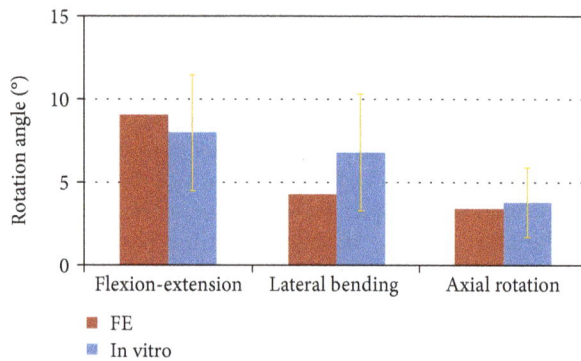

FIGURE 2: Comparison of the calculated intervertebral rotations of L4-L5 in the finite element (FE) model against experimental data [17] under a moment of 7.5 Nm for different loading cases.

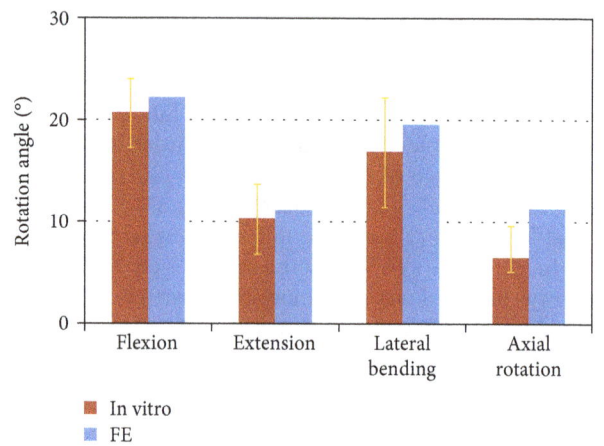

FIGURE 3: Comparison of the rotations in the finite element (FE) model and measured (Rohlmann et al. [18]) rotations in the lumbar spine under a moment of 7.5 Nm for different loading cases.

*2.3. Graded Facetectomy Model.* Starting from the intact model, different graded facetectomies were simulated by modifying the facet joint of L4-L5 with the facet capsular ligament: 50% unilateral facetectomy, total left unilateral facetectomy, and total bilateral facetectomy. Regarding 50% unilateral facetectomy, different portions could be removed, depending on the surgical approaches. Therefore, to study sensitivity, four different 50% unilateral facetectomies were simulated by removing the upper, lower, outer, and medial portions of the left facet joint of L4-L5, respectively.

*2.4. Boundary and Loading Conditions.* The inferior endplate of L5 was rigidly fixed as a boundary condition. Flexion, extension, right lateral bending, left lateral bending, right axial rotation, and left axial rotation of the upper body were investigated. All loads (Table 2) were chosen according to Rohlmann et al. [23, 24] and Dreischarf et al. [25, 26]. The

finite element program ABAQUS, version 6.13 (Dassault Systèmes, Versailles, France) was used for the simulations.

## 3. Results

*3.1. Validation.* The calculated IVR of the L4-L5 motion segment was within the range of in vitro experimental data [17] (Figure 2). Regarding the overall rotation, the estimated IVR was compared with in vitro data (Figure 3). The mobility of the model in flexion-extension and lateral bending was inside the range measured for seven lumbar specimens [18]. The mobility of the model in axial rotation was slightly outside, but the mobility for a single motion segment was still within the range of other published data [27]. Regarding the axial compressive load, the estimated IDP of L4-L5 in a standing position was 0.44 MPa. This is comparable to in vivo

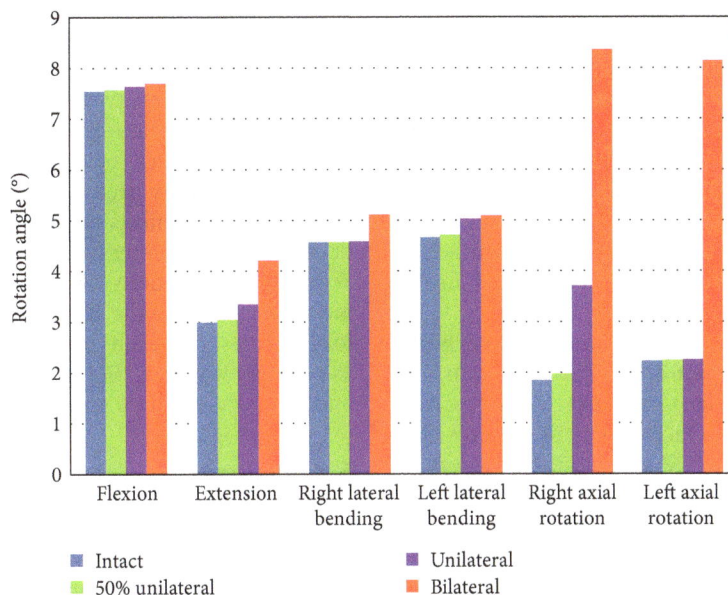

FIGURE 4: The values of rotation angles in each motion plane for the intact model and graded facetectomy models.

measurements by Wilke et al. [28], who recorded 0.50 MPa for spinal loading.

*3.2. Intervertebral Rotation.* The rotation angles in each motion plane for the intact model and graded facetectomy models are summarized in Figure 4. The values presented for the 50% unilateral facetectomy were the mean values calculated for the four different 50% unilateral facetectomies simulated. In flexion, graded facetectomy had only a minor effect. In extension, unilateral facetectomy increased IVR by 11.7% and bilateral facetectomy increased IVR by 40.7%. For right lateral bending, unilateral facetectomy and bilateral facetectomy increased the IVR by 0.3% and 11.9%, respectively, while for left lateral bending, this was 7.7% and 9.0%, respectively. In general, facetectomy had a large effect on the axial rotation. The 50% unilateral facetectomy, unilateral facetectomy, and the bilateral facetectomy increased the right axial rotation of the L4-L5 motion segment by 7.2%, 101.3%, and 354.3%, respectively, and by 0.6%, 1.1%, and 265.3%, respectively, for left axial rotation. For all loading types, the 50% facetectomy only increased the IVR by a maximum of 7.2%, which occurred under right axial rotation.

In most times, different types of partial resection resulted in similar IVR with a difference of less than 2%. Only for right axial rotation, removing the lower and outer portion of the left L4-5 facet joint increased the IVR by 6.4% (0.12°) and 19.2% (0.35°), respectively.

*3.3. Intradiscal Pressure and Facet Joint Force.* In most cases, facetectomy had only a minor influence on the IDP. In extension, the unilateral facetectomy and the bilateral facetectomy increased the IDP by 10.7% and 23.6%, respectively, and for left axial rotation, the bilateral facetectomy increased the IDP by 9.6%. The extension movement also produced the greatest facet joint force on the contralateral facet joint. For this loading case, the 50% unilateral facetectomy increased the contralateral facet joint force by

25% on average and the total unilateral facetectomy increased the force by 108.1%.

*3.4. Maximum von Mises Equivalent Stresses in the Annuli.* The four 50% unilateral facetectomy procedures only resulted in slightly different results for maximum von Mises stress in the annuli in comparison to the intact model. Unilateral facetectomy increased the maximum von Mises stress in the annuli by 13.1% in extension and 23.5% in right axial rotation. Bilateral facetectomy increased the maximum von Mises stress in the annuli by 32.3% in extension and 59.3% in axial rotation.

## 4. Discussion

An FE model of L3–L5 was constructed in this study, and the mobility of the model and the IDP were calculated for validation study. The effect of graded facetectomy on intervertebral rotations, intradiscal pressure, facet joint forces, and maximum von Mises equivalent stresses in the annuli was analyzed for all six loading conditions.

Regarding validation for the overall rotation, the calculated overall IVR of L3–L5 was justified. For example, the calculated axial rotation of L3–L5 was 6.54° in our FE model under a 7.5 Nm moment. According to Pearcy et al., the ratio between the rotation of L3–L5 and L1–L5 is 60% [19, 20]. The estimated axial rotation of L1–L5 in our model was 10.9° (6.54°/60%). Figure 3 showed the comparison between the justified IVR of L1–L5 and in vitro data [18]. All calculated data for the IDP, the IVR of L4-L5, and the overall IVR were inside the range of in vivo/in vitro data, respectively. Therefore, the load and mobility of the FE model were in the physiological range.

For the four 50% unilateral facetectomies simulated, there were no significant differences in results after resecting different portions of the vertebra compared with the intact model. Fusion or dynamic stabilization may not be necessary.

Similarly, Zhou et al. [5] also concluded that lumbar stability was not significantly affected if graded facetectomy was performed to remove less than 50% of bone, which is the same as our finding. In right axial rotation, removing the lower and outer portions of the left L4-5 facet joint increased the IVR by 6.4% and 19.2%, respectively. Although the absolute values were only 0.12° and 0.35°, retaining these portions of the bone may be beneficial. Choi et al. [29] also suggested that the resection should not involve the articular surface as preserving a larger articular surface is important for maintaining spinal stability.

This study demonstrated that total unilateral and bilateral facetectomy had little impact on the IVR in flexion and lateral bending, which is similar to in vitro results reported by Quint et al. [30]. These two facetectomy procedures also had a minor influence on the IDP and facet joint forces in flexion and lateral bending. For extension, total unilateral and bilateral facetectomy increased the IVR by 11.7% and 40.7%. After total unilateral facetectomy, the contralateral facet joint force increased by 108.1% in extension. This was the largest increase in contralateral facet joint force among all loading cases. At the same time, the increased IDP and the maximum von Mises stresses in the annuli in this model indicated a greater load through the intervertebral disc of L4-L5. This would inevitably lead to a greater risk of intervertebral disc degeneration and arthritis of the facet joints. Therefore, extension postures need to be achieved with care after total unilateral/bilateral facetectomy.

The facetectomy had a significant effect on IVR in axial rotation. Notably, after bilateral facetectomy, the IVR for right and left axial rotation increased by 354.3% and 265.3%. This is comparable to results from the literature [11]. Besides spinal instability, greater IDP of L4-L5 intervertebral disc and stress in the annuli will result in rupture of the annulus fibrosus. These remind us that axial rotation is another position needed to be treated carefully from the biomechanical point of view. Meanwhile, due to the change of stability, fusion or dynamic stabilization would be needed to reconstruct the lumbar stability from the biomechanical results. In this study, only the biomechanical aspects were regarded, but clinical experiences are inevitable as well; a cooperation of surgeons and bioengineers could induce the individual optimum for specific patients.

The majority of previous publications on spinal biomechanics constructed models based on the anatomy of European or American subjects [7, 10, 11]. However, differences in anatomy have been demonstrated between European or American people and Asian people, especially for the orientation of the facet joint. Grogan et al. [31] reported a mean facet joint angle of the lumbar spine from American subjects to be 37°. Yang and Wang reported this to be 47° for the lumbar spine of Chinese [32], while the value for Thais measured by Pichaisak et al. was 46° [33]. Given the vast and ever-growing Asian population, a concise FE analysis of graded facetectomy may be of great benefit across an array of disciplines and professions for Asians.

Some limitations of this study should be noted. In the case of spine, only a few parameters such as intervertebral

rotation and intradiscal pressure were measurable and thus suitable for validation. Therefore, facet joint forces and the maximum von Mises equivalent stresses in the annuli were presented only by relative ratios. The model used for simulation was from an asymptomatic volunteer. The effects of different pathological factors on the stability of spine after graded facetectomy need to be investigated in further study. In addition, the effects of muscle forces and bone mineral density on facetectomy need further study as well. Although several simplifications were made, the reported results are reliable because the same parameters were chosen for all loading cases. The results in the present study should be viewed as a comparative analysis between graded facetectomy models and an intact model for all six spinal loading conditions.

## 5. Conclusions

The results conclude that, after unilateral and bilateral facetectomy, care must be taken when placing the spine into extension and axial rotation posture from the biomechanical point of view.

## Competing Interests

The authors declare that there is no conflict of interest regarding the publication of this paper.

## Acknowledgments

This work was supported by the National Natural Science Foundation of China (Grant no. 81572138 and Grant no. 31300779) and the Shanghai Municipal Commission of Health and Family Planning (Project 20144Y0245).

## References

[1] C. Ammendolia, P. Cote, Y. R. Rampersaud et al., "The boot camp program for lumbar spinal stenosis: a protocol for a randomized controlled trial," *Chiropractic & Manual Therapies*, vol. 24, no. 1, p. 25, 2016.

[2] S. J. Atlas, R. B. Keller, D. Robson, R. A. Deyo, and D. E. Singer, "Surgical and nonsurgical management of lumbar spinal stenosis: four-year outcomes from The Maine Lumbar Spine Study," *Spine (Phila Pa 1976)*, vol. 25, no. 5, pp. 556–562, 2000.

[3] K. Abumi, M. M. Panjabi, K. M. Kramer, J. Duranceau, T. Oxland, and J. J. Crisco, "Biomechanical evaluation of lumbar spinal stability after graded facetectomies," *Spine (Phila Pa 1976)*, vol. 15, no. 11, pp. 1142–1147, 1990.

[4] A. Okawa, K. Shinomiya, K. Takakuda, and O. Nakai, "A cadaveric study on the stability of lumbar segment after partial laminotomy and facetectomy with intact posterior ligaments," *Journal of Spinal Disorders*, vol. 9, no. 6, pp. 518–526, 1996.

[5] Y. Zhou, G. Luo, T. W. Chu et al., "The biomechanical change of lumbar unilateral graded facetectomy and strategies of its microsurgical reconstruction: report of 23 cases," *Zhonghua Yi Xue Za Zhi*, vol. 87, no. 19, pp. 1334–1338, 2007.

[6] H. Li and Z. Wang, "Intervertebral disc biomechanical analysis using the finite element modeling based on medical images," *Computerized Medical Imaging and Graphics*, vol. 30, no. 6-7, pp. 363–370, 2006.

[7] T. Zander, A. Rohlmann, C. Klockner, and G. Bergmann, "Influence of graded facetectomy and laminectomy on spinal biomechanics," *European Spine Journal*, vol. 12, no. 4, pp. 427–434, 2003.

[8] K. K. Lee and E. C. Teo, "Effects of laminectomy and facetectomy on the stability of the lumbar motion segment," *Medical Engineering & Physics*, vol. 26, no. 3, pp. 183–192, 2004.

[9] C. S. Chen, C. K. Feng, C. K. Cheng, M. J. Tzeng, C. L. Liu, and W. J. Chen, "Biomechanical analysis of the disc adjacent to posterolateral fusion with laminectomy in lumbar spine," *Journal of Spinal Disorders & Techniques*, vol. 18, no. 1, pp. 58–65, 2005.

[10] A. Kiapour, D. Ambati, R. W. Hoy, and V. K. Goel, "Effect of graded facetectomy on biomechanics of Dynesys dynamic stabilization system," *Spine (Phila Pa 1976)*, vol. 37, no. 10, pp. E581–E589, 2012.

[11] D. U. Erbulut, "Biomechanical effect of graded facetectomy on asymmetrical finite element model of the lumbar spine," *Turkish Neurosurgery*, vol. 24, no. 6, pp. 923–928, 2014.

[12] W. T. Edwards, Y. Zheng, L. A. Ferrara, and H. A. Yuan, "Structural features and thickness of the vertebral cortex in the thoracolumbar spine," *Spine (Phila Pa 1976)*, vol. 26, no. 2, pp. 218–225, 2001.

[13] U. M. Ayturk and C. M. Puttlitz, "Parametric convergence sensitivity and validation of a finite element model of the human lumbar spine," *Computer Methods in Biomechanics and Biomedical Engineering*, vol. 14, no. 8, pp. 695–705, 2011.

[14] A. Shirazi-Adl, A. M. Ahmed, and S. C. Shrivastava, "Mechanical response of a lumbar motion segment in axial torque alone and combined with compression," *Spine (Phila Pa 1976)*, vol. 11, no. 9, pp. 914–927, 1986.

[15] V. K. Goel, Y. E. Kim, T. H. Lim, and J. N. Weinstein, "An analytical investigation of the mechanics of spinal instrumentation," *Spine (Phila Pa 1976)*, vol. 13, no. 9, pp. 1003–1011, 1988.

[16] A. Rohlmann, T. Zander, H. Schmidt, H. J. Wilke, and G. Bergmann, "Analysis of the influence of disc degeneration on the mechanical behaviour of a lumbar motion segment using the finite element method," *Journal of Biomechanics*, vol. 39, no. 13, pp. 2484–2490, 2006.

[17] B. Ilharreborde, M. N. Shaw, L. J. Berglund, K. D. Zhao, R. E. Gay, and K. N. An, "Biomechanical evaluation of posterior lumbar dynamic stabilization: an in vitro comparison between universal clamp and Wallis systems," *European Spine Journal*, vol. 20, no. 2, pp. 289–296, 2011.

[18] A. Rohlmann, S. Neller, L. Claes, G. Bergmann, and H. J. Wilke, "Influence of a follower load on intradiscal pressure and intersegmental rotation of the lumbar spine," *Spine*, vol. 26, no. 24, pp. E557–E561, 2001.

[19] M. J. Pearcy and S. B. Tibrewal, "Axial rotation and lateral bending in the normal lumbar spine measured by three-dimensional radiography," *Spine (Phila Pa 1976)*, vol. 9, no. 6, pp. 582–587, 1984.

[20] M. Pearcy, I. Portek, and J. Shepherd, "Three-dimensional x-ray analysis of normal movement in the lumbar spine," *Spine (Phila Pa 1976)*, vol. 9, no. 3, pp. 294–297, 1984.

[21] K. Ueno and Y. K. Liu, "A three-dimensional nonlinear finite element model of lumbar intervertebral joint in torsion," *Journal of Biomechanical Engineering*, vol. 109, no. 3, pp. 200–209, 1987.

[22] R. Eberlein, G. Holzapfel, and C. A. Schulze-Bauer, "An anisotropic model for annulus tissue and enhanced finite element analyses of intact lumbar disc bodies," *Computer Methods in Biomechanics and Biomedical Engineering*, vol. 4, no. 3, pp. 209–229, 2000.

[23] A. Rohlmann, T. Zander, M. Rao, and G. Bergmann, "Applying a follower load delivers realistic results for simulating standing," *Journal of Biomechanics*, vol. 42, no. 10, pp. 1520–1526, 2009.

[24] A. Rohlmann, T. Zander, M. Rao, and G. Bergmann, "Realistic loading conditions for upper body bending," *Journal of Biomechanics*, vol. 42, no. 7, pp. 884–890, 2009.

[25] M. Dreischarf, A. Rohlmann, G. Bergmann, and T. Zander, "Optimised loads for the simulation of axial rotation in the lumbar spine," *Journal of Biomechanics*, vol. 44, no. 12, pp. 2323–2327, 2011.

[26] M. Dreischarf, A. Rohlmann, G. Bergmann, and T. Zander, "Optimised in vitro applicable loads for the simulation of lateral bending in the lumbar spine," *Medical Engineering & Physics*, vol. 34, no. 6, pp. 777–780, 2012.

[27] F. Heuer, H. Schmidt, Z. Klezl, L. Claes, and H. J. Wilke, "Stepwise reduction of functional spinal structures increase range of motion and change lordosis angle," *Journal of Biomechanics*, vol. 40, no. 2, pp. 271–280, 2007.

[28] H. Wilke, P. Neef, B. Hinz, H. Seidel, and L. Claes, "Intradiscal pressure together with anthropometric data–a data set for the validation of models," *Clinical Biomechanics (Bristol, Avon)*, vol. 16, Suppl 1, pp. S111–S126, 2001.

[29] G. Choi, S. H. Lee, P. Lokhande et al., "Percutaneous endoscopic approach for highly migrated intracanal disc herniations by foraminoplastic technique using rigid working channel endoscope," *Spine (Phila Pa 1976)*, vol. 33, no. 15, pp. E508–E515, 2008.

[30] U. Quint, H. J. Wilke, F. Loer, and L. E. Claes, "Functional sequelae of surgical decompression of the lumbar spine–a biomechanical study in vitro," *Zeitschrift für Orthopädie und Ihre Grenzgebiete*, vol. 136, no. 4, pp. 350–357, 1998.

[31] J. Grogan, B. H. Nowicki, T. A. Schmidt, and V. M. Haughton, "Lumbar facet joint tropism does not accelerate degeneration of the facet joints," *American Journal of Neuroradiology*, vol. 18, no. 7, pp. 1325–1329, 1997.

[32] X. Yang and J. Wang, "The affections of the orientations and the severity of degeneration of facet joints to the degenerative lumbar pondylolisthesiss," *Chinese Journal of Spine and Spinal Cord*, vol. 19, no. 1, pp. 52–55, 2009.

[33] W. Pichaisak, C. Chotiyarnwong, and P. Chotiyarnwong, "Facet joint orientation and tropism in lumbar degenerative disc disease and spondylolisthesis," *Journal of the Medical Association of Thailand*, vol. 98, no. 4, pp. 373–379, 2015.

8

# Assessment of the Nurse Medication Administration Workflow Process

Nathan Huynh,[1] Rita Snyder,[2] José M. Vidal,[3] Omor Sharif,[1] Bo Cai,[4]
Bridgette Parsons,[3] and Kevin Bennett[5]

[1]Civil & Environmental Engineering, University of South Carolina, Columbia, SC 29208, USA
[2]College of Nursing, University of Arizona, Tucson, AZ 85721, USA
[3]Computer Science and Engineering, University of South Carolina, Columbia, SC 29208, USA
[4]Epidemiology and Biostatistics, University of South Carolina, Columbia, SC 29208, USA
[5]School of Medicine, University of South Carolina, Columbia, SC 29208, USA

Correspondence should be addressed to Nathan Huynh; nathan.huynh@sc.edu

Academic Editor: Feng-Huei Lin

This paper presents findings of an observational study of the Registered Nurse (RN) Medication Administration Process (MAP) conducted on two comparable medical units in a large urban tertiary care medical center in Columbia, South Carolina. A total of 305 individual MAP observations were recorded over a 6-week period with an average of 5 MAP observations per RN participant for both clinical units. A key MAP variation was identified in terms of unbundled versus bundled MAP performance. In the unbundled workflow, an RN engages in the MAP by performing only MAP tasks during a care episode. In the bundled workflow, an RN completes medication administration along with other patient care responsibilities during the care episode. Using a discrete-event simulation model, this paper addresses the difference between unbundled and bundled workflow and their effects on simulated redesign interventions.

## 1. Introduction

In recent years, concern about the impact of health care system interventions on clinical workflow processes has escalated primarily due to the implementation of electronic health records and computerized provider order entry systems [1–4]. The impact and unintended consequences of these system redesign interventions have underscored the lack of knowledge about high-risk clinical processes and the concomitant patient safety risks associated with system redesign that may destabilize these processes in dynamic care delivery environments [1]. Evidence about clinical workflow processes is quite limited. Their dynamic nature and the complexity of healthcare environments within which they occur make them difficult to assess with current observation methods and tools. There is a critical need for innovative methods and technologies that support a low-risk environment in which to visualize, examine, and manipulate

high-risk clinical processes to assess the potential impact of redesign interventions on multilevel systems, clinician, and patient outcomes [5, 6].

Medication errors remain a serious health care problem in the United States which result in approximately 7,000 deaths, cause harm to approximately 1.5 million people, and cost billions of dollars in hospital treatment annually [7–11]. Leape et al.'s [12] early research into medication errors highlighted the need to examine system factors associated with medication errors. This research used a systems analysis approach to examine all phases of the medication process, that is, physician ordering, transcription/verification, pharmacy dispensing, and nurse administration, to determine types of medication errors by stage of drug ordering and delivery. Findings indicated that, of the identified medication errors ($n = 334$), nurse medication administration errors (38%) were the second largest category of medication errors following physician medication order errors (39%) [12]. The

MAP is, predominantly, a nursing responsibility that has been estimated to consume approximately 40% of nursing practice time [13]. Since Leape et al.'s [12] early research on medication errors, the MAP has become increasingly complex due to escalating patient acuity, numerous generic and trade medication names, expanded medication delivery routes, increased use of new and diverse medication safety technologies, and an increased number of medication orders [13, 14]. The lack of standardization of the MAP is also a key contributing factor in medication administration complexity [13].

Typically, the MAP involves a Registered Nurse (RN) performing many tasks, including, but not limited to, (1) assessing the patient to obtain pertinent data, (2) gathering medications, (3) confirming the six rights (i.e., right dose, patient, route, medication, time, and documentation), (4) administering the medications, (5) documenting administration, and (6) observing for therapeutic and untoward effects [15]. Clinical observation has confirmed a significant degree of nurse-to-nurse variability in MAP tasks and task sequencing that is subject to environmental interruptions that result in medication administration practices that deviate from standard practice protocols. Empirical evidence, however, is lacking about MAP characteristics and the nature of RN and environmental characteristics and interruptions that influence it. This makes it very difficult to anticipate the impact of system redesign interventions undertaken to enhance medication safety, for example, introduction of medication safety technology and the potential consequences of redesign interventions. To this end, this study identified MAP workflow characteristics and developed a computer simulation model based on these characteristics to assess the impact of simulated MAP redesign interventions on selected MAP redesign outcomes. It builds on our previous work where we developed a mobile application for recording live MAP observations [16] and a discrete-event simulation model of the MAP [17].

## 2. Methods

*2.1. Setting.* The study was undertaken in a tertiary medical center in Columbia, South Carolina, United States. The medical center is a 414-bed modern complex that anchors a comprehensive network of 600-plus affiliated physicians, including six strategically located community medical and urgent care centers, an occupational health center, the largest extended care facility in the Carolinas, and an Alzheimer's Care Center. The medical center also supports an array of health and wellness classes. The hospital employs more than 5,200 people and offers a variety of community outreach programs and education and health screenings. A high surgical volume is supported with 29 state-of-the-art operating rooms that have cutting edge, state-of-the-art medical technology and procedures. Patient safety and security are top concerns and health care team work is stressed. Identification bands, proper cough etiquette, frequent hand-washing, protective wear, and public safety officers are integral parts of the medical center's commitment to patient safety and security.

The study was conducted on two comparable medical units that served adult patients with medical, surgical, neurological, oncology, orthopedic, and renal conditions. Patients were typically admitted for chronic care management, diagnostic studies, and medical interventions. The units were comparable in terms of size (range = 30–36 beds), average daily census (range = 26–31 patients), patient length of stay (range = 6.5–7 days), and number of RNs (range = 25–29 full-time equivalent), as well as numbers and types of technical and secretarial support staff. The term "average" refers to arithmetic mean hereafter. Both clinical units comprised single bed rooms along 4 hallways. Each patient room had an individual bathroom, an inside supply cabinet, and a locked medication cabinet. A wall-mounted locked documentation station with a drop-down writing platform was located outside each patient room. A nurses' station was centrally located with an adjacent dumbwaiter and various separate rooms, for example, medications, clean/soiled equipment, supplies, breaks, family consultation, and a manager office. An integrated electronic health record (EHR) was used on each unit for all documentation, including medication administration and management. Two rolling computer carts were available on each hallway and RNs used them during walking rounds to receive change-of-shift report, and to document all care, including medication administration. More acutely ill patients were routinely assigned to rooms closer to the nurses' station.

*2.2. Sample.* Since medication administration is predominantly a responsibility of RNs, the study sample comprised RNs. The study did not involve patients and no patient information was collected during the course of the study. Following protocol approvals from university and medical center Institutional Review Boards, RN volunteers were recruited from full-time RN populations for each study unit. All full-time RNs from Unit 1 ($N = 16$) and Unit 2 ($N = 20$) were invited to participate. Study recruitment information was distributed at unit staff meetings by unit managers and during unit recruitment visits by the study Principal Investigator (PI). Registered Nurses interested in volunteering for the study met with the PI in a unit conference room where the PI explained the study prior to them signing a consent form and completing a demographic information form. A total of 17 RNs participated in the study with 7 from Unit 1 (44%) and 10 from Unit 2 (50%). Demographic findings indicated that RN characteristics were comparable across the two units. Combined findings for all 17 RN volunteers indicated that the majority were white [$n = 15$ (88%)] women [$n = 16$ (94%)] who had been licensed as an RN an average of 11 years, had practiced as an RN an average of 10 years, and had worked at the medical center an average of 6 years with 60% or more of that time spent on their study unit. The majority of RNs reported that they had a totally supportive medication safety culture [$n = 11$ (65%)] on their unit and that they felt totally comfortable [$n = 10$ (59%)] with reporting medication safety practice variations. Most RNs also indicated that they thought about medication safety frequently [$n = 15$ (88%)] and that the quality of the medication safety process on their unit was extremely high [$n = 9$ (53%)]. Medication safety technology, such as smart intravenous infusion pumps, was readily available [$n = 13$ (76%)] on the units, and the majority

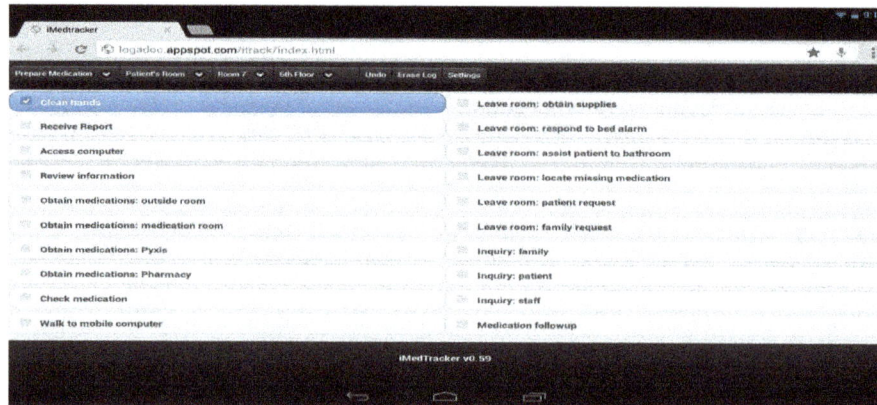

Figure 1: Screenshot of iMedTracker.

of the RNs used it frequently [$n = 16$ (94%)]. The majority of RNs had also completed 1 self-paced computer instructional program [$n = 15$ (88%)] on medication safety, with 7 (41%) completing this within one month prior to the study. The majority of RNs reported that they were very likely [$n = 11$ (65%)] to be interrupted while engaged in the medication administration process. Their self-reports, however, did not provide any specific interruption types or patterns.

### 2.3. MAP Observation Data Collection

*2.3.1. MAP Observation Recording Tool.* To record RN medication administration functions, tasks, and interruptions in a live clinical environment and to generate baseline data for the development of our computer simulation model, the research team developed the "iMedTracker" mobile application; it is an extension of the application we developed in our previous study [16]. The iMedTracker is a web-based application developed using the jQuery Mobile framework (http://jquerymobile.com/). The team chose to develop a web-based application instead of a native application because it would allow the application to run on any smartphone or tablet. The iMedTracker represents one of the first mobile applications designed specifically to record MAP workflows and one that can run on multiple mobile devices. Figure 1 provides a screenshot of the iMedTracker application running on a Nexus 10.

The first menu item of iMedTracker is the MAP function. Observers can change the function by tapping on the item. When the item is pressed, a drop-down list is displayed for users to choose from. The list of choices include "prepare medication" and "administer medication." There is a separate list of tasks associated with each function, and they change according to the function selected. To facilitate the recording process, the medication documentation tasks are listed under the administer medication function.

The three menu items to the right of "prepare medication" allow observers to record the location of the activity (e.g., patient's room, medication room, and kitchen), patient's room number, if applicable, and the clinical unit number (e.g., 6th and 7th). As their names imply, the "Undo" menu item undoes the last recorded activity, and the "Erase Log" menu

item erases the stored data. The last menu item "Settings" takes observers to another screen where they can input their name, input the code (instead of name) of the RN being shadowed, and e-mail the data to project investigators. No patient data are recorded.

On the iMedTracker, the left column lists the tasks, and the right column lists the interruptions. When a task or interruption is selected, the application automatically captures its start time and writes the record to the database. The application indicates that the activity is in operation by highlighting that item, as illustrated by the "clean hands" task in Figure 1. To record the end of an activity, observers would press on that item and the application would automatically capture the activity's end time. If a mistake is made, observers can tap on the Undo button to cancel the last action.

*2.3.2. MAP Observation Data Collection Protocol.* The MAP observational data collection protocol was field tested in this study using expanded methods and developed in our previous studies [16, 17]. Several steps were taken to ensure data recording consistency including (1) observer training in the use of the mobile device and iMedTracker application; (2) creation of common observation rules and data collection procedures; and (3) assessment of observer interrater reliability (IRR).

Three student observers participated in two 4-hour classroom training sessions that included (1) an introduction to the iMedTracker application, (2) group recording practice using iMedTracker and sample MAP videotapes from a previous study, and (3) four independent recording sessions using iMedTracker and sample MAP videotapes. Independent observer recordings were compared and discussed by the group to assess recording variations. Following classroom training, observers participated in a one-week orientation to the two study units. During this week, observers used iMedTracker to record live MAP observations for three data collection sessions and participate in debriefing conferences with study investigators at the conclusion of each session. Debriefing feedback was used to establish observation rules to enhance observer recording consistency and clarify data collection procedures (Table 1).

TABLE 1: MAP observation rules.

| Rule # | Description |
|--------|-------------|
| 1 | Each observation must begin with an "enter room" and end with a "move to next room." The "enter room" should be entered only once when the RN first entered the room and should occur before "greet patient." The "move to next room" should be recorded after the postdocumentation is done. Between the "move to next room" and "enter room" tasks, if the RN is performing activities related to the medication, then record all such activities. |
| 2 | The "other care" task is for direct/hands on patient care such as changing a wound dressing. |
| 3 | The "assess patient for other needs" task is for the final check of the patient's well-being; for example, is there anything else I can do for you? |
| 4 | For intravenous medication (IV) administration, the pre/post line flushes are part of administration. |
| 5 | For med administration, activities performed away from the bedside should be recorded as "prepare for medication admin" and at the bedside should be recorded as "administer medications." |
| 6 | When the RN does not complete med administration—moves to the next patient—then returns to the original patient to complete med administration, this is considered a new observation and thus a new set of "enter room" and "move to next room." |
| 7 | If the patient does not swallow oral medications, the end time of "administer medication" should not be recorded. |
| 8 | Products given to the patient during med administration that are not reviewed/documented on the patient's med record, for example, Orajel, are not considered medications. |
| 9 | The "perform assessment" task is for both mental and physical assessment. |
| 10 | Activities at the computer between scanning of meds are considered documentation. |
| 11 | Whenever the RN leaves the room during the med admin process, specify one of the "leave room" reasons, not "move to next room." |
| 12 | The "review patient computer record" task is used when the RN is looking at the computer screen listing of prescribed medications. The "review patient medication box" task is used when the RN is looking at the medications. Be careful when recording these tasks as they are next to each other. |
| 13 | When an RN goes to the medication room, change location accordingly and record the task as "obtain medications: medication room." If the RN accesses the pyxis, then record the task as "obtain medications: pyxis" while the other task is still active. Stop the "obtain medications: pyxis" task when the RN closes the pyxis, and stop the "obtain medications: medication room" task when the RN exits the medication room. |

Interrater reliability was assessed 3 times during the 6-week data collection period. For each IRR assessment, a total of 4 separate MAP observations were recorded. Each assessment involved all three observers simultaneously recording a study RN's MAP task sequence for each of her/his assigned patients. Edit distance ratios (EDRs), using the Demareau-Levenshtein approach, were calculated to assess IRR [19]. Edit distance is derived from information theory and is specifically used to assess IRR with uneven task sequences. It represents the difference or distance between two strings of characters in terms of the number of edit operations, that is, insertion, deletion, and/or substitution, needed to transform the first string into the second one [20, 21]. All EDRs met the standard minimum 0.70 agreement criterion for multiobserver pairwise comparisons with Time 1 EDR means of 0.78, 0.69, and 0.69; Time 2 means of 0.80, 0.71, and 0.73; and Time 3 means of 0.86, 0.72, and 0.73 [22].

*2.3.3. MAP Observations.* An observation was defined as an individual patient care episode that began with the first medication administration task performed and ended when the RN moved to the next patient. Trained student observers conducted a total of 54 MAP sessions over six weeks, during the hours of 7:00 to 11:00 AM on Mondays, Wednesdays, and Fridays in the months of June and July. A total of 305

individual MAP observations were recorded during the 54 MAP sessions with an average of 5 MAP observations per RN study participant for both clinical units.

*2.4. Data Analysis*

*2.4.1. Process Maps.* The first step of the data analysis was to develop process maps of the MAP. A process map is a pictorial representation of the sequence of actions that comprise a process. They were developed to provide baseline information on how the MAP was being performed and to understand its process characteristics. Analysis of the MAP data revealed that there were generally two distinct workflow processes: unbundled and bundled. In the unbundled workflow, an RN engaged in the MAP by performing only MAP tasks during a care episode (Figure 2). In the bundled workflow, an RN completed medication administration together with other patient care responsibilities during the care episode (Figure 3).

As shown in Figure 2, the unbundled MAP workflow typically started when the RN received and reviewed reports of patients she/he was assigned for that shift. After reviewing the reports, the RN then determined if any of her/his patients required special medications that were located in the medication room or Pyxis (a medication dispensing machine located inside the medication room). If so, she/he would

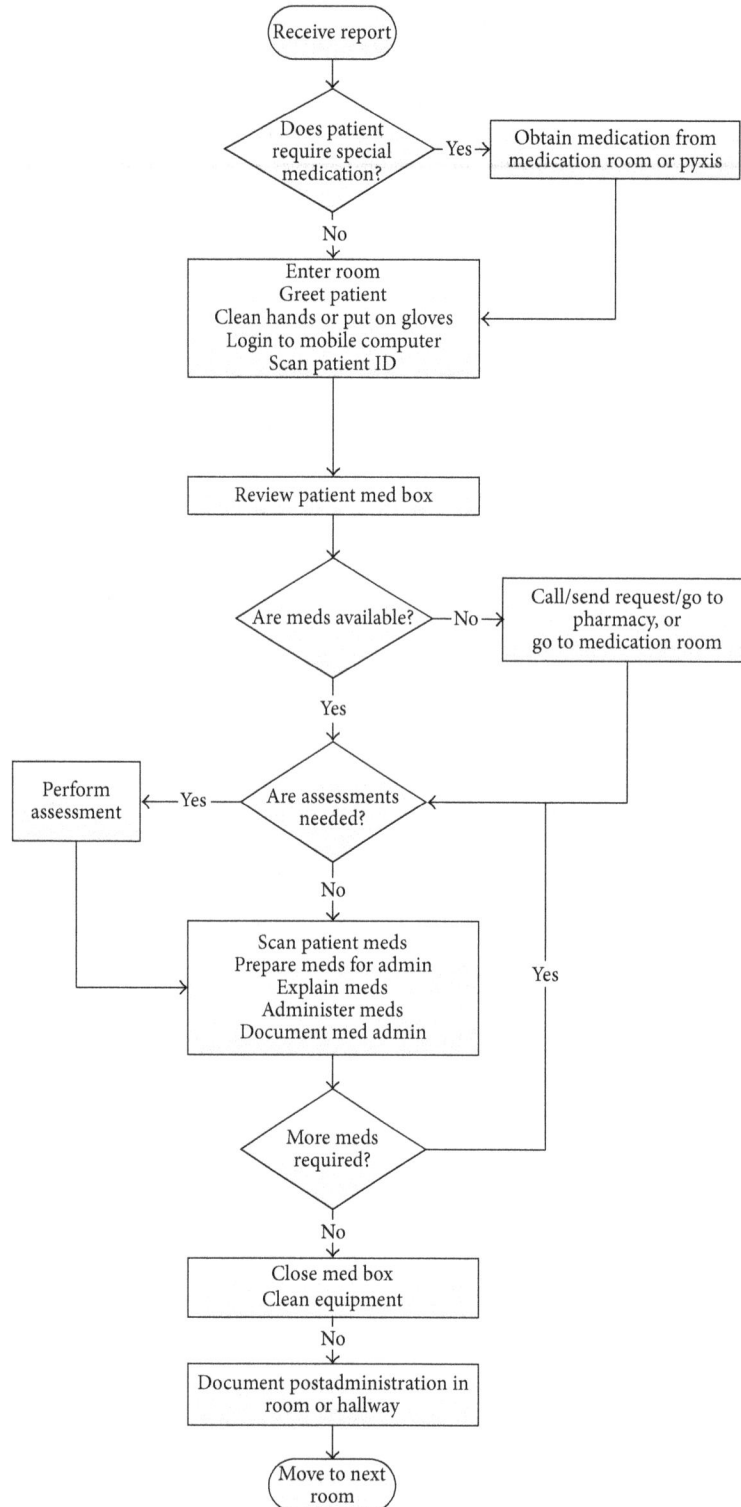

FIGURE 2: Unbundled MAP workflow.

retrieve them. The RN then visited each patient one at a time. The care episode or observation began when the RN entered the patient's room. This was often followed by a combination of tasks such as greet patient, clean hands or put on gloves, log in to mobile computer, and scan patient's ID. After reviewing the patient's medication list, the RN reviewed the medication box that was located in the patient's room to determine if all of the needed medications were available. If not, she/he needed to call the pharmacy, send a request to the pharmacy through the computer, or go to the pharmacy or medication room.

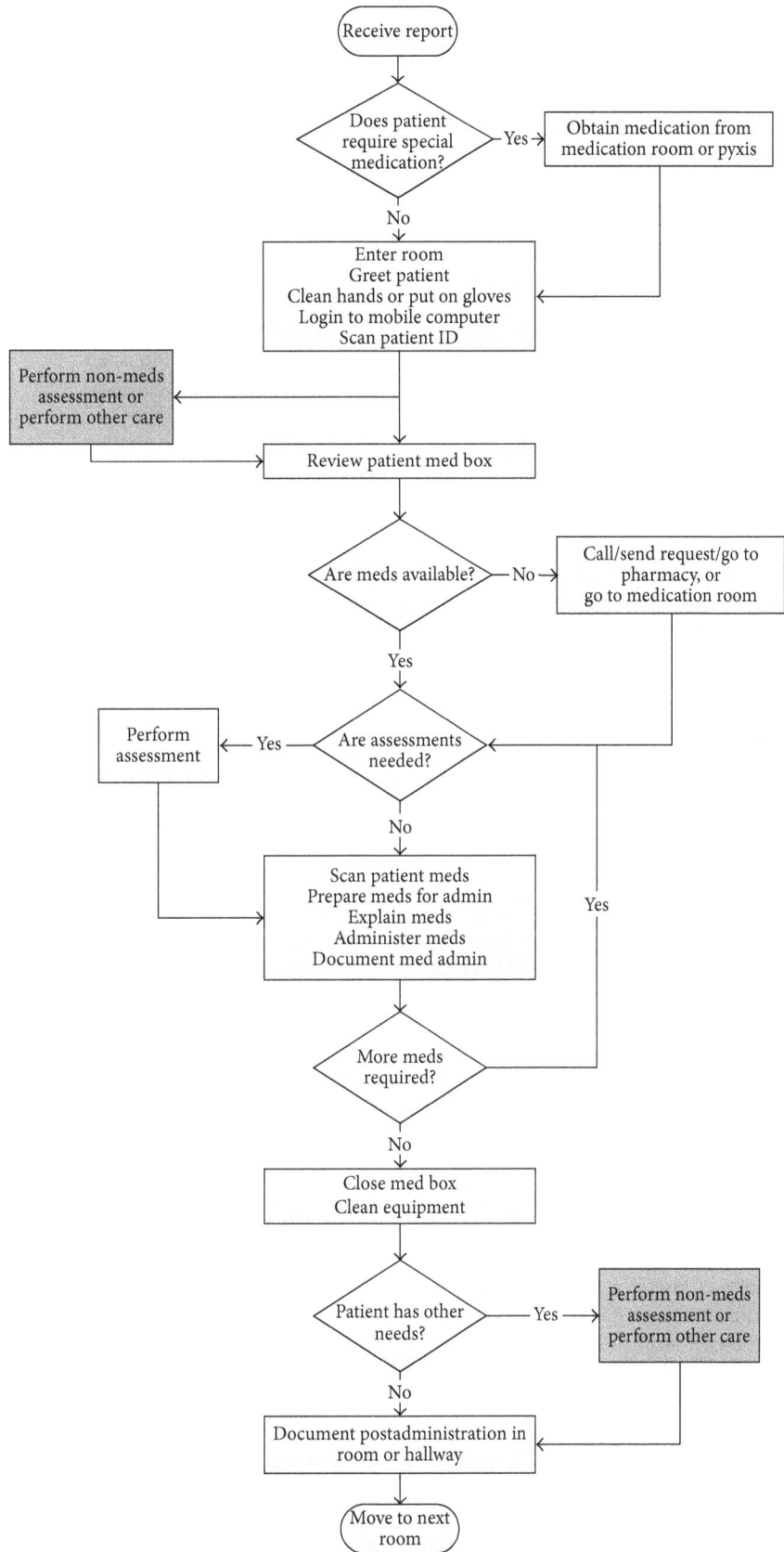

FIGURE 3: Bundled MAP workflow.

TABLE 2: Characteristics of unbundled versus bundled observations.

|  | Unbundled | Bundled |
| --- | --- | --- |
| Number of observations | 102 | 203 |
| Number of observations with interruptions | 84 | 187 |
| Probability of interruptions | 0.82 | 0.92 |
| Average duration of observation (minutes) | 14.11 | 26.06 |
| Standard deviation of observation duration (minutes) | 12.378 | 90.95 |

These events were considered patient-driven interruptions; an interruption is an event that requires the RN to momentarily break away from his/her current task. If the medications were available, then the RN would check to see if any of the medications to be given required an assessment (i.e., a pulse for a patient receiving Digoxin). Once assessments were done, if applicable, the RN then proceeded with the medication administration tasks: scanning patient medications, preparing medications for administration, explaining medications to the patient, administering the medication, and documenting the medication administration. The medication administration tasks were repeated for however many medications the patient needed. Once the RN completed the medication administration tasks, she/he then closed the medication box and cleaned her/his equipment. This was followed by the postadministration medication documentation task. Some RNs performed this task while they were still inside the patient's room, while others preferred to do it in the hallway. The care episode or observation ended when the RN moved to the next patient's room.

As highlighted in Figure 3 for the bundled MAP workflow, the key difference between the unbundled and bundled workflow was the added "nonmedication assessment or other care" tasks. These included tasks such as changing a wound dressing, assessing the physical and mental capacity of the patient (Rule #9, Table 1), or providing assistance with dietary needs. It was observed that these nonmedication tasks could take place before, during, or after medication administration.

*2.4.2. Process Characteristics.* Table 2 provides a summary of the differences between unbundled and bundled observations. Of the 305 observations, there were almost twice as many bundled observations as there were unbundled ones (203 versus 102). Bundled observations took nearly twice as long to complete (26 versus 14 minutes). The contrast in standard deviations indicated that the bundled observation was highly variable, with some observations taking nearly two hours to complete. Lastly, bundled observations were more likely to be associated with interruptions (patient-driven or time-driven) compared to unbundled observations (92% versus 82%). That is, the bundled MAP workflow had a 92% chance of having one or more interruptions. Patient-driven interruptions were defined as those that were triggered by patient-related care, whereas time-driven interruptions were

TABLE 3: MAP workflow interruptions.

| Patient-driven | Time-driven |
| --- | --- |
| Leave room to obtain supplies | Leave room due to bed alarm |
| Leave room to locate medication | Staff inquiry |
| Leave room due to patient request | Personal time |
| Leave room to assist patient to bathroom | Answer phone call |
| Leave room due to family request | Make phone call |
| Patient inquiry | Computer battery issue |
| Family inquiry | Unable to scan med |
| Medication follow-up | Other interruptions |
| Obtain supplies from utility room | |
| Obtain supplies from medication room | |
| Obtain supplies from kitchen | |
| Obtain supplies from front RN station | |
| Obtain supplies from back RN station | |

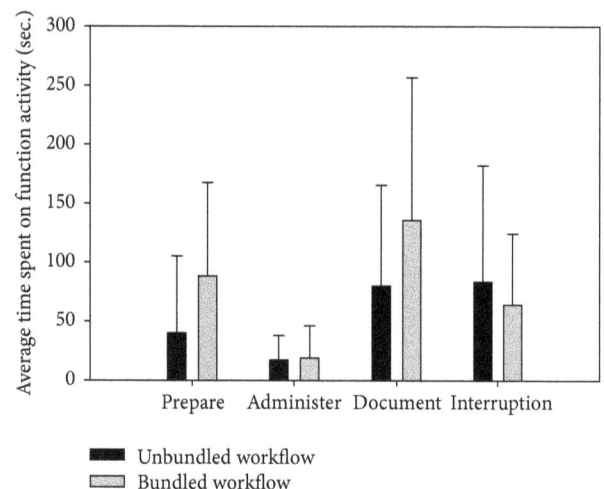

FIGURE 4: Average MAP task time (error bars indicate one standard deviation).

triggered by other sources (considered as random events) (Table 3).

Figure 4 shows the difference in the average amount of time between unbundled and bundled MAP workflows for an RN performing specific MAP tasks, for example, prepare medication, administer medication, and document medication. Additionally, Figure 4 shows the difference in the time spent on interruptions for the unbundled and bundled MAP workflows. The error bars in the graph denote one standard deviation. Results indicated that RNs spent more time preparing and documenting medication for the bundled MAP workflow. The time spent administering medications was comparable between the two MAP workflows. While the unbundled MAP workflow had a lower chance of incurring interruptions, the duration of interruptions was slightly

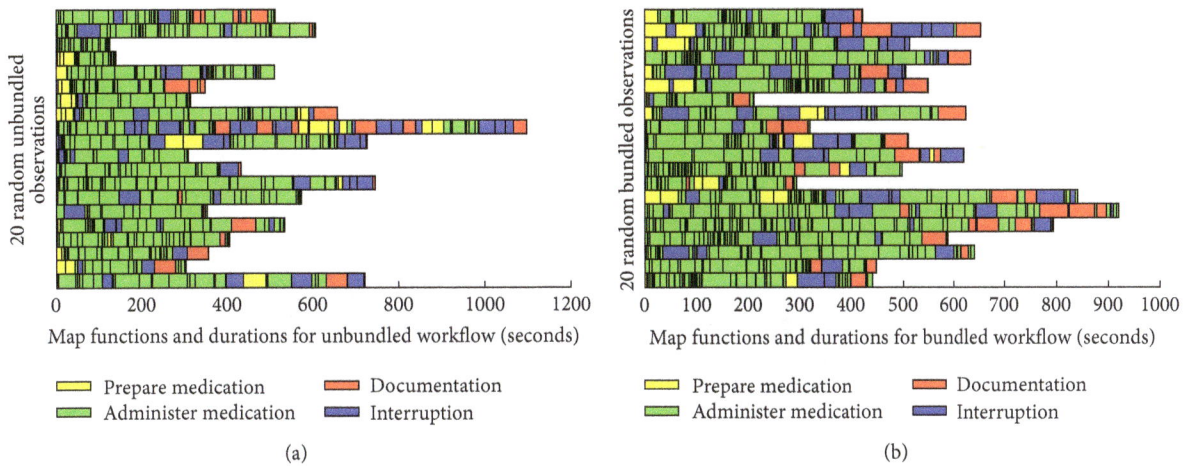

FIGURE 5: Timeline belt: (a) unbundled workflow; (b) bundled workflow.

longer than those that occurred during the bundled MAP workflow. This may indicate that patient-driven interruptions are more time consuming.

To assess MAP workflow fragmentation, a timeline belt comparable to that proposed by Zheng et al. [23] was developed for both the unbundled (Figure 5(a)) and bundled (Figure 5(b)) MAP workflows. Twenty (20) observations were randomly selected for each workflow type. Each timeline belt or row in Figure 5 represents one MAP workflow observation. For each observation, MAP tasks and interruptions were mapped into one of four functions: prepare medication (yellow), administer medication (green), document medication (red), and interruption (blue). The length of a colored segment is proportional to the duration (in seconds) of the task or interruption. Thus, the longer an observation is the longer the timeline belt is, and the more fragmented an observation is, the more colored segments there are. As visually depicted in Figure 5, RNs engaged in a bundled MAP workflow switched between MAP functions and tasks more frequently (higher number of segments), experienced more interruptions (more blue segments), and took longer to care for patients (longer timeline belt).

## 3. Model Development and Validation

This section presents the methodology utilized in developing the MAP simulation model that explicitly models the observed bundled and unbundled workflow processes. This is accomplished via the incorporation of the statistical model discussed in Section 3.1. In Section 3.2, the design and functionality of the simulation model are explained in detail, followed by the discussion of the model input parameters and values. Lastly, the model validation procedure and results are discussed. The potential use of the validated simulation model is demonstrated in Section 4 where it is used to assess redesign interventions.

*3.1. Statistical Model.* Empirically, the bundled versus unbundled MAP workflow processes seemed to be related to the RN's level of experience; that is, the more experienced the RN,

TABLE 4: Parameter estimates and standard errors of Poisson mixed model.

| Parameter | Bundled model | Unbundled model |
|---|---|---|
| Random effect variance | 0.143 (0.052)* | 0.170 (0.102) |
| Years of work in hospital | −0.048 (0.021)* | 0.004 (0.028) |

*$p$ value < 0.05. All models are adjusted for race, gender, years of licensure, and years of practice.

the more she/he bundled care tasks to enhance organization and efficiency. We, therefore, tested the hypothesis that nurses' work experience would have a significant impact on the number of patient-driven interruptions in unbundled and bundled cases. Since each RN was observed multiple times during the study, a mixed Poisson model was used to estimate the expected number of patient-driven interruptions during each observation. This model incorporated the random intercept into the model to accommodate the variations of measures within and between RNs. Using the mixed Poisson also accounted for overdispersion (conditional variance exceeds the conditional mean). Initially, we included all RN demographic variables in the model as covariates to assess the impact of moderator variables. A stepwise model selection procedure was used to remove the nonsignificant variables based on the $p$ values. In addition, we also removed the variables which failed to meet the convergence criteria during the approximation procedure. In the bundled observations (Table 4), the significant variance of random intercept indicated that heterogeneity existed in terms of RN patient-driven interruptions. The significant negative effect of "years of work in hospital" implied that experienced RNs were able to reduce the number of patient-driven interruptions. In contrast, there was no significant variation among RNs or effect of "years of work in hospital" in the unbundled observations. The analysis was conducted using SAS/STAT 9.2 [24].

*3.2. Computer Simulation Model.* Many health care studies have utilized discrete-event simulation (DES) to model the

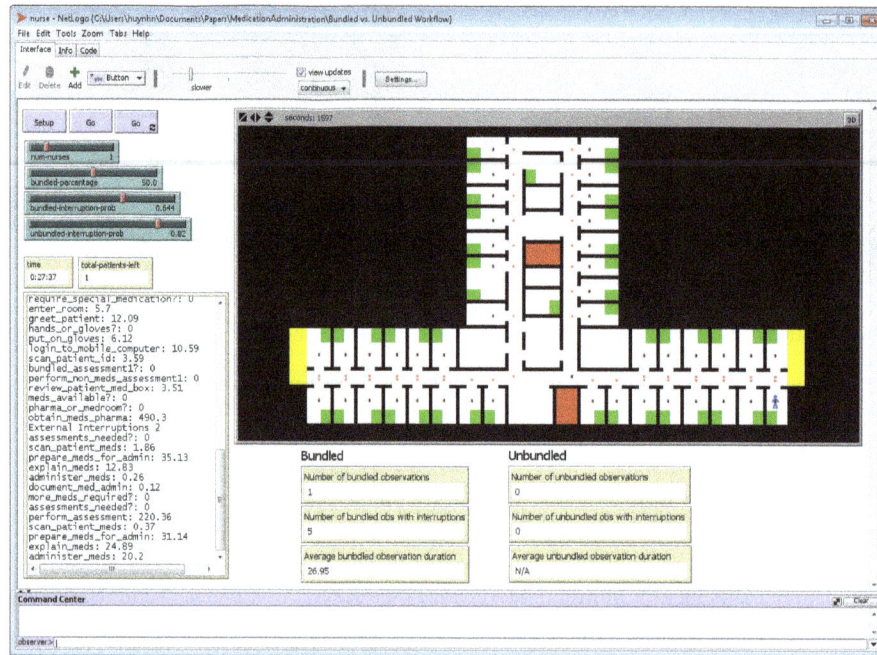

FIGURE 6: Graphical user interface of MAP simulation model.

operation of a system as a discrete sequence of events in time. The MAP workflows reflected a discrete set of events and were best modeled using DES. However, the RNs were not a homogenous set of agents with identical characteristics and this had an effect on their MAP workflows. In particular, the RNs' number of years worked in the hospital was correlated with the number of patient-driven interruptions for bundled workflows. For this reason, it was necessary to model RNs as individual agents with their own characteristics. Pseudocode 1 provides a high-level algorithmic view of the simulation model, which was implemented using Netlogo [25]. We chose Netlogo because of our prior experience with it.

As illustrated in Pseudocode 1, the simulation model has three key procedures: *setup*, *simulate*, and *do-task*. The *setup* procedure performed all the preliminary steps before the workflow is simulated. In this procedure, the model initialized the variables, drew the layout of the units (to show location of RNs), generated a user-specified number of RNs working on a unit and patients to be assigned to each RN (the ratio of RNs to patients is based on collected data), and assigned specific attributes to each RN. The model simulated RNs' movements according to the actual study clinical unit floor layout and patient room numbers. This was done to track the total RN walking distance as a proxy for fatigue, which has long been considered a contributory factor in patient care errors [23]. The RN attributes that were explicitly modeled included the workflow type (i.e., bundled or unbundled) and the "years of work in hospital." As discussed, the characteristic "years of work in hospital" was used to estimate the number of patient-driven interruptions each RN would encounter per observation. Time-driven interruptions were

calculated per 10-minute intervals using the probability determined from data.

The *simulate* procedure was responsible for controlling the program flow. It maintained a queue of RNs to simulate and RNs were selected from this queue based on the timing of the events to be simulated. For each RN, it determined if the RN had completed all the tasks for an observation. If so, the RN was moved to the next room (i.e., observation/patient). If not, it assigned the next task to the RN and the time it took to complete that task. This information was then placed in the priority queue and subsequently drawn when it got to the front of the queue. The task processing times were determined using best-fit distributions and parameters (determined based on sample data). Thus, the simulation model is a stochastic model due to the randomness in task processing times and number of interruptions. The *simulate* procedure ended when all RNs had completed their assignments.

The *simulate* procedure relied on the *do-task* function to determine the next task within the unbundled or bundled workflow. The "conditional" term in the *do-task* function denoted a decision point in the workflow (represented by diamond shapes in Figures 2 and 3). When a conditional was encountered, the model determined the branch it followed based on the observed probabilities. Thus, while MAP activities were structured based on the workflows, there was significant workflow variability due to a number of conditionals (i.e., special medications, medication availability, medication-related assessments, and other care).

Figure 6 shows a screenshot of the developed MAP simulation model. The graphical user interface includes the "setup" button that calls the *setup* procedure and the "go" button that calls the *simulate* procedure. Additionally, the

```
Setup procedure
  Initialize variables
  Draw floor layout of units
  Generate RN agents and patients for each unit
  Create RN characteristics
Simulate procedure
  (RN, RN.task) = pick from the front of priority queue
  if RN.task = 0 then go-to-next-room
    next-task = ask RN to do-task RN.task
  add (RN, next-task, duration-of next-task) to priority
  queue until no more patients left
do-task [task] function
  if task is a conditional
    result = run conditional
    next-task = pick based on result and workflow
  else
    next-task = pick based on workflow
  return next-task
```

Pseudocode 1: MAP computer simulation model high-level pseudocode.

GUI includes sliders that allow users to specify the number of RNs to simulate, the probability that an RN follows the bundled workflow, and the probabilities that they will encounter interruptions in the unbundled and bundled workflows. When the model is running, the GUI shows which rooms the RNs are in, their current activities, and relevant statistics.

*3.3. Input Parameters.* The simulation model uses a number of input parameters. The primary input is the list of tasks associated with unbundled and bundled workflows. Algorithm 1 provides a portion of the codes we implemented to model the bundled workflow. Each row in Algorithm 1 is an "edge" in the workflow graph. The first item is the "from" task of the edge. If there is no second item in the row then the first item in the next row is the "to" task. If the task ends in a ? then it is a conditional, to be executed at runtime. If the conditional statement evaluates to true (based on the observed probabilities) then we perform the second task in the row; otherwise, we perform the third task in the row. The task durations were drawn from the Gamma distribution with parameters $\alpha$ and $\lambda$, where $\alpha =$ mean $*$ mean/variance and $\lambda =$ mean/variance. The durations of the commonly encountered bundled tasks are shown in Table 5; there are over 60 tasks in each of the two workflows; thus, not all tasks are shown.

Values related to the number of patients assigned to a nurse, the number of patient-driven and time-driven interruptions, and the number of medications needed by a patient were drawn from a discrete empirical distribution constructed from the observed data. Table 6 shows the cumulative distribution function (CDF) values used by the simulation model to determine the values for these parameters. That is, a random number between 0 and 1 is generated and the CDF is used to determine the value for the corresponding parameter.

*3.4. Model Validation.* Model validation is the process of ensuring that the simulation model behaves in the way it

TABLE 5: Duration of bundled tasks.

| Task name | Average duration (sec) | Std. dev. (sec) |
|---|---|---|
| Clean hands (upon entering room) | 5.08 | 10.14 |
| Put on gloves | 13.82 | 6.38 |
| Enter room | 2.34 | 3.32 |
| Greet patient | 3.38 | 6.37 |
| Login to mobile computer | 7.51 | 4.65 |
| Review patient computer record | 17.65 | 25.99 |
| Scan patient ID | 6.52 | 4.90 |
| Perform assessment | 63.75 | 78.65 |
| Review patient med box | 17.04 | 16.42 |
| Scan patient meds | 4.24 | 6.16 |
| Document med admin | 6.43 | 7.64 |
| Administer meds | 68.94 | 88.72 |
| Other care | 61.65 | 99.21 |
| Explain meds | 13.63 | 14.35 |
| Prepare meds for admin | 34.47 | 37.19 |
| Close medication box | 4.67 | 6.66 |
| Clean equipment | 19.71 | 19.41 |
| Clean hands (upon leaving room) | 5.87 | 9.88 |
| Document post administration (in hallway) | 148.67 | 118.42 |
| Document post administration (in patient's room) | 76.06 | 106.43 |
| Obtain meds from pyxis | 42.92 | 27.92 |
| Obtain meds from medication room | 52.19 | 39.69 |
| Obtain meds from pharmacy | 489.00 | 162.53 |

was intended according to the modeling assumptions made. The MAP model validation was achieved by comparing

```
set bundled [
    "receive_report"
    ["require_special_medication?" "medroom_or_pyxis?" "enter_room"]
    ["medroom_or_pyxis?" "obtain_meds_medroom" "obtain_meds_pyxis"]
    ["obtain_meds_medroom" "enter_room"]
    ["obtain_meds_pyxis" "enter_room"]
    "enter_room"
    "greet_patient"
    ...
    ...
]
```

ALGORITHM 1: Bundled workflow data input to simulation model.

TABLE 6: Simulation model parameters.

| Model parameter | Discrete cumulative distribution function |
|---|---|
| Number of patients assigned to nurse $(1, 2, \ldots, 11)$ | DISC $(0, 0.23171, 0.14634, 0.08537, 0.14634, 0.17073, 0.08537, 0.10976, 0.01219, 0, 0, 0.01219)$ |
| Number of patient-driven interruptions (for unbundled workflow: $1, 2, \ldots, 11$) | DISC $(0, 0.37333, 0.22666, 0.22666, 0.10666, 0.01333, 0.01333, 0.02670, 0, 0, 0, 0.01333)$ |
| Number of patient-driven interruptions (for bundled workflow: $1, 2, \ldots, 11$) | DISC $(0, 0.225, 0.2375, 0.21875, 0.1375, 0.09375, 0.04375, 0.00625, 0.00625, 0.0125, 0.0125, 0.00625)$ |
| Number of time-driven interruptions (for unbundled workflow: $1, 2, \ldots, 6$) | DISC $(0, 0.61165, 0.26214, 0.05340, 0.04854, 0.01456, 0.00971)$ |
| Number of time-driven interruptions (for bundled workflow: $1, 2, \ldots, 8$) | DISC $(0, 0.57271, 0.27069, 0.09620, 0.04251, 0.01119, 0.00224, 0.00224, 0.00224)$ |
| Number of medications needed by a patient $(1, 2, \ldots, 16)$ | DISC $(0, 0.032787, 0.2, 0.118033, 0.12131, 0.10492, 0.07213, 0.09836, 0.06885, 0.02951, 0.05246, 0.02951, 0.01311, 0.01311, 0.01639, 0.01311, 0.01639)$ |

the model's observation duration with the actual MAP observation duration. Netlogo's Behavior Space tool was used to generate 1,000 observations (i.e., replications) and each observation was run until the nurse completes MAP for all of her/his assigned patients. Note that the duration of each replication is dependent on a number of random factors, including how many patients are assigned to the nurse and how many medications are needed by the patients. The model's average observation durations were compared against the actual average observation durations. Since the observation durations are not normally distributed, the Wilcoxon Rank-Sum Test was used to test the null hypothesis that the distribution of observation durations generated by the model was the same as that of the actual observation durations. The Wilcoxon test, using the statistical software R [26], yielded a $p$ value = 0.5341 for unbundled observations and a $p$ value = 0.7629 for bundled observations, and the null hypothesis could not be rejected.

## 4. Assessment of MAP Redesign Interventions

The validated MAP simulation model was used to assess the impact of two hypothetical redesign interventions in a simulated setting: (1) intervention 1 increased RNs' use of an unbundled MAP workflow and (2) intervention 2 reduced

TABLE 7: Results of intervention 1.

| Unbundled percentage (%) | Average number of interruptions per RN per shift (95% CI) | Average observation duration per RN per shift, min (95% CI) |
|---|---|---|
| 0 | 10.48 (10.24 to 10.71) | 16.58 (16.34 to 16.82) |
| 33.5 (base case) | 9.15 (8.93 to 9.37) | 15.14 (14.92 to 15.36) |
| 50 | 9.02 (8.81 to 9.24) | 14.92 (14.70 to 15.14) |
| 100 | 7.17 (7.0 to 7.34) | 12.74 (12.55 to 12.92) |

*Confidence intervals were calculated using Kelton et al.'s method [18].

MAP patient-driven interruptions. For intervention 2, the time-driven interruptions were not considered because they are random and RNs do not have control over them.

To assess the impact of intervention 1, the input to the MAP model was modified to have different percentages of RNs follow the unbundled workflow, that is, 0%, 33.5% (base case), 50%, and 100%. The experimentation was conducted using 1,000 replications and each replication was run until the nurse completes all of her/his assignments. Table 7 provides a summary of the results for intervention 1, and Figure 7 illustrates the impact of these scenarios on the average observation duration per RN per shift. The results indicated

TABLE 8: Results of intervention 2 for unbundled workflow.

| | Probability of incurring interruption | Interruption counts per RN per shift (95% CI) | Average observation duration per RN per shift, min (95% CI) |
| --- | --- | --- | --- |
| Base case | 0.82 | 7.46 (7.28 to 7.63) | 13.66 (13.23 to 14.09) |
| 10% reduction | 0.738 | 6.75 (6.58 to 6.92) | 13.38 (12.95 to 13.80) |
| 20% reduction | 0.656 | 5.86 (5.70 to 6.02) | 13.30 (12.88 to 13.72) |
| 30% reduction | 0.574 | 5.19 (5.05 to 5.34) | 13.23 (12.81 to 13.65) |

*Confidence intervals were calculated using Kelton et al.'s method [18].

TABLE 9: Results of intervention 2 for bundled workflow.

| | Probability of incurring interruption | Interruption counts per RN per shift (95% CI) | Average observation duration per RN per shift, min (95% CI) |
| --- | --- | --- | --- |
| Base case | 0.92 | 10.15 (9.93 to 10.37) | 18.40 (17.82 to 18.98) |
| 10% reduction | 0.828 | 9.73 (9.50 to 9.96) | 17.80 (17.23 to 18.36) |
| 20% reduction | 0.736 | 8.26 (8.06 to 8.46) | 18.02 (17.45 to 18.59) |
| 30% reduction | 0.644 | 7.49 (7.29 to 7.68) | 17.19 (16.64 to 17.73) |

*Confidence intervals were calculated using Kelton et al.'s method [18].

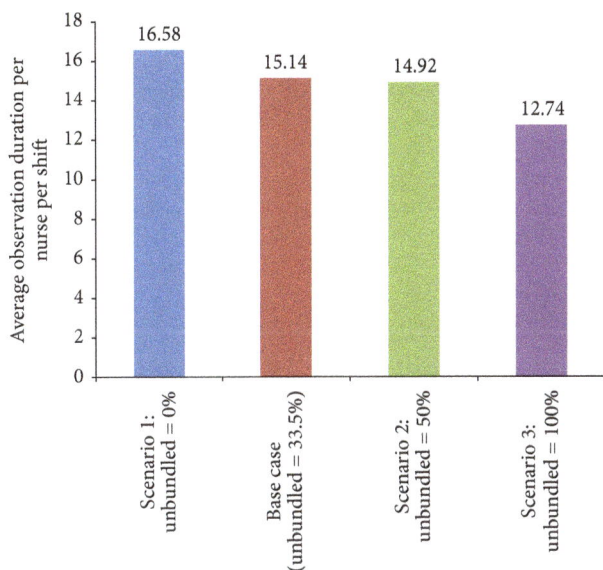

FIGURE 7: Impact of intervention 1 on average (mean) observation duration in minutes (note: base case and scenario 2 have a mixture of unbundled and bundled observations).

that as the percentage of RNs following the unbundled workflow increased, the average number of interruptions and observation duration decreased.

To assess the impact of intervention 2, the input to the MAP model was modified to assume a reduction of 10%, 20%, and 30% in patient-driven interruptions for both unbundled and bundled workflows. Tables 8 and 9 provide a summary of the results for the unbundled and bundled workflow, respectively. As shown in Table 8, for unbundled workflow, the results indicated that as the probability of interruptions decreased, so did the interruption counts and observation

duration. This result implied that if RNs could avoid situations that lead to interruptions, they would be more efficient. A similar result was observed for bundled workflow (Table 9), except that the average observation duration did not follow a decreasing trend. This was most likely due to other nonmedication tasks incorporated into the bundled workflow. Also, the patient-driven interruption time for bundled workflow tended to be lower than that of unbundled workflow. Thus, the fewer number of patient-driven interruptions had less of an impact on observation duration for bundled workflow than it did for unbundled workflow.

## 5. Discussion

Study findings indicated that there was a lack of consistent MAP workflow among RNs. Two predominant MAP workflow patterns, unbundled and bundled, emerged from the data. However, even within these two workflow patterns, additional variations were observed. For example, the number of patient-driven interruptions was associated with an RN's years of work in the hospital. Hence, it is possible that other RN characteristics might play a role in RN MAP workflow and additional research is needed in this area.

MAP timeline belts suggested that the bundled workflow is not desirable due to a higher incidence of MAP task switching (i.e., workflow fragmentation) and interruptions. Previous research findings have shown that frequent task switching often increases physical activities that can result in a higher likelihood of cognitive slips and mistakes that can lead to performance error [23]. Study qualitative findings from tape recorded comments pointed to a number of interruptions that were likely to occur from "other care" when RNs followed a bundled MAP workflow pattern. For example, RNs engaged in a bundled MAP workflow pattern often responded to patient requests for dietary assistance and other care requests such as toileting assistance (Table 10). While we

TABLE 10: Nonmedication related sources of interruptions.

| Category | Interruption source |
|---|---|
| Patient dietary assistance | Give patient requested food |
| | Get ice for patient |
| | Leave room to find apple sauce |
| | Leave room to dispose of patient's breakfast |
| Patient care assistance | Assist another patient |
| | Assist patient to the bathroom |
| | Get translator for patient |
| | Get towels from linen room |

classified these patient requests as interruptions, we recognize that they are necessary or essential to the patients' wellbeing. Moreover, we recognize that RNs cannot seek to be more efficient at the expense of the quality or completeness of care. Nevertheless, these "other care" interruptions raised a variety of nursing practice questions about the safety impact of the bundled MAP workflow pattern on medication administration error outcomes and other practice considerations such as use of aseptic technique in medication administration. Additional research is needed to address these and other emergent questions.

## 6. Conclusions

This study developed a computer simulation model to assess the performance of nursing unbundled versus bundled MAP workflows. It extended our previous work in several areas: (1) the iMedTracker was modified to work on iPad devices instead of iPod Touch to minimize scrolling and thereby facilitate the recording of live MAP observations, (2) data collection took place in an actual hospital setting instead of an academic simulation laboratory and thereby provided more realistic RN characteristics and MAP workflow observations, (3) the MAP agent-level DES simulation model was modified to incorporate RN and MAP characteristics to account for patient-driven and time-driven interruptions, and (4) statistical modeling techniques were used to compliment development of the MAP computer simulation model. While our methods and tools were validated in this study, key limitations should be considered when reviewing study results. These included (1) one study hospital, (2) only 2 medical units, (3) small number of RN participants ($n = 17$), (4) lack of patient contextual data, (5) small number of MAP observations ($n = 305$), and (6) data collected only during morning shifts of Mondays, Wednesdays, and Fridays. These limitations prohibited us from conducting an actual process redesign with the stakeholders. We plan to address these shortcomings in a larger proposed field study that is currently under review. Furthermore, in future work, we plan to develop an agent-based model of MAP that simulates the complex behavior of RNs through the use of agents. Specifically, we wish to model the autonomous behavior of the nurse agents and the interactions between the agents themselves and their environment. To accomplish

this goal, we are currently expanding the capabilities of the iMedTracker to provide data for the agent-based model development and validation.

## Competing Interests

The authors indicated no potential competing interests.

## Acknowledgments

The authors greatly appreciate the support of the study hospital nursing staff and managers. This study could not have been completed without them. The authors also extend sincere thanks to study research assistants, Caroline Mulatya, Matthew Fleming, Krishma Naik, and Bradley Huffman, for their dedication to the project. The study was supported by funds from Dr. Snyder's SmartState Endowed Chair in Health Informatics Quality and Safety Evaluation during her tenure at the University of South Carolina. The SmartState Endowed Chair Program is funded by the South Carolina Commission on Higher Education.

## References

[1] J. S. Ash, D. F. Sittig, E. G. Poon, K. Guappone, E. Campbell, and R. H. Dykstra, "The extent and importance of unintended consequences related to computerized provider order entry," *Journal of the American Medical Informatics Association*, vol. 14, no. 4, pp. 415–423, 2007.

[2] Z. Niazkhani, H. Pirnejad, M. Berg, and J. Aarts, "The impact of computerized provider order entry systems on inpatient clinical workflow: a literature review," *Journal of the American Medical Informatics Association*, vol. 16, no. 4, pp. 539–549, 2009.

[3] J. M. Walker and P. Carayon, "From tasks to processes: the case for changing health information technology to improve health care," *Health Affairs*, vol. 28, no. 2, pp. 467–477, 2009.

[4] J. Grossman, R. Gourevitch, and D. A. Cross, "Hospital experiences using electronic health records to support medication reconciliation," Research Brief Number 17, National Institute for Health Care Reform (NIHCR), Washington, DC, USA, 2014.

[5] P. Carayon, A. Schoofs Hundt, B.-T. Karsh et al., "Work system design for patient safety: the SEIPS model," *Quality and Safety in Health Care*, vol. 15, supplement 1, pp. i50–i58, 2006.

[6] Institute of Medicine, *Keeping Patients Safe: Transforming the Work Environment of Nurses*, National Academies Press, Washington, DC, USA, 2004.

[7] S. B. Lee, L. L. Lee, R. S. Yeung, and J. T. Chan, "A continuous quality improvement project to reduce medication error in the emergency department," *World Journal of Emergency Medicine*, vol. 4, no. 3, pp. 179–182, 2013.

[8] K. G. Burke, "Executive summary: the state of the science on safe medication administration symposium," *The American Journal of Nursing*, vol. 105, no. 3, pp. 4–9, 2005.

[9] R. G. Hughes and E. Ortiz, "Medication errors: why they happen, and how they can be prevented," *American Journal of Nursing*, vol. 105, no. 3, pp. 14–24, 2005.

[10] C. Sullivan, K. M. Gleason, D. Rooney, J. M. Groszek, and C. Barnard, "Medication reconciliation in the acute care setting: opportunity and challenge for nursing," *Journal of Nursing Care Quality*, vol. 20, no. 2, pp. 95–98, 2005.

[11] S. H. Sanchez, S. S. Sethi, S. L. Santos, and K. Boockvar, "Implementing medication reconciliation from the planner's perspective: a qualitative study," *BMC Health Services Research*, vol. 14, no. 1, article 290, 2014.

[12] L. L. Leape, D. W. Bates, D. J. Cullen et al., "Systems analysis of adverse drug events," *Journal of the American Medical Association*, vol. 274, no. 1, pp. 35–43, 1995.

[13] K. McBride-Henry and M. Foureur, "Medication administration errors: understanding the issues," *Australian Journal of Advanced Nursing*, vol. 23, no. 3, pp. 33–42, 2006.

[14] H. Pirinen, L. Kauhanen, R. Danielsson-Ojala et al., "Registered Nurses' experiences with the medication administration process," *Advances in Nursing*, vol. 2015, Article ID 941589, 10 pages, 2015.

[15] S. K. Garrett and J. B. Craig, "Medication administration and the complexity of nursing workflow," in *Proceedings of the 21st Annual Society for Health Systems Conference and Expo*, Chicago, Ill, USA, April 2009.

[16] R. Snyder, N. Huynh, B. Cai, and A. S. Tavakoli, "Evaluation of medication administration process: tools and techniques," *Journal of Healthcare Engineering*, vol. 2, no. 4, pp. 527–538, 2011.

[17] N. Huynh, R. Snyder, J. M. Vidal, A. S. Tavakoli, and B. Cai, "Application of computer simulation modeling to medication administration process redesign," *Journal of Healthcare Engineering*, vol. 3, no. 4, pp. 649–662, 2012.

[18] W. D. Kelton, R. P. Sadowski, and D. A. Sadowski, *Simulation with ARENA*, McGraw-Hill, New York, NY, USA, 6th edition, 2014.

[19] R. A. Wagner and R. Lowrance, "An extension of the string-to-string correction problem," *Journal of the ACM*, vol. 22, pp. 177–183, 1975.

[20] R. O. Duda, P. E. Hart, and D. G. Stork, *Pattern Classification*, John Wiley & Sons, New York, NY, USA, 2nd edition, 2001.

[21] J. J. Liu, Y. L. Wang, and G. S. Huang, *Solving some Sequence Problems on Run-Length Encoded Strings: Longest Common Sequences*, Edit Distances, and Squares, VDM Verlag Dr. Müeller, Saarbrücken, Germany, 2008.

[22] M. A. Pett, *Nonparametric Statistics for Health Care Research*, Sage, Thousand Oaks, Calif, USA, 1997.

[23] K. Zheng, H. M. Haftel, R. B. Hirschl, M. O'Reilly, and D. A. Hanauer, "Quantifying the impact of health IT implementations on clinical workflow: a new methodological perspective," *Journal of the American Medical Informatics Association*, vol. 17, pp. 454–461, 2010.

[24] SAS Institute, *SAS/STAT® 9.2 User's Guide*, SAS Institute, Cary, NC, USA, 2008.

[25] U. Wilensky, *NetLogo*, Center for Connected Learning and Computer-Based Modeling, Northwestern University, Evanston, Ill, USA, 1999, http://ccl.northwestern.edu/netlogo/.

[26] R Development Core Team, *R: A Language and Environment for Statistical Computing*, R Foundation for Statistical Computing, Vienna, Austria, 2013, http://www.R-project.org/.

# 9

# Modelling pH-Optimized Degradation of Microgel-Functionalized Polyesters

**Lisa Bürgermeister,[1] Marcus Hermann,[2] Katalin Fehér,[3] Catalina Molano Lopez,[4] Andrij Pich,[4] Julian Hannen,[5] Felix Vogt,[6] and Wolfgang Schulz[1,2]**

[1]Fraunhofer Institute for Laser Technology, Steinbachstrasse 15, 52074 Aachen, Germany
[2]Nonlinear Dynamics of Laser Processing, RWTH Aachen University, Steinbachstrasse 15, 52074 Aachen, Germany
[3]Institute of Textile Technology, RWTH Aachen University, Otto-Blumenthal-Strasse 1, 52074 Aachen, Germany
[4]Functional and Interactive Polymers, DWI, RWTH Aachen University, Forckenbeckstrasse 50, 52074 Aachen, Germany
[5]Innovation, Strategy and Organization Group, RWTH Aachen University, Kackertstrasse 7, 52072 Aachen, Germany
[6]Department of Cardiology, RWTH Aachen University, Pauwelsstrasse 30, 52074 Aachen, Germany

Correspondence should be addressed to Lisa Bürgermeister; lisa.buergermeister@ilt.fraunhofer.de

Academic Editor: Hendra Hermawan

We establish a novel mathematical model to describe and analyze pH levels in the vicinity of poly(N-vinylcaprolactam-co-acetoacetoxyethyl methacrylate-co-N-vinylimidazole) (VCL/AAEM/VIm) microgel-functionalized polymers during biodegradation. Biodegradable polymers, especially aliphatic polyesters (polylactide/polyglycolide/polycaprolactone homo- and copolymers), have a large range of medical applications including delivery systems, scaffolds, or stents for the treatment of cardiovascular diseases. Most of those applications are limited by the inherent drop of pH level during the degradation process. The combination of polymers with VCL/AAEM/VIm-microgels, which aims at stabilizing pH levels, is innovative and requires new mathematical models for the prediction of pH level evaluation. The mathematical model consists of a diffusion-reaction PDE system for the degradation including reaction rate equations and diffusion of acidic degradation products into the vicinity. A system of algebraic equations is coupled to the degradation model in order to describe the buffering action of the microgel. The model is validated against the experimental pH-monitored biodegradation of microgel-functionalized polymer foils and is available for the design of microgel-functionalized polymer components.

## 1. Introduction

Cardiovascular diseases are the number one cause of death worldwide, globally claiming 17 million lives each year and accounting for 29% of all deaths [1]. Through the introduction of minimally invasive procedures like percutaneous coronary intervention (PCI) and the use of intravascular stents, the treatment of many cardiovascular diseases such as coronary artery disease, the obstruction of a coronary artery due to development of atherosclerosis, has been revolutionized [2, 3].

Nevertheless, efficacy and safety of available stents are limited in part as suitable autologous tissue engineered stents are lacking [4]. Mostly, nondegradable synthetic materials are

substituted to repair the injured cardiovascular tissue. Meant to prevail at the implantation site, these foreign and therefore inherently thrombogenic materials can be associated with several risks, including calcification and acute or late stent thrombosis, which require prevention by antiplatelet therapy [5].

In contrast, tissue engineered bioresorbable stents provide temporary scaffolding for the formation of autologous tissue with the capacity to regenerate and grow. After the degradation process of the stent, only the restored vessel remains which might reduce the risk of late stent thrombosis.

The most frequently used resorbable polymers for biomedical implants including bioresorbable stents are the aliphatic polyesters polylactic acid (PLA) and polyglycolic acid (PGA) and their copolymers. The mechanism of polyester degradation has been well investigated. Polymer chains are degraded by hydrolytic scission of ester linkages in the polymer backbone and thereby create carboxylic end groups. These acidic carboxyl end groups diffuse into the vicinity of the polymer and decrease the pH level there [6–10].

This pH drop is one of the main drawbacks of using aliphatic polyesters for implants as a low pH may cause tissue reactions like inflammation [11–13].

Still, biodegradable stents have marked potential long-term advantages [4, 14]. In order to overcome the disadvantage of acidic pH levels during degradation of biodegradable stents, we investigate the fabrication of polylactic acid (PLA) fibers for cardiovascular stents with pH-optimized degradation behavior using VCL/AAEM/VIm (8 mol%)-microgels as insoluble buffers [15].

Microgels are defined as hydrogel particles with a dimension from 10 nanometers up to the micrometer range. Hydrogels in general are novel components that arouse special interest in the biomedical field and nanotechnology [16, 17].

Depending on the molecular building units and the synthesis procedure, it is possible to synthesize colloidal hydrogels with controlled particle size. Those can be defined as polymer networks with smart properties such as water-uptake capacity, degree of swelling, and responsiveness to external stimuli. Furthermore, these nanoparticles show high colloidal stability, a well-defined structure, and a high surface area. Through variation of the monomer type and/or introduction of comonomers, responsiveness to temperature, pH, magnetic field, or light intensity can be tailored. This property, in combination with the swelling features, makes the utilization of microgels as biocompatible materials for pharmaceutical applications possible [16, 18–23].

Monomers like N-isopropylacrylamide (NIPAAm) and N-vinylcaprolactam (VCL) have been used for the synthesis of thermoresponsive microgels because they can form water-soluble polymers with lower critical solution temperature (LCST) [18, 20, 24, 25]. Other interesting components such as N-vinylimidazole (VIm) can be used to achieve pH-sensitivity due to its protonation/deprotonation process at different pH levels. Pich et al. [26] have successfully synthesized VCL/VIm-based microgels, which show both temperature and pH-responsiveness. In this study, the swelling could be controlled by the VIm content in the microgel.

However, cardiovascular stents require for the degradation period to last over months, making their experimental research as well as their design and optimization rather time-intensive. This study aims at developing a mathematical model able to predict the pH level resulting from polymer degradation and taking into account the buffering action of eventually incorporated microgels. This mathematical model will be validated against the experimental pH-monitored biodegradation of microgel-functionalized polymer foils and will be available for the design of microgel-functionalized polymer stents and other components.

Computational methods to model the degradation of biodegradable polymers have been proposed by a quantity of research teams. Siparsky et al. [27] described the kinetics of hydrolysis reaction by rate equations and their analytic solutions. Han [28] used Monte Carlo methods to predict the degradation of PLA, PGA, and some copolymers. He also investigated the influence of chemical buffers on the degradation process and the pH level. Wang et al. [29] presented a reduced model for polymer degradation using two rate equations for the concentrations of carboxylic end groups and ester bonds in the PLA phase. Pan et al. [30] included a model for chemical buffers in such a reduced model for biodegradation. Moreover, rate equations for the concentrations of different molecules sizes, which the polymer undergoes in its degradation process, were built up and analyzed by Lazzari et al. [31]. The buffering action of the poly(N-vinylimidazole) hydrogel was modelled and analyzed by Horta et al. [32, 33]. To the best of the authors' knowledge, so far no published model for the biodegradation of polymers buffered with VCL/AAEM/VIm-microgels exists.

Investigating microgel-functionalized resorbable polymers with pH-regulatory potential, a recent study of Fehér et al. [15] employs a publication-based keyword search strategy to investigate the existing knowledge base underpinning the topic. The authors find that only a marginal number of studies is dedicated to investigate the pH-regulative potential of microgel containing degradable polymers. This clearly demonstrates an underinvestigated topic. Given the potential scope of application, ranging from drug-coated, pH-regulating degradable textiles to stents, this paper is aligned to the apparent research gap.

## 2. Materials and Methods

*2.1. VCL/AAEM/VIm (8 mol%)-Microgel.* The synthesis of VCL/AAEM/VIm (8%)-microgel is well described in Fehér et al. [15]. The description is not repeated here.

*2.2. Polymer VCL/AAEM/VIm (8 mol%)-Microgel Foils.* Poly(L-lactide-co-glycolid) PLG 8523 by Purac and the microgel are weighed separately. Both samples are then filled up with a solvent in a way that the mass fraction of polymer $w_{Pol}$ and microgel $w_{MG}$ amount to 0.15, respectively. The sealed samples are stirred at 250 rpm for 24 hours in a magnetic stirrer. The resulting microgel and polymer solutions are mixed thoroughly to ensure a homogeneous solution. The solutions are evenly spread on a petri dish and thereby infused to a foil. After 48 hours within the distractor hood, the solvent is fully evaporated, allowing for the foil to be peeled from the glass.

*2.3. Degradation Experiment.* The degradation experiments are carried out according to ISO 13781 [34]. Each sample contains 0.1 g of the produced foil and is supplemented with distilled water (specific conductivity < 0.1 $\mu$S/cm at 25°C) at the ratio of 1 : 100. The samples are prepared in 20 mL glass containers and sealed during degradation periods. The containers are only opened for pH measurement.

Throughout the degradation process, the samples are stored in an oven at 37°C. pH measurement is conducted daily within the first 20 days followed by weekly readings for a total time period of at least 30 days. To determine the pH level, the samples are withdrawn from the oven. Due to the high temperature sensitivity of the pH level, the samples are cooled down to ambient temperature (20°C) prior to the measurement. Each measurement is repeated twice and the three results are averaged. To increase the experiment's significance, each sample is prepared twice and the average is calculated from the results. To ensure a homogeneous distribution of hydron H$^+$ during measuring, the samples are swiveled prior to the measurement. The pH-meter "SevenEasy™ S20" with an uncertainty of ±0.01 by Mettler Toledo, Gießen, Germany, is used. The electrode of the pH-meter is calibrated beforehand using buffer solutions with pH levels of 4.01, 7.00, and 9.21.

*2.4. Physical Model Reduction and Mathematical Modelling.* In order to analyze the pH level in a vicinity of a degrading polyester component, we predict the concentration of hydron [H$^+$] resulting from dissociation of carboxyl groups of the degrading polymer. As the dissociation of the carboxyl groups COOH to COO$^-$ and hydron H$^+$ in aqueous solution takes place on a very short timescale, we make use of the equilibrium constant $K_{COOH} = [COO^-][H^+]/[COOH]$ for the dissociation reaction and insert it into the balance of mass and charge to calculate the concentration of hydron [H$^+$]:

$$[H^+] = \frac{K_w}{[H^+]} + \frac{K_{COOH}[M]}{[H^+] + K_{COOH}} \qquad (1)$$

with the equilibrium constant for the dissociation of H$_2$O to OH$^-$ and H$^+$: $K_w = [H^+][OH^-]$. The brackets [X] mark the concentration of the corresponding species X. We used the fact that the concentration of oligomers [M] corresponds to the concentration of carboxyl groups [COOH]. The concentration of H$_2$O is not part of the equation as we assume it to be constant because the water penetration into the polymer is on a very short timescale.

The concentration of carboxyl groups increases with the progressing scission of polymer chains by hydrolysis reaction and is thus time dependent. Hydrolysis of polyesters proceeds partly as spontaneous reaction and partly catalyzed by hydron H$^+$. The reaction is called autocatalytic as the reaction products hydroxyl alcohol and carboxylic acid end groups—also referred to as oligomers [28]—dissociate and acidize the environment and as a result accelerate the rate of hydrolysis [27]. The hydrolysis reaction is explained in detail elsewhere [35].

We implement a phenomenological model for the degradation of biodegradable polymers initially introduced by Wang et al. [29]. As a result, we predict the evolution in time of oligomer concentration [M]$_{init}$ after degradation and before buffering as well as the evolution in time of concentration of ester bonds [E] inside the calculation area by two rate equations:

$$\frac{d[E]}{dt} = -k[E] - k^{cat}[E][H^+], \qquad (2)$$

$$\frac{d[M]_{init}}{dt} = -\frac{d[E]}{dt} \qquad (3)$$

with the rate coefficients $k$ and $k^{cat}$ for spontaneous and catalytic scission of ester bonds inside the polymer, respectively. Using the equilibrium constant $K_{COOH}$, we transform (2) to

$$\frac{d[E]}{dt} = -k[E] - k^{cat}\sqrt{K_{COOH}}[E]\sqrt{[M]}. \qquad (4)$$

[M] refers to the concentration of oligomers available for the autocatalytic scission.

After dissociation of oligomers, the hydrons are buffered by the VIm groups of the microgel. Microgel and polymer form a two-phase system. The hydrons diffuse inside the microgel and are bound to the VIm. The dissociation products COO$^-$ bound to the oligomers will also diffuse inside the microgel and remain there unbound due to electrostatic forces. The diffusion processes will continue until the thermodynamic equilibrium between the two phases is reached. Using the assumption that the buffer reaction is fast compared to the degradation processes, we use the equilibrium constant of the buffer reaction $K_P = [P][H^+]/[PH^+]$ with the concentration of free buffer molecules [P] and occupied buffer molecules [PH$^+$], respectively, and find a system of algebraic equations describing the buffering action of the microgel. The derivation is explained in detail for poly(N-vinylimidazole) by Horta and Piérola [33]:

$$[COO^-]_{gel}$$
$$= \frac{[H^+]_{gel}^3 + [H^+]_{gel}^2(K_P + [P]_0) - [H^+]_{gel} \cdot K_w - K_P \cdot K_w}{[H^+]_{gel} \cdot ([H^+]_{gel} + K_P)},$$

$$[COO^-]_{gel}$$
$$= -\left([H^+] - \frac{K_w}{[H^+]}\right) \cdot \frac{V_{bath}}{V_{gel}} + \left([H^+]_{init} - \frac{K_w}{[H^+]_{init}}\right) \qquad (5)$$
$$\cdot \frac{V_{init}}{V_{gel}},$$

$$[H^+] = \sqrt{[H^+]_{gel}[COO^-]_{gel} + K_w},$$

where [X]$_{gel}$ represents the concentration of the species X in the microgel phase, [X]$_{init}$ represents the concentration in the polymer before the buffering reaction, $V_{init/gel/bath}$ are the volumes occupied by the polymer without the gel, the volume of the microgel, and the volume of the polymer including the microgels, respectively, and [P]$_0$ is the initial concentration of buffer molecules in the system. Using (1), we calculate from [H$^+$] the concentration of oligomers [M]$_{bath}$ after the buffering action of the microgel and complete the ODE system ((2) + (3)) by a rate equation for the concentration of oligomers [M] after buffering which allows for diffusion of the oligomers:

$$\frac{d[M]}{dt} = \frac{[M]_{bath}}{[M]_{init}}\left(-\frac{d[E]}{dt}\right) + D_0\Delta[M] \qquad (6)$$

with $D_0$ being a constant diffusivity of oligomers.

The calculation area and initial and boundary conditions are chosen appropriate for the degradation experiment

TABLE 1: Parameters used for simulation.

| Symbol | Value | Unit | Description | Source |
|---|---|---|---|---|
| $K_{COOH}$ | $10^{-3,87}$ | mol/L | Equilibrium constant of dissociation reaction of COOH at $37°$C | [28] |
| $K_w$ | $1.8 \cdot 10^{-14}$ | (mol/L)$^2$ | Equilibrium constant of dissociation reaction of $H_2O$ at $37°$C | [36] |
| $k$ | 0.005 | 1/week | Rate constant of spontaneous ester bond scission | Fit to experiments |
| $k^{cat} \cdot \sqrt{K_{COOH}}$ | $0.5 \cdot 10^{-3}$ | $\sqrt{m^3/mol}$/week | Rate constant for autocatalyzed ester bond scission | Fit to experiments |
| $K_p$ | $1 \cdot 10^{-10}$ | mol/L | Equilibrium constant for buffer reaction at $20°$C | Fit to experiments |
| $[P]_0$ | 0.3487 | mol/L | Initial buffer concentration | Fit to experiments |
| $V_{gel}/V_{init}$ | $9.42 \cdot 10^{-6}$ | — | Fraction of volumes occupied by gel and polymer | Derived from experimental procedure |
| $V_{bath}/V_{init}$ | $1 - V_{gel}/V_{init}$ | — | Fraction of volumes occupied by polymer + gel and polymer | — |
| $D_{0,p}$ | $2 \cdot 10^{-9}$ | m$^2$/week | Diffusion constant of oligomer in the polymer | [28] |
| $D_{0,w}$ | $2 \cdot 10^{-8}$ | m$^2$/week | Diffusion constant of oligomer in water | [37] |
| $d_p$ | 0.15 | mm | Thickness of polymer foil | Derived from experimental procedure |
| $d_w$ | 19.6 | mm | Thickness of water column above polymer foil | Derived from experimental procedure |

described above. As a consequence of the typical extensions of a polymer foil, diffusion will be dominant in one dimension. Thus, we set up a 1D diffusion model and use $x$ as the coordinate in space. The calculation area consists of two components: the (microgel containing) polymer with the thickness $d_p$ and the surrounding water with the thickness $d_w$. At time $t = 0$, ester bonds have the initial concentration $[E]_0$ in the polymer foil ($0 \leq x \leq d_p$) and 0 in the water volume ($x > d_p$) and the initial concentrations of oligomers $[M]_{init}$ and $[M]$ are 0 everywhere:

$$[E] (t = 0)|_{0 \leq x \leq d_p} = [E]_0,$$
$$[E] (t = 0)|_{x > d_p} = 0, \quad (7)$$
$$[M] (t = 0) = [M]_{init} (t = 0) = 0.$$

The boundaries at $x = 0$ and $x = d_w$ are isolated and do not allow for diffusion of oligomers. At the boundary $x = d_p$ continuity of oligomers is required:

$$\left.\frac{d[M]}{dx}\right|_{x=0} = \left.\frac{d[M]}{dx}\right|_{x=d_w} = 0,$$
$$[M]\left(x = d_p^-\right) = [M]\left(x = d_p^+\right). \quad (8)$$

A schematic representation of experimental set-up and the calculation area is depicted in Figure 1.

The diffusivity of oligomers $D_{0,p}$ and $D_{0,w}$ is considered to be constant in the polymer and the water layer, respectively. In order to simulate the swiveling of the samples in the experimental procedure, we increase the diffusion constant $D_{0,w}$ in (6) by a factor of $10^3$ for a very short period on every simulated measurement event.

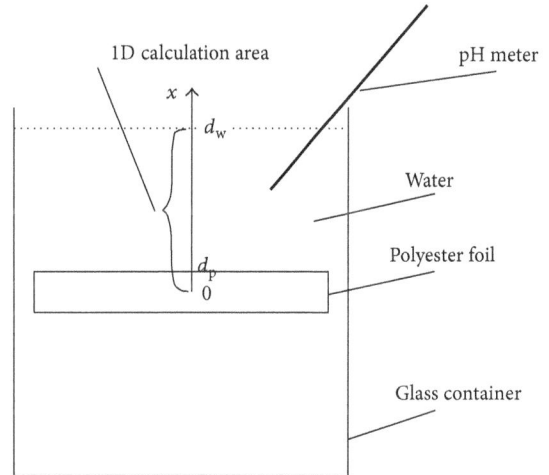

FIGURE 1: Schematic representation of the 1D simulation area, where $x$ depicts the coordinate in space and $d_p$ and $d_w$ are the positions of the boundary of polymer foil and water layer, respectively.

The parameters which have been used to carry out the simulation experiments, discussed in the following chapter, are listed in Table 1.

## 3. Results and Discussion

*3.1. Buffering Action of VCL/AAEM/VIm-Microgels.* As the buffering model (5) was originally applied to a poly(N-vinylimidazole) gel [33], we investigate its appropriateness for the VCL/AAEM/VIm-microgels in a preliminary study.

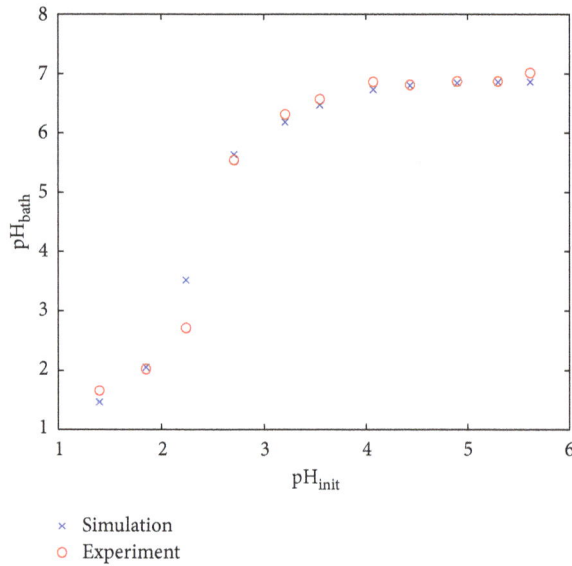

FIGURE 2: pH level ($pH_{bath}$) of different initial concentrations of hydrochloric acid ($pH_{init}$) after buffering with 0.1 g microgel.

× Simulation
○ Experiment

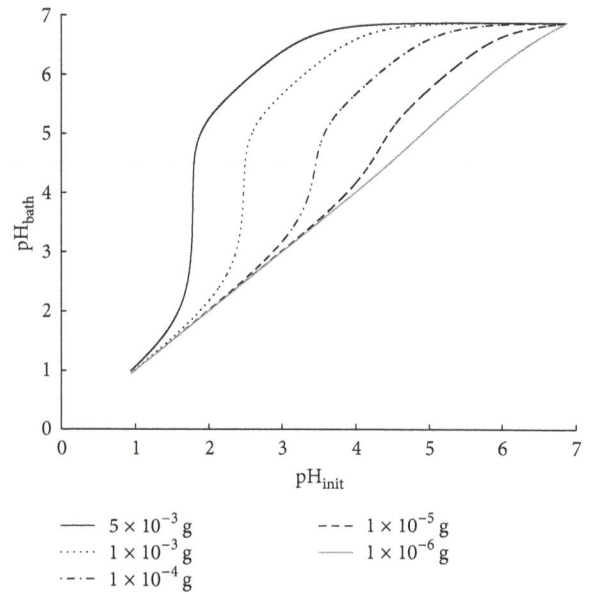

—— $5 \times 10^{-3}$ g     – – – $1 \times 10^{-5}$ g
······· $1 \times 10^{-3}$ g     —— $1 \times 10^{-6}$ g
·–·– $1 \times 10^{-4}$ g

FIGURE 3: Predicted pH-value ($pH_{bath}$) after buffering different initial pH levels ($pH_{init}$) with different constant microgel amount.

Therefore, we adjust hydrochloric acid to different initial pH levels $pH_{init}$, add 0.1 g of VCL/AAEM/VIm-microgel, and measure the pH level of the common bath $pH_{bath}$. We calculate the resulting pH levels $pH_{bath}$ using (5) and the same initial pH levels as in the experiment. The simulation result in comparison to the experiment is plotted in Figure 2. We consider the unknown equilibrium constant for the buffer reaction $K_p$ and the amount of VIm molecules per microgel unit $\sigma$ as fitting parameters and use the withdrawn values of $K_p = 1 \cdot 10^{-10}$ mol/L and $\sigma = 1{,}522 \cdot 10^{20}$ 1/g for further simulation. The preliminary study shows a threshold behavior for the buffering effect. Initial pH levels above 4 ($pH_{init} \geq 4$) are buffered by VCL/AAEM/VIm-microgel to a neutral pH level. For initial pH levels below this value, the buffering action of VCL/AAEM/VIm-microgel in the used concentration is not sufficient to receive a neutral pH level.

Furthermore, we analyze the amount of VCL/AAEM/VIm-microgel necessary for successful buffering action to a neutral pH level. The result is shown in Figure 3. Initial pH levels of 3.75 and higher can be buffered to neutral level by a total amount of 0.005 g microgel (solid black line in Figure 3). This corresponds to a microgel mass fraction $w_{MG}$ of 0.05 in the polymer foils (for preparation, see above). A threshold below which very strong decay of pH level arises is seen at $pH_{init} = 1.78$ for the 0.005 g VCL/AAEM/VIm-microgel. Lower VCL/AAEM/VIm-microgel amounts (non-solid and gray lines in Figure 3) lead to higher threshold pH levels. Thus, the curves in Figure 3 are shifted to the right with decreasing VCL/AAEM/VIm-microgel amount. The threshold behavior is less distinct for lower microgel amounts. Hence, the curves in Figure 3 are also flattened with decreasing VCL/AAEM/VIm-microgel amount. Nearly no buffering action is predicted for a mass of $1 \cdot 10^{-6}$ g VCL/AAEM/VIm-microgel.

This analysis is valid for the ideal case when considering a homogenous VCL/AAEM/VIm-microgel distribution inside the polymer, where diffusion of oligomers to reach the VIm-molecules is not necessary and no barriers, for example, electrostatic reasons, occur.

3.2. Degradation Studies. The experimental results from the degradation studies of polymer foils with VCLVCL/AAEM/VIm-microgel mass fractions of $w_{MG} = 0.00$ and $w_{MG} = 0.05$, respectively, are depicted in Figure 4 via the mean and the standard deviation of the two measurement series (see above). Without microgel, a drop in pH level arises as expected leading to pH = 5.4 after 35 days. As the pH level is measured in the water component of the experimental set-up ($d_p \leq x \leq d_w$ in Figure 1), the pH level in the core of the polymer foil ($x = 0$) will be lower. This lowest pH level is relevant to choosing the appropriate VCL/AAEM/VIm-microgel content.

We use the experimental results of polymer foils with a microgel mass fraction of $w_{MG} = 0.00$ to determine the rate constants in the degradation model (2) in order to find a good agreement between simulation and experimental measurements. The simulation result as average pH level in the water component ($d_p \leq x \leq d_w$ in Figure 1) is plotted as a solid line in Figure 4. The influence of the simulated swiveling process can be seen clearly as steps in the pH level curve. The obtained degradation rates as all other model parameters are listed in Table 1.

The pH level in the center of the polymer foil ($x = 0$ in Figure 1) is evaluated and plotted over time in Figure 5. The pH level drops to 1.42 after 35 days using a mass fraction of $w_{MG} = 0.00$ (solid line). Applying a VCL/AAEM/VIm-microgel buffer with a mass fraction of $w_{MG} = 0.05$ to the resulting solution ($pH_{init} = 1.42$) will not be sufficient to buffer the pH to a neutral level but only to a pH level of approximately $pH_{bath} = 2$ according to Figure 3. Nevertheless, in the center of the foil after 35 days only a small decrease

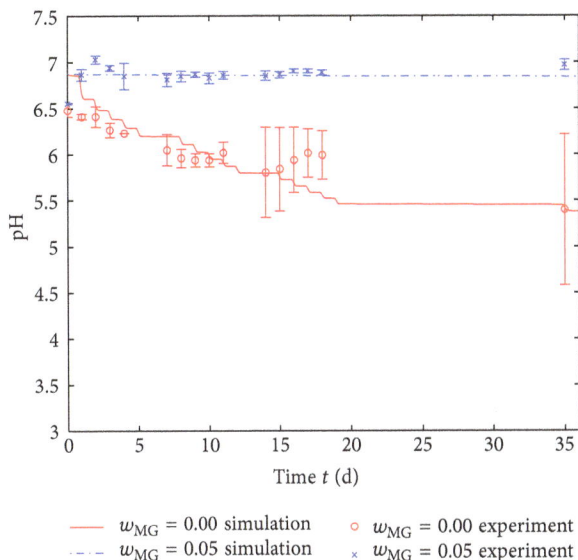

FIGURE 4: pH level over time during degradation experiment of polymer foils with a VCL/AAEM/VIm-microgel mass fraction $w_{MG}$ of 0.00 and 0.05, respectively, in comparison to the simulation (for evaluation in water component, see Figure 1). The model parameters are given in Table 1.

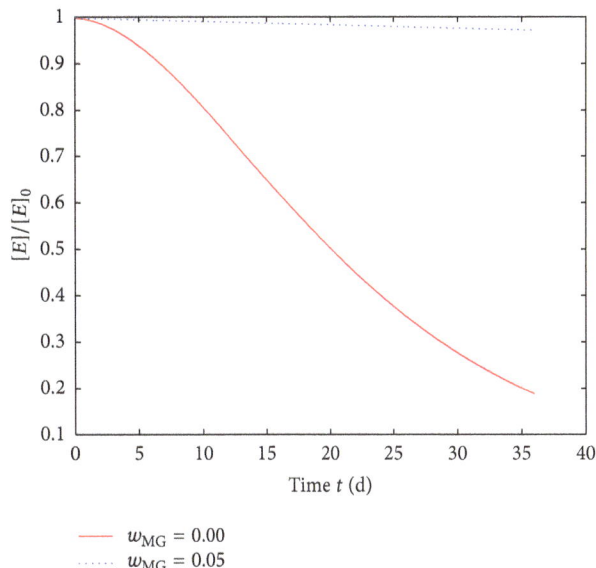

FIGURE 6: Simulated normalized ester bond concentration [E]/[E]$_0$ over time for polymer foils with a VCL/AAEM/VIm-microgel mass fraction of $w_{MG} = 0.00$ and $w_{MG} = 0.05$, respectively. The concentration was evaluated as an average of the polymer foil ($0 < x < d_p$ in Figure 1). The model parameters are given in Table 1.

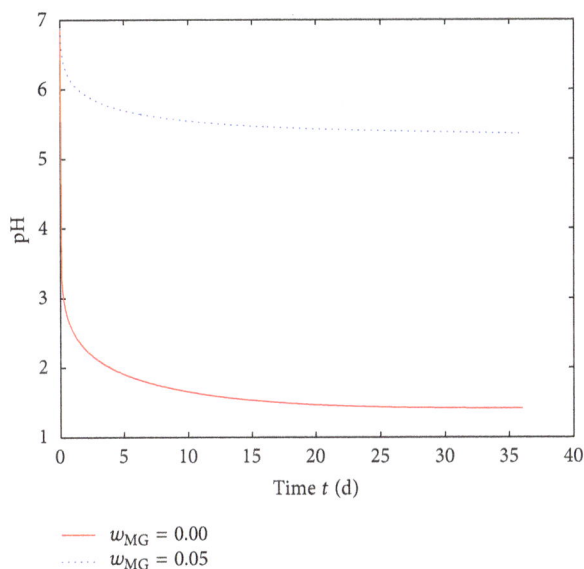

FIGURE 5: Simulated pH level over time for polymer foils with a VCL/AAEM/VIm -microgel mass fraction of $w_{MG}$ = 0.00 and $w_{MG} = 0.05$, respectively. The pH level was evaluated at the center of the polymer foil ($x = 0$ in Figure 1). The model parameters are given in Table 1.

in pH level (~5.37) is predicted for a microgel mass fraction of $w_{MG} = 0.05$ (dotted line in Figure 5). This discrepancy results from the deceleration of the degradation process through VCL/AAEM/VIm-microgel. The deceleration can be explained via the reduction of the autocatalyzed degradation. The normalized concentration of ester bonds in the polymer component over time is depicted in Figure 6. It illustrates

the reduction of overall degradation rate by incorporation of VCL/AAEM/VIm-microgel. Thus, a VCL/AAEM/VIm-microgel mass fraction of $w_{MG} = 0.05$ will possibly be sufficient to buffer the pH to a neutral level. Figure 4 confirms this expectation in theory and experiment. The predicted decrease of pH level in the water component is smaller than in the center of the foil and is in good accordance with the measurements.

In order to briefly demonstrate the influence of the experimental procedure on the development of pH level, three different swiveling procedures are simulated and the resulting average pH levels in the water phase are plotted in Figure 7 (no swiveling: dashed line, swiveling at discrete measurement events: solid line, and continuous swiveling: dotted line). The strong deviation in simulated pH levels shows the importance of standardized experimental procedures.

3.3. Limitations of the Study. The rate equation system for degradation of polymers ((1)–(3) and (6)) is a very reduced model. Any difference between scission of ester bonds at molecule ends and that of bonds in the middle of the polymer molecules is neglected as well as the effects of crystallinity, of diffusivity varying in time, and others. Nevertheless, a very similar model is already considered very useful for the prediction of size and shape effects on biodegradation [29]. One has to perform reference experiments without incorporation of VCL/AAEM/VIm-microgels to determine the rate coefficients of the presented degradation model. With these references our model can be used for investigating the pH levels in the vicinity of polymer components and for analyzing buffering behavior. The reference experiments will have different results using different polymers and therefore have to be performed for every material that is investigated.

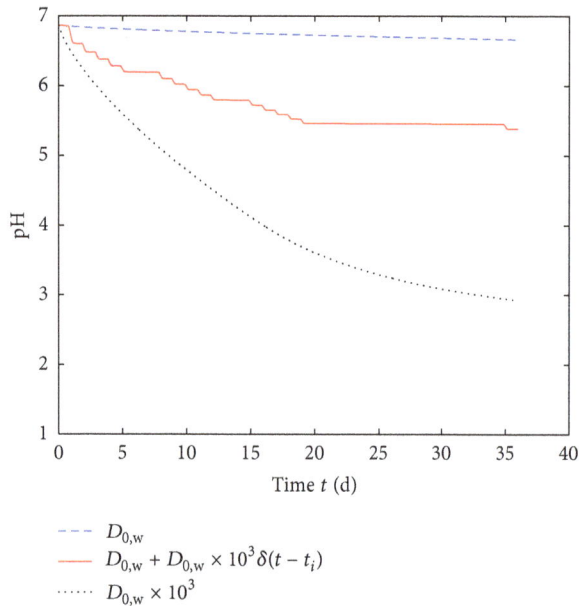

FIGURE 7: Simulated pH level over time for polymer foils without any VCL/AAEM/VIm-microgel content. The diffusivity was changed from a low value ($D_{0,w}$) to a higher value ($D_{0,w} \cdot 10^3$) to a low value with several peaks $i$ ($D_{0,w} + D_{0,w} \cdot 10^3 \delta(t - t_i)$) with the Kronecker delta $\delta$). The pH level was evaluated as an average of the water phase ($d_p < x < d_w$ in Figure 1). The model parameters are given in Table 1.

The simulated model task consisting of a 1D calculation area is a simplified task and deviations from experimental measurements are expectable. It is adequate for a first benchmark of the model with experiments and appropriate for model development as very short computation time results from the simple task.

Model refinements and extensions are necessary in order to investigate the influence of microgel distribution inside the polymer and buffering reaction kinetics. For this purpose, new specific experiments have to be conducted.

We study the degradation behavior of polymer foils in a preclinical set-up according to ISO 13781. Any biological influences like enzymes, vascularization, buffering in body fluids, or patient individual factors cannot be investigated in degradation experiments of this kind. As can be seen from simulation results (Figure 7), conditions (e.g., flow of liquid medium) during degradation experiments have an important influence on the degradation results. Thus, the authors suggest building up a more complex test bench for degradation experiments simulating blood flow amongst others before beginning with clinical studies.

## 4. Conclusions

VCL/AAEM/VIm-microgel-functionalized fibers with pH-optimized degradation behavior are a promising approach for a wide range of medical applications. In particular, the treatment of many cardiovascular diseases such as coronary artery disease will benefit from biodegradable material for stents

without the drawback of acidic pH levels as a consequence of degradation.

Within this study, a mathematical model is presented, which can deal as an important tool to design components with pH-optimized degradation behavior. Iterative design of suitable degradation behavior based on mathematical modelling is shown to exploit the potentials of the medical application and will save engineering costs and time for degradable polymer devices and can contribute to reducing animal studies.

The mathematical model consists of a reduced degradation model based on a rate equation system including diffusion of acidic degradation products into the vicinity of the component. This degradation model is coupled with a set of algebraic equations modelling the buffering action of VCL/AAEM/VIm-microgel. Both models (rate equations for degradation and algebraic buffering model) are evaluated separately in comparison to experimental measurements of pH level and show good agreement with them.

The pH level during the degradation of polymer foils is monitored during 35 days and serves as reference to fit the rate constants of the mathematical degradation model. Additionally, initial pH levels are buffered with a constant amount of VCL/AAEM/VIm-microgel to calibrate the model for the buffer reaction.

A VCL/AAEM/VIm-microgel mass fraction of $w_{MG} = 0.05$ is found to deliver a sufficient buffering action within at least 35 days of degradation of polymer foils. Simulation as well as experimental studies confirmed this buffering effect.

## Competing Interests

The authors declare that there is no conflict of interests regarding the publication of this paper.

## Acknowledgments

The current research project "pHaser" is funded by the Excellence Initiative of the German federal and state governments.

## References

[1] WHO, "Cardiovascular diseases (CVDs): fact sheet N∘317," 2016, http://www.who.int/mediacentre/factsheets/fs317/en/.

[2] R. L. Mueller and T. A. Sanborn, "The history of interventional cardiology: cardiac catheterization, angioplasty, and related interventions," *American Heart Journal*, vol. 129, no. 1, pp. 146–172, 1995.

[3] P. W. Serruys, M. J. B. Kutryk, and A. T. L. Ong, "Coronary-artery stents," *The New England Journal of Medicine*, vol. 354, no. 5, pp. 483–495, 2006.

[4] M. Generali, P. E. Dijkman, and S. P. Hoerstrup, "Bioresorbable scaffolds for cardiovascular tissue engineering," *European Medical Journal Interventional Cardiology*, vol. 1, pp. 91–99, 2014.

[5] P. W. Serruys, J. A. Ormiston, Y. Onuma et al., "A bioabsorbable everolimus-eluting coronary stent system (ABSORB): 2-year outcomes and results from multiple imaging methods," *The Lancet*, vol. 373, no. 9667, pp. 897–910, 2009.

[6] A. Weiler, H.-J. Helling, U. Kirch, T. K. Zirbes, and K. E. Rehm, "Foreign-body reaction and the course of osteolysis after polyglycolide implants for fracture fixation: experimental study in sheep," *The Journal of Bone and Joint Surgery B*, vol. 78, no. 3, pp. 369–376, 1996.

[7] F. W. Cordewener, M. F. Van Geffen, C. A. P. Joziasse et al., "Cytotoxicity of poly(96L/4D-lactide): the influence of degradation and sterilization," *Biomaterials*, vol. 21, no. 23, pp. 2433–2442, 2000.

[8] S. W. Shalaby, *Biomedical Polymers: Designed-to-Degrade Systems*, Hanser Publishers, New York, NY, USA; Hanser/Gardner Publications, Toronto, Canada, 1994.

[9] M. S. Taylor, A. U. Daniels, K. P. Andriano, and J. Heller, "Six bioabsorbable polymers: in vitro acute toxicity of accumulated degradation products," *Journal of Applied Biomaterials*, vol. 5, no. 2, pp. 151–157, 1994.

[10] C. M. Agrawal and K. A. Athanasiou, "Technique to control pH in vicinity of biodegrading PLA-PGA implants," *Journal of Biomedical Materials Research*, vol. 38, no. 2, pp. 105–114, 1997.

[11] E. J. Bergsma, F. R. Rozema, R. R. M. Bos, and W. C. de Bruijn, "Foreign body reactions to resorbable poly(L-lactide) bone plates and screws used for the fixation of unstable zygomatic fractures," *Journal of Oral and Maxillofacial Surgery*, vol. 51, no. 6, pp. 666–670, 1993.

[12] O. M. Böstman, "Osteolytic changes accompanying degradation of absorbable fracture fixation implants," *Journal of Bone and Joint Surgery B*, vol. 73, no. 4, pp. 679–682, 1991.

[13] O. Böstman and H. Pihlajamäki, "Clinical biocompatibility of biodegradable orthopaedic implants for internal fixation: a review," *Biomaterials*, vol. 21, no. 24, pp. 2615–2621, 2000.

[14] A. Colombo and E. Karvouni, "Biodegradable stents: 'Fulfilling the mission and stepping away," *Circulation*, vol. 102, no. 4, pp. 371–373, 2000.

[15] K. Fehér, T. Romstadt, C. A. Böhm et al., "Microgel-functionalised fibres with pH-optimised degradation behaviour—a promising approach for short-term medical applications," *BioNanoMaterials*, vol. 16, no. 4, pp. 259–264, 2015.

[16] S. Saxena, C. E. Hansen, and L. A. Lyon, "Microgel mechanics in biomaterial design," *Accounts of Chemical Research*, vol. 47, no. 8, pp. 2426–2434, 2014.

[17] A. S. Hoffman, "Hydrogels for biomedical applications," *Advanced Drug Delivery Reviews*, vol. 54, no. 1, pp. 3–12, 2002.

[18] V. Aseyev, H. Tenhu, and F. M. Winnik, "Non-ionic thermoresponsive polymers in water," in *Self Organized Nanostructures of Amphiphilic Block Copolymers II*, A. H. E. Müller and O. Borisov, Eds., vol. 242 of *Advances in Polymer Science*, pp. 29–89, Springer, Berlin, Germany, 2011.

[19] S. Nayak and L. A. Lyon, "Soft nanotechnology with soft nanoparticles," *Angewandte Chemie—International Edition*, vol. 44, no. 47, pp. 7686–7708, 2005.

[20] V. Boyko, A. Pich, Y. Lu, S. Richter, K.-F. Arndt, and H.-J. P. Adler, "Thermo-sensitive poly(N-vinylcaprolactam-co-acetoacetoxyethyl methacrylate) microgels: 1—synthesis and characterization," *Polymer*, vol. 44, no. 26, pp. 7821–7827, 2003.

[21] K. Raemdonck, J. Demeester, and S. De Smedt, "Advanced nanogel engineering for drug delivery," *Soft Matter*, vol. 5, no. 4, pp. 707–715, 2009.

[22] L. A. Lyon, Z. Meng, N. Singh, C. D. Sorrell, and A. St John, "Thermoresponsive microgel-based materials," *Chemical Society Reviews*, vol. 38, no. 4, pp. 865–874, 2009.

[23] R. Pelton, "Temperature-sensitive aqueous microgels," *Advances in Colloid and Interface Science*, vol. 85, no. 1, pp. 1–33, 2000.

[24] B. Taşdelen, N. Kayaman-Apohan, O. Güven, and B. M. Baysal, "Swelling and diffusion studies of poly(N-isopropylacrylamide/itaconic acid) copolymeric hydrogels in water and aqueous solutions of drugs," *Journal of Applied Polymer Science*, vol. 91, no. 2, pp. 911–915, 2004.

[25] X. Zhou, F. Su, Y. Tian, and D. R. Meldrum, "Dually fluorescent core-shell microgels for ratiometric imaging in live antigen-presenting cells," *PLoS ONE*, vol. 9, no. 2, Article ID e88185, 2014.

[26] A. Pich, A. Tessier, V. Boyko, Y. Lu, and H.-J. P. Adler, "Synthesis and characterization of poly(vinylcaprolactam)-based microgels exhibiting temperature and pH-sensitive properties," *Macromolecules*, vol. 39, no. 22, pp. 7701–7707, 2006.

[27] G. L. Siparsky, K. J. Voorhees, and F. Miao, "Hydrolysis of polylactic acid (PLA) and polycaprolactone (PCL) in aqueous acetonitrile solutions: autocatalysis," *Journal of Environmental Polymer Degradation*, vol. 6, no. 1, pp. 31–41, 1998.

[28] X. Han, "Degradation models for polyesters and their composites," 2011.

[29] Y. Wang, J. Pan, X. Han, C. Sinka, and L. Ding, "A phenomenological model for the degradation of biodegradable polymers," *Biomaterials*, vol. 29, no. 23, pp. 3393–3401, 2008.

[30] J. Pan, X. Han, W. Niu, and R. E. Cameron, "A model for biodegradation of composite materials made of polyesters and tricalcium phosphates," *Biomaterials*, vol. 32, no. 9, pp. 2248–2255, 2011.

[31] S. Lazzari, F. Codari, G. Storti, M. Morbidelli, and D. Moscatelli, "Modeling the pH-dependent PLA oligomer degradation kinetics," *Polymer Degradation and Stability*, vol. 110, pp. 80–90, 2014.

[32] A. Horta, M. J. Molina, M. R. Gómez-Antón, and I. F. Piérola, "The pH inside a swollen polyelectrolyte gel: poly(N-vinylimidazole)," *The Journal of Physical Chemistry B*, vol. 112, no. 33, pp. 10123–10129, 2008.

[33] A. Horta and I. F. Piérola, "Poly(N-vinylimidazole) gels as insoluble buffers that neutralize acid solutions without dissolving," *The Journal of Physical Chemistry B*, vol. 113, no. 13, pp. 4226–4231, 2009.

[34] ISO, "Poly(L-lactide) resins and fabricated forms for surgical implants—in vitro degradation testing," ISO 13781:1997, 1997.

[35] N. Lucas, C. Bienaime, C. Belloy, M. Queneudec, F. Silvestre, and J.-E. Nava-Saucedo, "Polymer biodegradation: mechanisms and estimation techniques—a review," *Chemosphere*, vol. 73, no. 4, pp. 429–442, 2008.

[36] 2016, http://www.chemie.de/lexikon/Dissoziationskonstante .html.

[37] A. C. F. Ribeiro, V. M. M. Lobo, D. G. Leist et al., "Binary diffusion coefficients for aqueous solutions of lactic acid," *Journal of Solution Chemistry*, vol. 34, no. 9, pp. 1009–1016, 2005.

# 10

# Comparison of Healthcare Workers Transferring Patients Using Either Conventional Or Robotic Wheelchairs: Kinematic, Electromyographic, and Electrocardiographic Analyses

**Hiromi Matsumoto,**[1] **Masaru Ueki,**[2] **Kazutake Uehara,**[2] **Hisashi Noma,**[3] **Nobuko Nozawa,**[2] **Mari Osaki,**[1] **and Hiroshi Hagino**[1,4]

[1]*Rehabilitation Division, Tottori University Hospital, Nishi-cho 36-1, Yonago, Tottori 683-8504, Japan*
[2]*Center for Promoting Next-Generation Highly Advanced Medicine, Tottori University Hospital, Nishi-cho 36-1, Yonago, Tottori 683-8504, Japan*
[3]*Department of Data Science, The Institute of Statistical Mathematics, Midori-cho 10-3, Tachikawa, Tokyo 190-8562, Japan*
[4]*School of Health Science, Faculty of Medicine, Tottori University, Nishi-cho 86, Yonago, Tottori 683-8503, Japan*

Correspondence should be addressed to Hiromi Matsumoto; h.matsumoto@med.tottori-u.ac.jp

Academic Editor: Feng-Huei Lin

*Objectives.* The aim of this study was to compare the musculoskeletal and physical strain on healthcare workers, by measuring range of motion (ROM), muscle activity, and heart rate (HR), during transfer of a simulated patient using either a robotic wheelchair (RWC) or a conventional wheelchair (CWC). *Methods.* The subjects were 10 females who had work experience in transferring patients and another female adult as the simulated patient to be transferred from bed to a RWC or a CWC. In both experimental conditions, ROM, muscle activity, and HR were assessed in the subjects using motion sensors, electromyography, and electrocardiograms. *Results.* Peak ROM of shoulder flexion during assistive transfer with the RWC was significantly lower than that with the CWC. Values for back muscle activity during transfer were lower with the RWC than with the CWC. *Conclusions.* The findings suggest that the RWC may decrease workplace injuries and lower back pain in healthcare workers.

## 1. Introduction

Musculoskeletal and physical strain caused by patient handling are prevalent among healthcare workers. In particular, musculoskeletal pain and lower back muscle injuries in nurses working in the geriatric setting are very high because of the significant number of patient transfers to wheelchairs that involve lifting [1–4]. It has been reported that physical therapists working in rehabilitation settings who perform 6–10 patients transfers per day are 2.4 times more likely to develop lower back injuries than therapists who do not perform transfers [5]. A previous study on occupational and physical therapists showed that transferring or lifting patients was associated with 26.6% of all injuries during work-related activities [6]. Moreover, a study on various nursing work activities showed that during the transfer of patients, the

nurses' heart rate (HR) increased to approximately 125 beats/ min (bpm) and they had higher levels of neuromuscular fatigue [4]. Therefore, the transfer of patients to wheelchairs produces increased burden on the musculoskeletal and cardiovascular systems through changes in joint range of motion (ROM), muscle activity, and HR. Therefore, there is a higher probability of musculoskeletal and physical strain in healthcare workers who transfer patients.

Several interventions have been reported to decrease musculoskeletal injuries in healthcare workers [7–9]. In fact, the implementation of safe patient handling and movement policies by the nursing profession has dramatically decreased work-related injuries and chronic pain [9]. Nurses who are more skilled in patient transfer increase the patients' perceptions of safety and comfort during transfers [8]. Some previous literature reported the efforts to decrease musculoskeletal injuries; however, strong evidence for the effectiveness of intervention is lacking.

On the other hand, following the adoption of no-lift policies, transfer robotic devices have emerged as tools that have the potential to prevent injuries in healthcare workers [10]. Robotic lift and powered devices may decrease both the patients' effort and the clinicians' physical burden. One tool emerging from these initiatives is a battery-powered sit-to-stand transfer device that safely lifts and lowers patients between the seated and standing positions [11, 12]. Transfer of patients with disabilities who are unable to contribute their own effort depends on powered robotic devices. However, the patients' physical activity or motivation may increase if the patients can transfer themselves using these assistance devices.

Recently, a new robotic wheel chair (RWC) has been developed which enables patients to be transferred directly in the sitting position using their own effort and the assistance of a healthcare worker [13]. The manual transfer of disabled patients from the bed to a conventional wheelchair (CWC) is demanding and involves complex movements. Patient-handling tasks involved with a CWC can be classified into 3 groups: lifting of the patient, repositioning or turning from the bed towards the direction of the wheelchair, and seating the patient safely in the chair. However, the RWC involves only 1 transfer step, which is that the assistant pushes the patient sitting on a bed forward in the same position to the seat of the RWC. Therefore, the RWC may decrease the complexity of transfer and decrease physical load during transfer for healthcare workers.

The purpose of this experimental study was to investigate the burden on healthcare workers by measuring ROM, muscle activity, and HR during transfer of a simulated patient using either the RWC or a CWC.

## 2. Methods

*2.1. Participants.* Ten females adults were recruited from an acute hospital and included 6 nurses and 4 rehabilitation therapists who had work experience in transferring patients (mean age: 32.2 ± 9.3 years; range: 23–47 years; body weight: 48.8 ± 4.7 kg; height: 157.2 ± 6.7 cm; BMI: 19.7 ± 1.3 kg/m$^2$). Another female adult (age: 27 years; body weight: 49.0 kg; height: 153.0 cm; BMI: 20.9 kg/m$^2$) participated in the study acting as the simulated patient who was transferred from bed to the wheelchairs. The simulation was assumed to be a right hemiplegia patient whose right upper extremity was fixed in a sling. Instructions for this procedure were provided by a researcher as, "please do not encourage movement of your right lower extremity during transfer to the wheelchair" [13]. The subjects had no musculoskeletal or neurological impairments. All the participants provided written, informed consent, and the study was approved by the local ethics committee of the Faculty of Medicine, Tottori University (number 2292).

*2.2. Instrumentation.* Three-dimensional (3D) motion analysis (MyoMotion Analysis System; Noraxon USA Inc., Arizona, USA) consists of combined motion sensors, surface

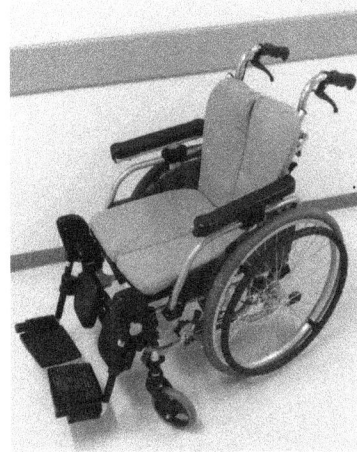

FIGURE 1: Conventional wheelchair (CWC).

electromyography (EMG), and synchronized video recordings. Signals of the subjects from these systems were digitally recorded (200 Hz and 1500 Hz and 30 Hz, resp.). In addition, the HR of each subject was measured via a wireless chest-strap electrocardiogram (ECG) monitor (Dynascope; Fukuda Denshi Co., Ltd., Tokyo, Japan). The motion sensor used Inertial Measurement Units, which are widely recognized as a means to overcome the disadvantages of existing optical motion capture systems [14]. The device can measure various kinematic parameters, such as object orientation and velocity, using accelerometers, gyroscopes, and magnetometers. The system has a measurement accuracy of 0.4 degrees for static measurements and 1.2 degrees for dynamic measurements.

*2.3. Device.* A standard CWC (Matsunaga, Co., Ltd., Gifu, Japan) was used in the study (Figure 1). The arm and foot supports could swing out upwards (seat width, 40 mm; front height, 42 cm; total length, 95.5 cm; weight, 18 kg). The RWC used in the study (Rodem, Tmsuk, Co., Ltd., Fukuoka, Japan) has an electric powered seat and a powered wheelchair. The seat moves back and forth and has an elevating mechanism to adjust the height of the patient (width, 720 mm; length, 750 mm; minimum turning radius, 360 mm; weight, approximately 80 kg; battery, lithium-ion battery) (Table 1 and Figure 2).

*2.4. Experimental Procedure.* The motion sensors used for ROM measurements during transfer of the simulated patient were placed on the seventh cervical, seventh thoracic, and fifth lumbar vertebrae and bilaterally on the upper arm, forearm, thigh, shank, and forefoot (Figure 3). Calibration of the motion sensors was performed before the measurements using the segment model in the standing position. EMG electrodes were secured over the muscle bellies of both sides of the biceps, vastus medialis, upper back, and lower back muscles using standard techniques. Following practice, an EMG signal was recorded during maximum isometric manual testing of each muscle [15]. HR was assessed using a 3-electrode EKG (modified V5 lead). The signals from the motion sensors, EMG, and HR were recorded simultaneously in both

TABLE 1: Specifications of the robotic wheelchair (RWC).

| | |
|---|---|
| Range of motion of seat | 425 mm (up and down and/or front and back) |
| Speed of motion of seat | 28 mm/s (up and down and/or front and back) |
| Speed | Advance: max. speed 4.5 km/h, min. speed 2.5 km/h |
| | Reverse: 2.0 km/h |
| Minimum turning radius | 360 mm |
| Driving time | 20 km |
| Weight | 80 kg |
| Size | Length × width × height: 750 mm × 720 mm × 1,000 mm |
| Rear wheel size | 16 inch |
| Number of wheels | Drive wheel × 2, training wheels × 3 |
| Motor output | 24 V 120 W × right and left side (AC motor) |

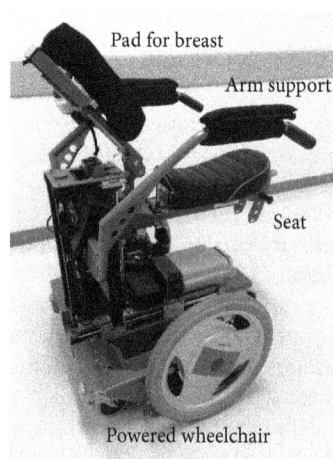

FIGURE 2: Robotic wheel chair (RWC). The seat in the RWC leans forward; thus, it makes the patients incline forward rather than lean back on the RWC. Patients are supported with a breast pad during sitting or driving. This device received a CE marking for safety and maneuverability. The criterion for using this device is the patients who have the ability to stand with assistance, and the exclusion criterion is the patients who have the inability to sit by oneself.

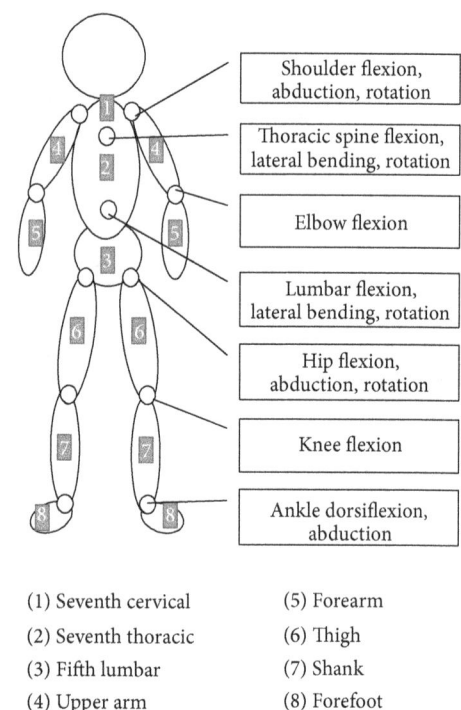

(1) Seventh cervical        (5) Forearm
(2) Seventh thoracic        (6) Thigh
(3) Fifth lumbar            (7) Shank
(4) Upper arm               (8) Forefoot

FIGURE 3: Placement of motion sensors and analysis of joint motion.

experimental conditions (i.e., transfer using either the RWC or the CWC), while the subjects performed the following tasks, once in each situation and in random order: (1) CWC: the subjects supported the trunk of the simulated patient sitting on a bed and lifted the patient to a standing position, converted the patient's position toward the direction of the wheelchair, and seated the patient safely; (2) RWC: the subjects, located on the right side of the simulated patient who was sitting on a bed, supported the pelvis of the patient and pushed the patient directly onto the seat of the RWC. Transfer of the simulated patient was assisted until the patient was positioned on the seat (Figure 4). The RWC was located at the front of the patient with the height of the seat adjusted to the patient's sitting position using the robotic elevation system.

*2.5. Data Analysis.* Visual 3D motion analysis software (MR3; Noraxon USA Inc., Arizona, USA) was used to analyze the signal processing of the motion sensors, EMG, and video

recordings. In both experimental conditions, the onset and cessation of ROM analysis, EMG, and ECG were defined as the start of assistance until the end of assistance to transfer the simulated patient and were determined by visual interpretation of the video recordings. ROM of the upper extremity, trunk, and lower extremity segments were calculated during both experimental conditions. In both situations, real-time ROM during patient transfer was analyzed using data obtained between 2 motion sensors; for example, right elbow-joint motion was analyzed using integrated signals of the accelerometers, gyroscopes, and magnetometers between the right upper arm and right forearm sensors, and the peak ROM was identified. For each muscle, the EMG data was integrated over 0.01 s intervals during each experimental condition and then normalized for each muscle's EMG signal of maximum voluntary contraction (MVC) which was

(a)

(b)

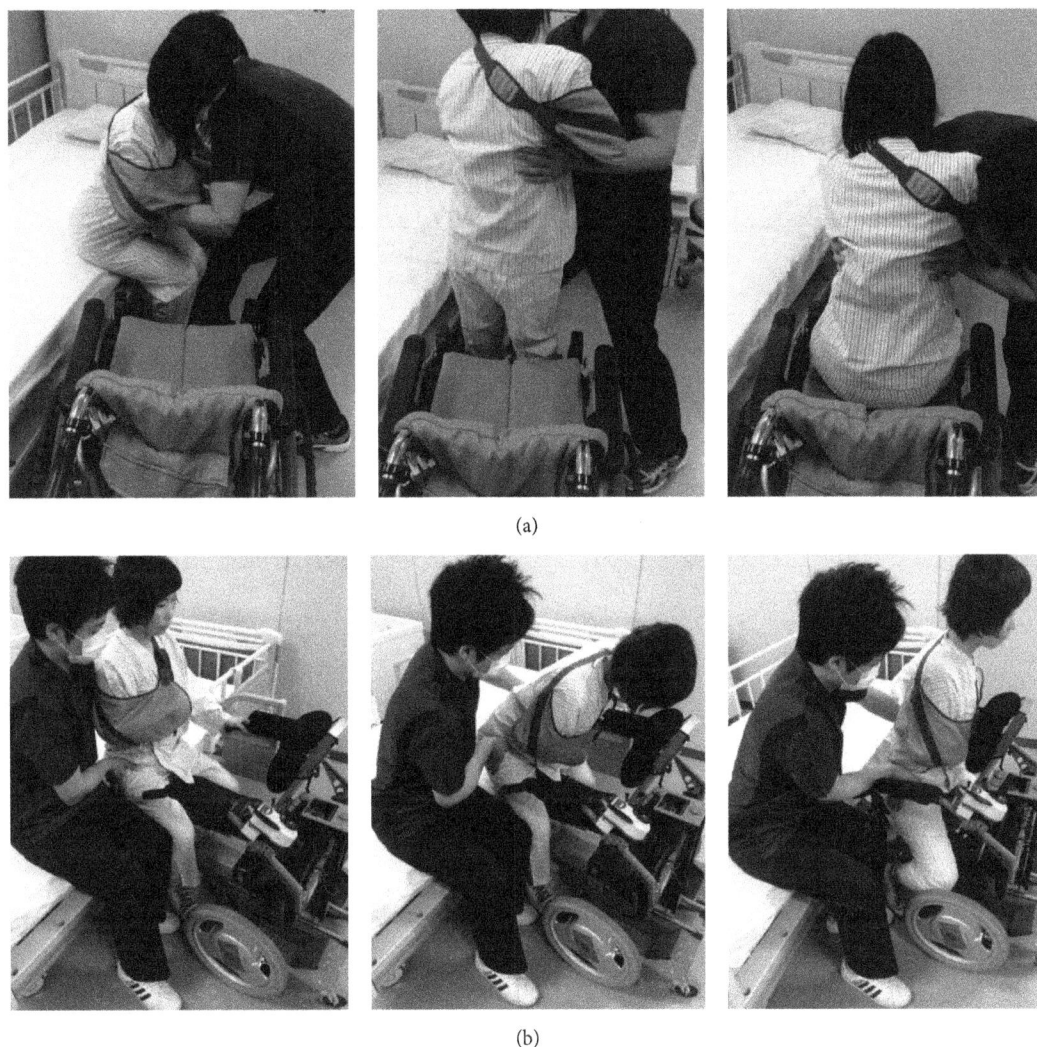

FIGURE 4: Transfer to the CWC and RWC. (a) Patient-handling tasks involved with a CWC can be classified into 3 groups: lifting of the patient, repositioning or turning from the bed towards the direction of the wheelchair, and seating the patient safely in the chair. (b) The RWC involves only 1 transfer step, which is that the assistant pushes the patient sitting on a bed forward in the same position to the seat of the RWC.

recorded during maximum isometric manual test. Mean muscle activity, expressed as %MVC, and mean HR were calculated during both experimental conditions.

*2.6. Statistical Analysis.* All data were expressed as mean ± standard deviation (SD). Differences between the 2 experimental conditions were determined using paired *t*-tests. All statistical analyses were performed using SPSS for Windows Version 22 (IBM, Co., Ltd., Tokyo, Japan) and R ver. 3.0.3 (R Foundation for Statistical Computing, Vienna, Austria).

## 3. Results

*3.1. Peak ROM on Motion Analysis.* Table 2 shows the comparison of the motion analyses for CWC and RWC transfer. The peak ROM of both shoulder flexion and left ankle abduction during assistive transfer to the RWC were significantly lower than with the CWC. Left shoulder abduction, right

shoulder rotation, and left knee flexion were significantly higher with the RWC than with the CWC.

*3.2. %MVC on EMG Analysis.* Table 3 shows the comparison of the muscle activation analysis for CWC and RWC transfer. The %MVC of the right biceps, the left upper back muscles, the left lower back muscles, and the right vastus medialis muscle were significantly lower with the RWC than with the CWC. The %MVC of the left biceps was significantly higher with the RWC than with the CWC.

*3.3. ECG.* There was a significant difference in mean HR during transfer between the 2 conditions (RWC, 87.1 ± 10.9 bpm versus CWC, 99.2 ± 13.2 bpm; $p = 0.006$).

*3.4. Statistical Power Analysis for Sample Size.* We performed power diagnoses for the tests with relevant outcomes and

TABLE 2: Peak ROM on motion analysis during transfer.

| | | CWC | | RWC | | 95% CI | | | $p$ |
|---|---|---|---|---|---|---|---|---|---|
| | | Mean | SD | Mean | SD | | | | |
| Lumbar flexion | | 35.6 | 12.7 | 35.8 | 12.6 | −5.332 | − | 5.012 | 0.946 |
| Lumbar lateral flexion | | 15.0 | 12.3 | 13.0 | 4.7 | −7.508 | − | 11.646 | 0.637 |
| Lumbar rotation | | 5.9 | 2.6 | 7.9 | 3.6 | −5.960 | − | 1.920 | 0.276 |
| Thoracic spine flexion | | 12.7 | 5.9 | 18.5 | 9.5 | −12.824 | − | 1.282 | 0.097 |
| Thoracic spine lateral flexion | | 13.7 | 7.4 | 13.7 | 3.4 | −5.998 | − | 5.880 | 0.983 |
| Thoracic spine rotation | | 12.6 | 5.4 | 13.0 | 5.2 | −6.479 | − | 5.523 | 0.861 |
| Elbow flexion | Left | 61.9 | 28.8 | 57.7 | 14.3 | −10.540 | − | 18.880 | 0.537 |
| | Right | 63.1 | 19.5 | 79.8 | 13.7 | −38.339 | − | 4.899 | 0.114 |
| Shoulder flexion | Left | 72.7 | 16.1 | 57.1 | 12.7 | 1.780 | − | 29.380 | 0.031 |
| | Right | 65.9 | 11.1 | 52.4 | 12.4 | 2.254 | − | 24.866 | 0.024 |
| Shoulder abduction | Left | 24.3 | 11.5 | 48.3 | 12.1 | −35.345 | − | −12.503 | 0.001 |
| | Right | 35.6 | 18.2 | 30.7 | 12.8 | −11.773 | − | 21.409 | 0.528 |
| Shoulder rotation | Left | 48.0 | 16.2 | 53.4 | 48.6 | −38.067 | − | 27.267 | 0.717 |
| | Right | 34.5 | 14.3 | 63.0 | 16.7 | −44.785 | − | −12.135 | 0.003 |
| Hip flexion | Left | 71.6 | 10.4 | 83.9 | 19.9 | −28.408 | − | 3.848 | 0.119 |
| | Right | 77.1 | 9.1 | 79.8 | 20.1 | −17.129 | − | 11.629 | 0.675 |
| Hip abduction | Left | 28.5 | 10.4 | 19.8 | 15.4 | −5.508 | − | 22.816 | 0.200 |
| | Right | 24.6 | 8.5 | 24.5 | 7.5 | −7.859 | − | 7.999 | 0.985 |
| Hip rotation | Left | 29.8 | 11.5 | 22.9 | 13.5 | −0.946 | − | 14.628 | 0.078 |
| | Right | 28.8 | 11.6 | 22.0 | 14.8 | −9.111 | − | 22.663 | 0.360 |
| Knee flexion | Left | 63.2 | 9.1 | 97.1 | 7.5 | −44.803 | − | −22.977 | 0.000 |
| | Right | 71.0 | 15.5 | 83.9 | 29.4 | −39.001 | − | 13.153 | 0.291 |
| Ankle dorsiflexion | Left | 20.1 | 7.7 | 20.0 | 12.3 | −9.885 | − | 9.953 | 0.994 |
| | Right | 27.2 | 12.9 | 29.4 | 12.3 | −16.824 | − | 12.306 | 0.734 |
| Ankle abduction | Left | 27.5 | 10.3 | 15.8 | 8.3 | 1.718 | − | 21.574 | 0.026 |
| | Right | 23.4 | 8.7 | 19.3 | 6.6 | −4.326 | − | 12.386 | 0.304 |

ROM, range of motion; CWC, conventional wheel chair; RWC, robotic wheel chair.

TABLE 3: %MVC on EMG analysis during transfer.

| | CWC | | RWC | | 95% CI | | | $p$ |
|---|---|---|---|---|---|---|---|---|
| | Mean | SD | Mean | SD | | | | |
| Biceps muscle right side | 65.6 | 31.6 | 34.9 | 29.8 | 13.167 | − | 48.179 | 0.003 |
| Biceps muscle left side | 62.7 | 37.0 | 90.1 | 44.0 | −53.197 | − | −1.603 | 0.040 |
| Upper back muscles right side | 59.6 | 25.5 | 66.9 | 33.4 | −30.139 | − | 15.459 | 0.485 |
| Upper back muscles left side | 66.9 | 34.4 | 35.2 | 20.6 | 17.214 | − | 46.102 | 0.001 |
| Lower back muscles right side | 48.4 | 18.9 | 56.7 | 22.0 | −22.898 | − | 6.438 | 0.236 |
| Lower back muscles left side | 53.9 | 25.0 | 29.4 | 18.9 | 16.699 | − | 32.331 | 0.000 |
| Vastus medialis muscle right side | 41.9 | 33.3 | 15.2 | 16.1 | 0.391 | − | 53.016 | 0.047 |
| Vastus medialis muscle left side | 53.0 | 50.2 | 37.5 | 48.4 | −18.916 | − | 50.010 | 0.334 |

%MVC, % maximum voluntary contraction; CWC, conventional wheel chair; RWC, robotic wheel chair.

checked that most of them would have sufficient statistical power, for example, shoulder flexion (left 62.4%, right 67.6%), shoulder abduction (left 98.7%, right 8.5%), upper back muscles (left 99.2%, right 10.0%), lower back muscles (left 99.9%, right 20.5%), and HR (88.6%). Therefore, our statistician considers that the sample size was valid from a statistical perspective.

## 4. Discussion

Our study showed that transferring a simulated patient from bed to the RWC decreased the ROM on shoulder flexion, back muscle activity, and HR in the subjects compared to using a CWC. These findings suggest that the RWC may have the advantage of decreased muscle activity of the leg or back muscles during transfer compared with the CWC. This is because the RWC enables healthcare workers to push the patient forward in the sitting position; they may not have to lift the patients. This may decrease the musculoskeletal and physical strain on healthcare workers during transfer. In addition, transferring patients using a CWC involves 3 steps: lifting the patient, turning towards the direction of the wheelchair, and seating the patient safely in the chair. This adds complexity and requires the clinician to use more technical methods when transferring the patient. In contrast, the RWC does not involve lifting the patient, who instead can be transferred in 1 step using their own effort to push forward onto the seat of the RWC. It is simpler to assist in these movements. It may also be more comfortable for patients. During transfer to the RWC, the patient does not need to change direction while in the standing position as is the case with the CWC. Therefore, transferring to the front using the RWC may decrease the physical load on healthcare workers who often have to perform many patient transfers during a single working day.

The peak ROM values in the motion analysis of the subjects during transfer to the RWC showed lower shoulder flexion and left ankle abduction compared with transfer to the CWC. Transfer of patients from bed to the RWC does not involve lifting and also the foot position while sitting is neutral. In contrast, the technique for transfer to a CWC places higher demand on the shoulder flexion required to lift the patient, and a stride standing position and lower extremity abduction to maintain standing balance. It is not necessary to increase these ROM values when transferring a patient to a RWC. On the other hand, ROM of left shoulder abduction, right shoulder rotation, and right knee flexion were higher with the RWC. During transfer to the RWC, healthcare workers flex their knees to transfer the patient in the sitting position compared with a standing transfer. Shoulder abduction and rotation occur during transfer to the RWC because of the need to hold the pelvis of the patients using both arms. We suggest that the RWC has the benefit of possibly lowering ROM during transfers. However, pushing the patient forward in the RWC may place a burden on the upper extremities. It is therefore important to recognize the potential of shoulder abduction and rotation muscle overload during transfers using the RWC.

With the RWC, lower back muscle activity and lower mean HR during transfers were observed on EMG and ECG

analyses. In the present study, analysis of the left back muscles during transfer from bed to the CWC showed 48%–66% MVC demand in the subjects. In a previous study, EMG analysis of the lower back muscles during transfer of patients to a CWC showed approximately 40% MVC in subjects [13]. We observed similar findings in our study, with the RWC decreasing left back muscle activity to a greater extent (i.e., %MVC of 29%–35%). It is also possible that HR increases because of increased muscle activity with a CWC compared to a RWC. In fact, a previous study showed that nurses rated patient lifting, transfer, and turning as the most physically demanding activities. Those tasks also correspond to the highest HRs recorded under clinical working conditions [4]. We suggest that this is an important advantage of the RWC compared to the CWC because of the need to decrease back muscle injury and cardiovascular stress during clinical work [4, 6]. Transfer from bed to the RWC requires healthcare workers to bend rather than rotate their trunks, without lifting the patients. This may decrease workplace injuries that occur during patient handling. This suggests that the RWC provides a simple transfer technique in which it is possible to transfer the load to the upper extremity when transferring patients with higher body weight.

The clinical implication of the RWC is that it represents a motorized device for older adults who are physically frail with weakness of the lower extremities and enables them to stand and turn to the wheelchair during transfer. In addition, we hypothesize that transfer using the RWC is advantageous for patients with Parkinsonism who cannot change their direction when standing. In this situation, we suggest that the RWC needs a robotic function or a sling to carry the patient in the sitting position to a seat. This would decrease the load on the upper extremities of the healthcare workers. We believe that riding the RWC is suitable for patients with pressure ulcers on the sacral area because the RWC does not have a back support; patients are supported by the breast support and do not have pressure on the sacrum. However, there is no available evidence regarding the pressure of the breast support or the seat. The weakness of the RWC is that this device does not have a back support, although the seat leans forward so that subjects do not fall backwards on the RWC. Thus, the use of this device is limited to those who have the ability to sit or stand with assistance. Additionally, transferring from the RWC to the CWC or bed is a weak point of this device because subjects who ride on the RWC must turn around and look behind in order to return to the bed. The RWC may need a rearview mirror or an automatic navigation system to correct this problem.

This study had several limitations. The patient was a simulated model. Therefore, the values obtained in our data analysis may not be applicable to the transfer of patients with paralysis, dysfunction of the lower extremities, or fractures. In addition, the sample size ($n = 10$) might not have been sufficiently large. However, we performed power diagnoses for the tests with relevant outcomes and checked that most of them would have sufficient statistical power. Also, as a result of the detailed experimental measurements that we made for all subjects, sufficient objective data for various indices and evidence that transfer of patients in the sitting positon clearly caused less physiological burden were obtained although repetitive load was not studied. The group of patients that would benefit most from transfers in the RWC and the associated implications are not addressed in the present study. Lastly, the study did not investigate muscle activity and psychological burden in the simulated patient. Future studies are therefore necessary to analyze these factors.

## 5. Conclusions

Shoulder flexion ROM, activity of the back muscles, and HR were decreased in the subjects when transferred from bed to the RWC. The RWC enables patients to be transferred in the sitting position directly to the frontal position. It is possible that the RWC will decrease workplace injuries and lower back pain in healthcare workers. Using an assisted device to transfer patients without manual lifting has obvious benefits in healthcare and rehabilitation settings.

## Competing Interests

All authors declare that they have no competing interests; each author certifies that there are no commercial relationships (e.g., consultancies, stock ownership, equity interests, and patent/licensing arrangements), which might pose conflict of interests in connection with this paper. Following the experiments described in this paper, their institution decided to develop the new robotic wheel chair with Tmsuk R&D Inc. in Japan, and they entered into a joint research agreement.

## Acknowledgments

The authors wish to sincerely acknowledge the staff members of the hospitals involved in this study. The authors also acknowledge Eri Kobayashi, Risa Otsuki, Tomomi Wada, Kyohei Nakata, Taro Omori, Kenjiro Naruse, and Takashi Yamakawa for their support. This study was performed between April 2014 and December 2014 in Tottori University Hospital. This study was supported by a Ministry of Education, Culture, Sports, Science and Technology grant.

## References

[1] N. Blay, C. M. Duffield, R. Gallagher, and M. Roche, "A systematic review of time studies to assess the impact of patient transfers on nurse workload," *International Journal of Nursing Practice*, vol. 20, no. 6, pp. 662–673, 2014.

[2] C.-K. Feng, M.-L. Chen, and I.-F. Mao, "Prevalence of and risk factors for different measures of low back pain among female nursing aides in Taiwanese nursing homes," *BMC Musculoskeletal Disorders*, vol. 8, article 52, 2007.

[3] K. Kjellberg, M. Lagerström, and M. Hagberg, "Work technique of nurses in patient transfer tasks and associations with personal factors," *Scandinavian Journal of Work, Environment and Health*, vol. 29, no. 6, pp. 468–477, 2003.

[4] L. Hui, G. Y. F. Ng, S. S. M. Yeung, and C. W. Y. Hui-Chan, "Evaluation of physiological work demands and low back neuromuscular fatigue on nurses working in geriatric wards," *Applied Ergonomics*, vol. 32, no. 5, pp. 479–483, 2001.

[5] M. Campo, S. Weiser, K. L. Koenig, and M. Nordin, "Work-related musculoskeletal disorders in physical therapists: a prospective cohort study with 1-year follow-up," *Physical Therapy*, vol. 88, no. 5, pp. 608–619, 2008.

[6] A. R. Darragh, M. Campo, and P. King, "Work-related activities associated with injury in occupational and physical therapists," *Work*, vol. 42, no. 3, pp. 373–384, 2012.

[7] T. R. Black, S. M. Shah, A. J. Busch, J. Metcalfe, and H. J. Lim, "Effect of transfer, lifting, and repositioning (TLR) injury prevention program on musculoskeletal injury among direct care workers," *Journal of Occupational and Environmental Hygiene*, vol. 8, no. 4, pp. 226–235, 2011.

[8] K. Kjellberg, M. Lagerström, and M. Hagberg, "Patient safety and comfort during transfers in relation to nurses' work technique," *Journal of Advanced Nursing*, vol. 47, no. 3, pp. 251–259, 2004.

[9] K. Siddharthan, A. Nelson, H. Tiesman, and F. F. Chen, "Advances in patient safety cost effectiveness of a multifaceted program for safe patient handling," in *Advances in Patient Safety: From Research to Implementation*, K. Henriksen, J. B. Battles, E. S. Marks, and D. I. Lewin, Eds., vol. 3, pp. 348–358, Agency for Healthcare Research and Quality, Rockville, Md, USA, 2005.

[10] H. Wang, C.-Y. Tsai, H. Jeannis et al., "Stability analysis of electrical powered wheelchair-mounted robotic-assisted transfer device," *Journal of Rehabilitation Research and Development*, vol. 51, no. 5, pp. 761–774, 2014.

[11] J. M. Burnfield, B. McCrory, Y. Shu, T. W. Buster, A. P. Taylor, and A. J. Goldman, "Comparative kinematic and electromyographic assessment of clinician- and device-assisted sit-to-stand transfers in patients with stroke," *Physical Therapy*, vol. 93, no. 10, pp. 1331–1341, 2013.

[12] J. M. Burnfield, Y. Shu, T. W. Buster, A. P. Taylor, M. M. McBride, and M. E. Krause, "Kinematic and electromyographic analyses of normal and device-assisted sit-to-stand transfers," *Gait and Posture*, vol. 36, no. 3, pp. 516–522, 2012.

[13] S. Takasugi, T. Ueshima, R. Kusaba et al., "Robotic wheelchair device assist safety transfer and driving," *Clinical Rehabilitation*, vol. 19, pp. 1114–1117, 2010 (Japanese).

[14] K. Itami, K. Fujita, K. Yokoi et al., "A study of wheelchair transfer assistance using simulated patients trained to portray hemiplegic patients: patients safety, comfort and independence V.S. prevention of low back pain among nurses," *Ningen Kangogaku Kenkyu*, vol. 3, pp. 19–28, 2004 (Japanese).

[15] H. Christin, B. Klaus, and D. Tim, "Ergonomic evaluation of upper limb movements in the automobile production measured by means of motion capturing," in *Proceedings of the 3rd International Digital Human Modeling Symposium*, Tokyo, Japan, May 2014.

# 11

# Dynamic Changes in Heart Rate Variability and Nasal Airflow Resistance during Nasal Allergen Provocation Test

**Tiina M. Seppänen,**[1,2] **Olli-Pekka Alho,**[2,3,4] **and Tapio Seppänen**[1,2]

[1]*Center for Machine Vision and Signal Analysis, University of Oulu, Oulu, Finland*
[2]*Medical Research Center Oulu, Oulu University Hospital and University of Oulu, Oulu, Finland*
[3]*Department of Otorhinolaryngology, Oulu University Hospital, Oulu, Finland*
[4]*Research Unit of Otorhinolaryngology and Ophthalmology, University of Oulu, Oulu, Finland*

Correspondence should be addressed to Tiina M. Seppänen; tiina.seppanen@ee.oulu.fi

Academic Editor: Mohamad Sawan

Allergic rhinitis is a major chronic respiratory disease and an immunoneuronal disorder. We aimed at providing further knowledge on the function of the neural system in nasal allergic reaction. Here, a method to assess simultaneously the nasal airflow resistance and the underlying function of autonomic nervous system (ANS) is presented and used during the nasal provocation of allergic and nonallergic subjects. Continuous nasal airflow resistance and spectral heart rate variability parameters show in detail the timing and intensity differences in subjects' reactions. After the provocation, the nasal airflow resistance of allergic subjects showed a positive trend, whereas LF/HF (Low Frequency/High Frequency) ratio and LF power showed a negative trend. This could imply a gradual sympathetic withdrawal in allergic subjects after the allergen provocation. The groups differed significantly by these physiological descriptors. The proposed method opens entirely new opportunities to research accurately concomitant changes in nasal breathing function and ANS.

## 1. Introduction

Allergic rhinitis is a major global health problem affecting about 10–20% of the population in all countries, ethnic groups, and ages. Using a conservative estimate, it occurs in over 500 million people and its prevalence is increasing in most countries. It is a major chronic respiratory disease that weakens quality of life, school/work productivity, and performance. Additionally, it is a substantial economic burden to societies. Allergic rhinitis is an inheritable systemic inflammatory condition which links, for example, with asthma [1]. However, it is very commonly underdiagnosed and undertreated, because of which specific programs and guidelines on the problem have been released, for example, by World Health Organization and European Union [1–3].

Allergic rhinitis is diagnosed when specific antigens are detected in the blood and the patient has symptoms that correspond with exposure to the sensitizing allergen. It is characterized by one or more symptoms, including nasal obstruction, rhinorrhea, sneezing, nasal itching, and eye irritation [4]. Nasal provocation tests can be used to verify the presence of allergy. Subjects are challenged with the suspected allergen and changes in the symptoms are recorded and possibly the amount of secretions and the respiratory function of the nose are measured. Nasal provocation tests are the standard procedure to evaluate the clinical response of the nasal mucosa to allergens with high specificity and sensitivity [5]. It is of special relevance in the detection of patient with local allergic rhinitis and has been used for the clinical monitoring of antiallergic drugs and allergen-specific immunotherapy and also provides information on the etiology of occupational respiratory diseases of allergic origin. To rule out nonspecific nasal hyperreactivity, nasal provocation tests are usually started with challenging the nasal mucosa with a control solution.

Nasal breathing function is difficult to quantify directly by the patient's own comprehension, history, and clinical examination, which calls for objective measurement methods.

Examples of these include acoustic rhinometry, peak nasal inspiratory flow measurement (PNIF), and rhinomanometry [6, 7]. Acoustic rhinometry assesses nasal geometry by measuring cross-sectional area of the nose as a function of the distance from the nostril. PNIF is a method that measures the nasal airflow during maximal forced nasal inspiration. Rhinomanometer measures the simultaneous nasal pressure and airflow from the values of which nasal airflow resistance is determined [8]. The resistance is characteristically described as a number that derives from one or more breathing cycles of data. Additionally, nasal cavities are measured one at a time and the total nasal resistance is calculated based on unilateral resistances. Thus, it is not possible to get accurate instantaneous values. In practice, there are several minutes between the consecutive resistance values that a rhinomanometer can provide. In nasal provocation tests, the major response to measure is the rise in nasal airflow resistance, which can be rapid (seconds or minutes), and the timing differs in different individuals. This makes it difficult to be detected with the above-mentioned methods. One possibility is to determine the resistance with the rhinomanometer in certain time intervals, but this cannot be done very rapidly and it has been indicated to give inconsistent and variable results with low reproducibility [9–11]. Thus, there is a need for a measurement giving accurate and continuous measurement data about the nasal breathing function.

The nose is armed with a complex nervous system that includes parasympathetic, sympathetic, and sensory nerves. Through the nervous system, the nose communicates with the cardiovascular apparatus, the lungs, and the gastrointestinal tract. Through neural interactions, events that are initiated in the nose can be transmitted to other organs and vice versa. The allergic response comprises changes at all levels of the neural arc: central nervous system integration, sensory nerve function, and autonomic/enteric neuroeffector cell function. Central sensitization can lead to the parasympathetic dominance which originated from the central nervous system. Neural hyperresponsiveness is believed to play a pivotal role in the allergic rhinitis. It would appear that the nervous system itself is altered and is rendered hyperactive in many allergic patients [12, 13].

Heart rate variability (HRV) analysis is an indirect noninvasive way to assess autonomic nervous system (ANS) modulation. It quantifies the degree of fluctuation of the beat-to-beat differences in cardiac rhythm [14]. The interactions between respiration, heart rate, and blood pressure fluctuations, which reflect the cardiovascular and cardiorespiratory couplings, are considered to be of paramount importance for the study of the ANS [15]. Relatively few studies have examined the association between the allergic rhinitis and autonomic nervous system, especially using HRV analysis. Lan et al. evaluated the effect of position on the autonomic nervous system of allergic and control volunteers by HRV analysis. They concluded that patients with allergic rhinitis may have poor sympathetic modulation in the sitting position [16]. Taşcilar et al. measured 24-hour ECG recordings from pediatric allergic rhinitis patients with allergic rhinitis and healthy controls. Their HRV analysis' results implied sympathetic withdrawal and parasympathetic predominance in

pediatric allergic rhinitis patients with allergic rhinitis [17]. Yokusoglu et al. in their turn measured 24-hour ambulatory ECG recordings from adults with allergic rhinitis and healthy controls. They found out that HRV indices predicting the parasympathetic predominance were increased in patients with allergic rhinitis [18].

Recently, we presented a novel method to assess nasal airflow resistance continuously and accurately [19]. The pressure signal is measured with a thin nasopharyngeal catheter inserted into the nasopharynx and the airflow signal with the rib cage and abdominal effort belts calibrated with our new method [20]. The resistance is calculated for each signal sample at any sampling frequency. This makes it possible to discover rapid changes in nasal airflow resistance, which is essential, for example, during provocation tests. In this study, the continuous nasal airflow resistance is produced using the above-mentioned methods and dynamically changing autonomic nervous system parameters are computed to study their simultaneous changes during an allergen provocation test. To our knowledge, this kind of study has not been done before, apparently because it has not been possible to produce nasal airflow resistance curves in this precision. Our objectives are to examine, firstly, whether there are associations between the dynamic reactions of nasal airflow resistance and autonomic nervous system parameters during the allergic reaction and, secondly, whether there are differences between the birch pollen allergic and the nonallergic groups.

## 2. Methods

*2.1. Materials.* An experimental study design was used. The study protocol was approved by the Regional Ethics Committee of the Northern Ostrobothnia Hospital District. In Finland, the birch pollen is one of the most common causes of the intermittent seasonal allergic symptoms; for this very reason, it was chosen as a provocation substance. For this preliminary study, ten (three females) birch pollen allergic and ten (three females) nonbirch pollen allergic adult volunteers were recruited. The diagnostic criteria for birch pollen allergic rhinitis were evidence of sensitization to birch pollen measured by the presence of allergen-specific IgE in the serum and a history of nasal symptoms during the birch pollen season [21]. All the volunteers gave written informed consent for participation in the study. The mean (SD) age of the allergic and nonallergic subjects was 24 (1) and 24 (3) years, respectively. The subjects had to be nonpregnant and free of surgical operations of nose, brain circulatory disorders, and heart diseases. Medication that affects the nose was not allowed to be used during a specific time period before the measurement. The subjects had to be free of any acute respiratory symptoms during the prior two weeks to the measurement. Before measurement, subjects refrained from having a smoke for at least four hours and heavy meal, caffeine, or other stimulants for at least two hours.

Measurements were made outside the birch pollen season. The subjects were examined by an ear, nose, and throat specialist. Before measurements, the specific IgE for birch pollen was determined from blood for all of them. Based on the blood samples, antibody levels of allergic subjects varied from moderate to very high.

ECG, pressure, and respiratory effort belt signals were recorded with the commercial polygraphic recorder (Embletta Gold, Denver, Colorado, USA). It had inductive respiratory effort belts for rib cage and abdomen with the sampling rate of 50 Hz. The sampling rates of pressure and ECG were 50 Hz and 200 Hz, respectively. For calibrating the rib cage and abdominal effort belt signals, simultaneous respiratory airflow signal was recorded with a spirometer (SpiroStar USB M9460, Medikro Oy, Kuopio, Finland) with the sampling rate of 100 Hz.

*2.2. Challenge Protocol.* A water-based immunologically standardized commercial 1 : 10000 SQU/mL birch extract (Allergologisk Laboratorium A/S, Copenhagen, Denmark) was used in the provocation. The diluent solution (Allergologisk Laboratorium A/S, Copenhagen, Denmark) of the allergen extract was used as a control solution. Both solutions were administered bilaterally into the nasal cavities by pump spray.

At the beginning of measurement, the rib cage effort belt was placed on the xiphoid process and the abdominal effort belt was placed near the umbilicus. Next, the subjects sat peacefully for a period of 30 min prior to the measurement to adapt themselves to the environment and to allow heart rate and blood pressure to stabilize. During the actual measurements, they were instructed to sit in back upright position avoiding speaking and movements. First, respiratory effort belt signals were recorded along with the spirometer signal for one minute. The data was used for calibrating the rib cage and abdominal effort belt signals to flow signals, as described in Section 2.3. After calibration, the spirometer was removed from the subject and a thin catheter (diameter: 1 mm) was inserted 8 cm deep along the floor of nasal cavity into the nasopharynx, with the tip of the catheter lying 1 cm anterior from the back wall of nasopharynx. Figure 1 shows the setup for the nasal pressure measurement with the catheter.

To inhibit the nasal secrete blocking, the nasal catheter air was blown with the syringe through the catheter before each measurement protocol phase and every time that the catheter blocking was detected.

The measurement protocol consisted of the three phases. At the first protocol phase, the ECG, pressure, and respiratory effort belt signals were recorded for 10 min to get the baseline situation. At the second phase, to rule out the nonspecific nasal hyperreactivity, the nasal mucosa was challenged with a control solution. It was sprayed carefully on the anterior mucosa of both nasal cavities, after which the ECG, pressure, and respiratory effort belt signals were recorded for 5 min. At the third phase, the birch pollen solution was sprayed carefully on the anterior nasal mucosa of both nasal cavities. After that, the ECG, pressure, and respiratory effort belt signals were recorded for 20 min. After spraying the solution, the recording was initiated as soon as possible but first waiting for the immediate reactions such as sneezing and snuffling to settle.

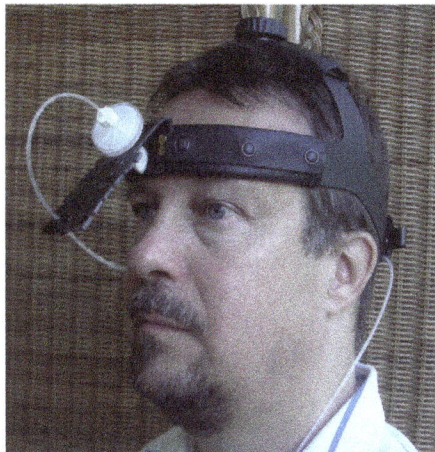

Figure 1: Measurement setup of nasal pressure signal with nasopharyngeal catheter.

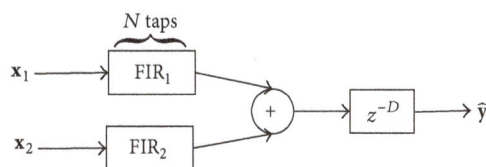

Figure 2: Improved respiratory effort belt calibration method.

Before analysis, all the signals were validated manually by using specially made visualization software. All the detected disturbances, which originated, for example, from moving, snuffling, sneezing, and blowing of air with the syringe through the catheter, were deleted from signals before analysis. Additionally, special care was taken to maintain the correct synchrony between the signals.

*2.3. Calculation of the Continuous Nasal Airflow Resistance.* In this study, we use our previously published novel method to estimate continuous nasal airflow resistance using pressure signal from the nasopharyngeal catheter inserted transnasally into the nasopharynx and calibrated rib cage and abdominal effort belt signals [19]. Recently, we published an improved respiratory effort belt calibration method [20], which reduces waveform errors considerably and is robust to breathing style changes. It is based on an optimally trained FIR (Finite Impulse Response) filter bank constructed as a MISO (Multiple-Input Single-Output) system between respiratory effort belt signals and the spirometer and a delay element ($z^{-D}$); see Figure 2. The method extends the traditional multiple linear regression method by using a number $N$ of consecutive signal samples and linear filtering for each prediction.

With the respiratory effort belts used in this study, the following realization of the filter bank was used:

$$y[j] = \boldsymbol{\alpha}_1^T \mathbf{x}_1[j] + \boldsymbol{\alpha}_2^T \mathbf{x}_2[j] + \varepsilon[j], \tag{1}$$

where $\boldsymbol{\alpha}_1^T$ and $\boldsymbol{\alpha}_2^T$ denote the $N$ tap coefficients of filters $\mathrm{FIR}_1$ and $\mathrm{FIR}_2$, respectively. Superscript $T$ indicates the matrix transpose in the formula, and $j$ denotes the time index of the signals. Variable $y$ indicates the respiratory airflow from spirometer. Vectors $\mathbf{x}_1$ and $\mathbf{x}_2$ include $N$ consecutive signal samples from the rib cage signal and abdomen signal, respectively: $\mathbf{x}_k[j] = [x_k[j], x_k[j-1], \ldots, x_k[j-N+1]]^T$, where $k = 1, 2$ and $j = N, \ldots, n$. With this measurement data, the variable $n$ was 3000, which was the number of observations used in the calibration.

During the calibration, tap coefficients $\boldsymbol{\alpha}_1^T$ and $\boldsymbol{\alpha}_2^T$ are estimated with the method of least squares from the available data. The least-squares estimator of the parameter vector $\boldsymbol{\alpha} = [\boldsymbol{\alpha}_1^T, \boldsymbol{\alpha}_2^T]^T$ is given by

$$\widehat{\boldsymbol{\alpha}} = \left(\mathbf{X}^T \mathbf{X}\right)^{-1} \mathbf{X}^T \mathbf{y}, \tag{2}$$

where $\mathbf{X}$ is $(n - N + 1) \times (2 \times N)$ matrix formed from the vectors $\mathbf{x}_1$ and $\mathbf{x}_2$:

$$\mathbf{X} = \begin{bmatrix} \mathbf{x}_1^T[N] & \mathbf{x}_2^T[N] \\ \mathbf{x}_1^T[N+1] & \mathbf{x}_2^T[N+1] \\ \vdots & \vdots \\ \mathbf{x}_1^T[n] & \mathbf{x}_2^T[n] \end{bmatrix}. \tag{3}$$

The length of the vector $\widehat{\boldsymbol{\alpha}}$ is $2 \times N$. Thus, the flow signal predicted from the rib cage and abdominal effort belt signals through the FIR filter bank is

$$\widehat{\mathbf{y}} = \mathbf{X}\widehat{\boldsymbol{\alpha}}. \tag{4}$$

In our previous study [22], the 0.3 sec length of FIR filters was found to produce the best airflow prediction with the same respiratory effort belts. Thus, we used $N$ value of 16 in this study.

Mathematical model of Broms et al. [23] offers parametric means to describe the nonlinear pressure/flow relationship; see Figure 3. In the model, the pressure/flow relationship is established as follows:

$$v_r = v_0 + cr, \tag{5}$$

where $v_r$ is the angle with radius $r$, $v_0$ is the angle in the origin, and $c$ is the curvature parameter. The resistance in radius $r$, denoted by $R_r$, is given by

$$R_r = x \tan v_r. \tag{6}$$

The constant $x$ is a normalization factor defined in [19].

However, the Broms model expects the data to be stationary, while the nasal system is nonstationary. Our method to estimate continuous nasal airflow resistance is a least-mean-square (LMS) extension to the Broms model [23] so that it can be used for calculating a continuous nasal airflow resistance through model adaptation to time-varying characteristics of the nasal functioning. In the extended model, an instantaneous nasal airflow resistance can be calculated after estimating the model parameters at each time instant from the input signals. The normalized [19] pressure signal, $P'$, and the estimate of flow signal, $F'$, are the LMS filter

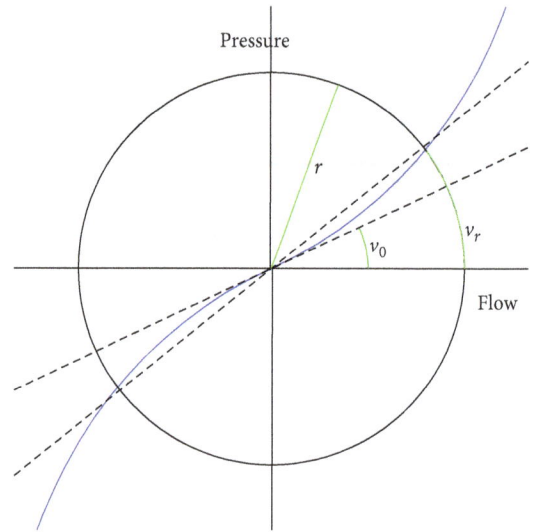

FIGURE 3: A graph of Broms model of resistance.

inputs. The filter length of one time sample has proven to be sufficient. The update formulas of parameters $v_0$ and $c$ are

$$v_0(i+1) = v_0(i) + \mu(i)\left\{v_r(i) - \left[v_0(i) + c(i)r(i)\right]\right\},$$
$$c(i+1) = c(i) \tag{7}$$
$$+ \mu(i)r(i)\left\{v_r(i) - \left[v_0(i) + c(i)r(i)\right]\right\},$$

where

$$v_r(i) = \tan^{-1}\left(\frac{P'(i)}{F'(i)}\right),$$
$$r(i) = \sqrt{P'^2(i) + F'^2(i)}. \tag{8}$$

The learning rate parameter $\mu$ and the initial values for $v_0$ and $c$ are defined in [19].

Hence, the instantaneous resistance values are calculated over the whole measurement data at any sampling frequency allowing for analysis of dynamic changes in the continuous nasal airflow resistance.

*2.4. Heart Rate Variability Analysis.* At first, the baseline fluctuation of the measured ECG signals was removed with a Savitzky-Golay filter (polynomial order 2). R-peaks were automatically detected from the filtered ECG signals based on the expected time between adjacent R-waves and amplitude threshold. The results were verified visually and corrected manually for false alarms and missed peaks. Tachogram was derived from the R-R intervals and converted to equidistantly sampled series by interpolation, in this case to the frequency of 4 Hz.

The tachogram was filtered with the bandpass Finite Impulse Response (FIR) filters with the cutoff frequencies corresponding to LF and HF bands. The LF band was set between 0.04 Hz and 0.15 Hz and HF band was set between 0.15 Hz and 0.4 Hz, as recommended by the Task Force [14].

The variance, which is the correlate of the signal power, was then computed in 3 min windows from the filtered signals. Thereafter, the window was shifted ahead by 18 sec (overlap of 90%) and the variance was computed again, which produced the LF and HF power signals. Typically, LF component is considered to reflect mostly the sympathetic modulation, HF component is considered to reflect mostly the parasympathetic modulation, and LF/HF ratio is considered to reflect mostly the sympathovagal balance, although this interpretation is not fully agreed among researches [14].

*2.5. Statistics.* Statistical significance of the changes in nasal airflow resistance, LF, HF, and LF/HF ratio and their trends in the subjects was assessed by Wilcoxon signed-rank test. Statistical significance between the subject groups in its turn, was assessed by Mann-Whitney test (Wilcoxon rank-sum test). The null hypothesis was that there are no differences in the medians of given data sets. The results were reported as statistically significant if a two-sided $p$ value was less than 0.05. Additionally, logistic regression was used to determine the best factors for predicting whether the subject is birch pollen allergic or not.

# 3. Results

ECG, respiratory effort signals, and pressure were recorded according to the measurement protocol described in Section 2.2. At first, the rib cage and abdominal effort belt signals were calibrated to flow of spirometer from the calibration recording. Then, continuous nasal airflow resistance signals were computed from the nasal pressure and calibrated respiratory effort belt signals. LF, HF, and LF/HF ratio signals were computed from the ECG signal. In this paper, we studied only the third protocol phase, where the allergic reactions for the birch pollen challenge were expected to appear.

Interestingly, it was observed that there is a linear trend in the resistance signals and the HRV signals in all allergic subjects. Thus, linear line fitting was performed to the trends to determine the slopes and their differences. For the allergic subjects, those parts of the nasal airflow resistance curves were selected to the trend analysis, where the resistance increased from the start of the protocol phase until some saturation point. However, individual variation of the time span of the resistance increase was large and for such reason analysis window varied between the subjects.

Importantly, it was observed that the trends in ANS parameters turned out not to be the same in length as trends in resistance. To our knowledge, this is the first time this kind of differences in timing between continuous nasal airflow resistance and ANS function is found out. We therefore selected different time windows for trend analysis for HRV signals in order to guarantee that only linear segments are considered. The starting time for the window was always the same as with the resistance signal for each subject, but the ending time depended on the actual end of the trend.

For the nonallergic subjects, no obvious trends were observed. Thus, the whole nasal airflow resistance, LF, HF, and LF/HF ratio signals from the third protocol phase were chosen to the trend analysis, excluding first the artefacts and the possible nonspecific nasal hyperreactivity at the beginning of the phase.

An example case of concomitant dynamic changes in the nasal airflow resistance, LF, HF, and LF/HF ratio curves of birch pollen allergic subject after allergen provocation is shown in Figure 4. A clear upward trend can be observed in the nasal airflow resistance curve and downward trends can be seen in the LF and LF/HF ratio curves. A robust line fitting algorithm was applied to the curves to quantify the extent of slopes.

A representative case of concomitant nasal airflow resistance, LF, HF, and LF/HF ratio curves of nonallergic subject after allergen provocation is shown in Figure 5. A gap at the beginning of resistance curve can be seen due to removing of artifacts during manual validation.

Table 1 presents the slopes and changes of nasal airflow resistance, LF, HF, and LF/HF ratio curves for each birch pollen allergic subject, together with their average values and standard deviations (SD) over the subject group. As can be seen from Table 1, LF and LF/HF ratio decreased consistently during the increase of nasal airflow resistance for all the birch pollen allergic subjects ($p = 0.000$), while the HF power changes had both positive and negative slopes. There was a statistically significant change in the resistance ($p = 0.002$), LF ($p = 0.002$), and LF/HF ratio ($p = 0.002$). There was no statistically significant change in HF ($p = 0.432$).

Table 2 presents the slopes and changes of resistance, LF, HF, and LF/HF ratio curves for each nonallergic subject, together with their average values and standard deviations over the subject group. In this group, LF and LF/HF ratio increased for 9/10 subjects. There was only one subject with decreasing LF and one subject with decreasing LF/HF ratio. A noticeable issue is that these two were different subjects and there was no subject with the simultaneous decreasing LF and decreasing LF/HF ratio. There was a statistically significant change in the LF ($p = 0.037$) and LF/HF ratio ($p = 0.006$) and no statistically significant change in resistance ($p = 0.865$) and HF ($p = 0.432$).

Between the groups, a statistically significant difference was found in several parameters, the slope of resistance ($p < 0.001$), resistance at the end ($p = 0.029$), change of resistance ($p < 0.001$), slope of LF ($p < 0.001$), change of LF ($p < 0.001$), slope of LF/HF ratio ($p < 0.001$), and change of LF/HF ratio ($p < 0.001$), between the birch pollen allergic and nonallergic groups. However, there was no statistically significant difference in the resistance at the beginning ($p = 0.579$), slope of HF ($p = 0.529$), and change of HF ($p = 0.912$) between the two groups.

Logistic regression was applied to determine parameters, which predict the allergy status (allergic or nonallergic) of the subjects most reliably. When the used parameter was the slope of LF/HF ratio, the logistic regression model predicted correctly 9/10 birch pollen allergic and 9/10 nonallergic subjects. When the parameter used was the slope of LF, the model predicted correctly 10/10 birch pollen allergic and 9/10 nonallergic subjects. The best result was achieved when both parameters, the slope of LF and the slope of LF/HF ratio, were

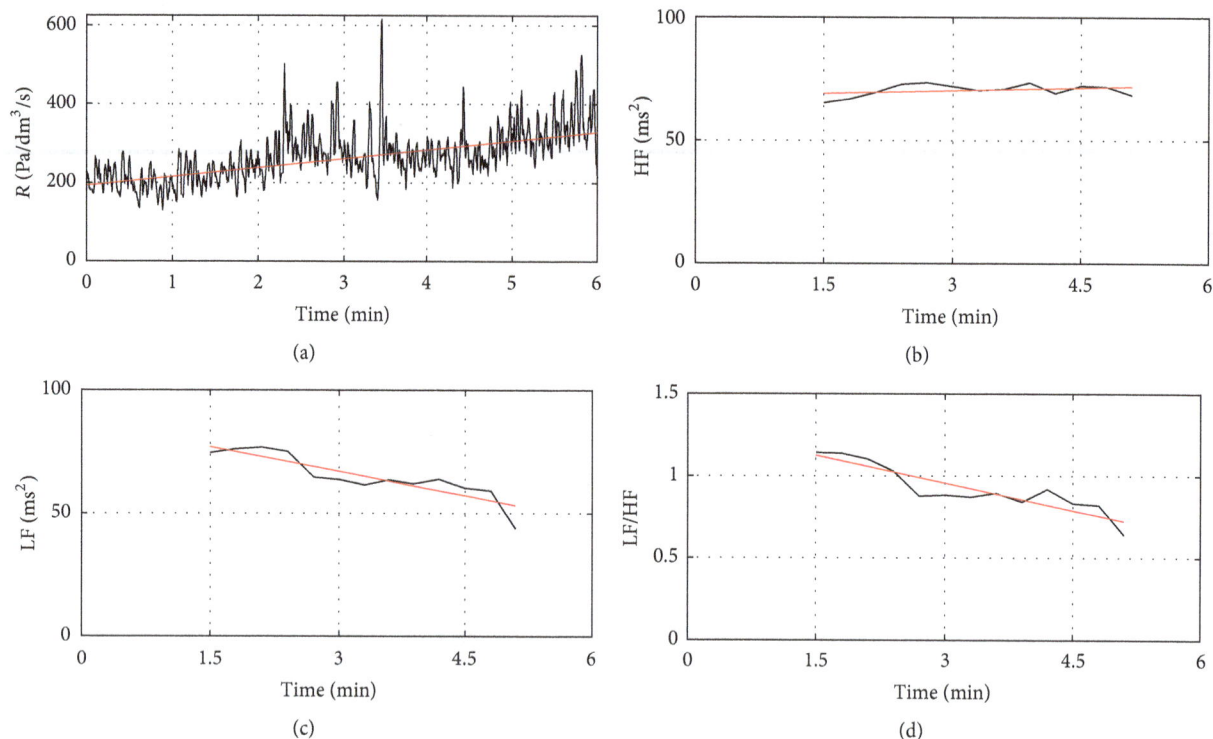

FIGURE 4: An increase of nasal airflow resistance and related LF, HF, and LF/HF ratio curves for birch pollen allergic subject 1. (a) Resistance curve (black) and robust fit of the resistance curve (red). (c) LF curve (black) and robust fit of the LF curve (red). (b) HF curve (black) and robust fit of the HF curve (red). (d) LF/HF ratio curve (black) and robust fit of the LF/HF ratio curve.

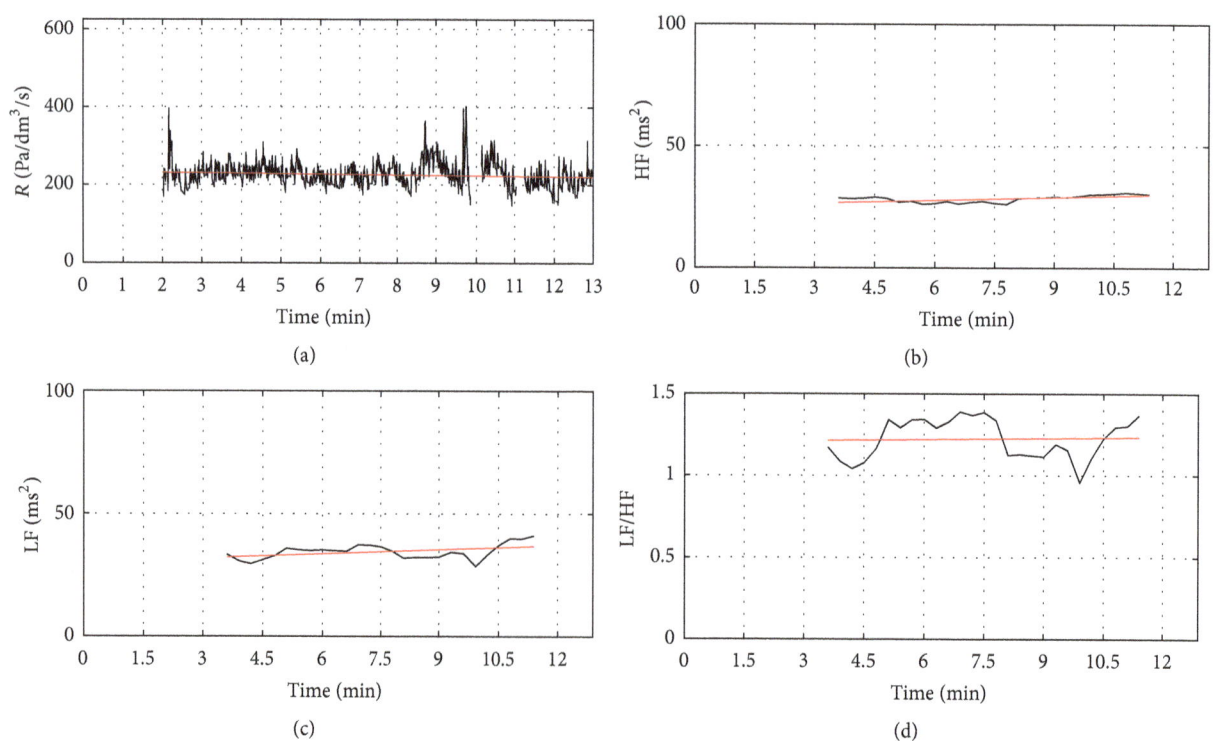

FIGURE 5: Nasal airflow resistance and related LF, HF, and LF/HF ratio curves for nonallergic subject 3. (a) Resistance curve (black) and robust fit of the resistance curve (red). (c) LF curve (black) and robust fit of the LF curve (red). (b) HF curve (black) and robust fit of the HF curve (red). (d) LF/HF ratio curve (black) and robust fit of the LF/HF ratio curve.

TABLE 1: Nasal airflow resistance, LF, HF, and LF/HF ratio results for birch pollen allergic subjects.

| Subject | Slope of resistance | Change of resistance [Pa/dm$^3$/s] | Slope of LF | Change of LF | Slope of HF | Change of HF | Slope of LF/HF ratio | Change of LF/HF ratio |
|---|---|---|---|---|---|---|---|---|
| 1 | 0.0121 | 135 | −259.9 | −3118 | 32.5 | 390 | −0.063 | −0.75 |
| 2 | 0.0108 | 110 | −28.6 | −1115 | −3.9 | −51 | −0.024 | −0.94 |
| 3 | 0.0045 | 67 | −25.0 | −300 | 1.1 | 13 | −0.262 | −3.14 |
| 4 | 0.0159 | 266 | −11.4 | −262 | 10.2 | 235 | −0.021 | −0.49 |
| 5 | 0.0087 | 113 | −359.8 | −1799 | 60.1 | 300 | −0.238 | −1.19 |
| 6 | 0.0087 | 73 | −10.6 | −117 | 22.2 | 244 | −0.016 | −0.17 |
| 7 | 0.0132 | 269 | −12.3 | −172 | 0.7 | 10 | −0.041 | −0.58 |
| 8 | 0.0019 | 41 | −12.7 | −481 | 1.3 | 49 | −0.075 | −2.84 |
| 9 | 0.0037 | 34 | −25.7 | −154 | −110.2 | −661 | −0.002 | −0.01 |
| 10 | 0.0002 | 9 | −14.2 | −798 | −0.9 | −51 | −0.018 | −1.03 |
| Average ± SD | 0.0080 ± 0.0052 | 112 ± 91 | −76.0 ± 125.6 | −832 ± 965 | 1.3 ± 44.0 | 48 ± 294 | −0.076 ± 0.094 | −1.11 ± 1.05 |

TABLE 2: Nasal airflow resistance, LF, HF, and LF/HF ratio results for nonallergic subjects.

| Subject | Slope of resistance | Change of resistance [Pa/dm$^3$/s] | Slope of LF | Change of LF | Slope of HF | Change of HF | Slope of LF/HF ratio | Change of LF/HF ratio |
|---|---|---|---|---|---|---|---|---|
| 1 | 0.0001 | 3 | 17.3 | 623 | 0.7 | 27 | 0.045 | 1.62 |
| 2 | 0.0001 | 4 | 5.7 | 262 | −1.1 | −52 | 0.024 | 1.09 |
| 3 | −0.0005 | −11 | 12.2 | 318 | 7.0 | 181 | 0.002 | 0.05 |
| 4 | 0.0005 | 14 | 62.3 | 2805 | 36.7 | 1653 | 0.009 | 0.40 |
| 5 | −0.0031 | −92 | 1.7 | 71 | −1.0 | −41 | 0.026 | 1.09 |
| 6 | 0.0014 | 33 | 54.5 | 1800 | 57.8 | 1907 | 0.018 | 0.59 |
| 7 | 0.0000 | 1 | 20.3 | 753 | 14.3 | 530 | −0.005 | −0.17 |
| 8 | 0.0004 | 12 | 26.9 | 994 | −14.5 | −535 | 0.015 | 0.56 |
| 9 | −0.0005 | −16 | 0.4 | 21 | −10.7 | −556 | 0.007 | 0.36 |
| 10 | −0.0001 | −3 | −15.4 | −861 | −4.4 | −245 | 0.010 | 0.55 |
| Average ± SD | −0.0002 ± 0.0012 | −5 ± 33 | 18.6 ± 24.2 | 679 ± 1020 | 8.5 ± 22.5 | 287 ± 851 | 0.015 ± 0.014 | 0.61 ± 0.53 |

used, in which case the model predicted correctly 10/10 birch pollen allergic and 10/10 nonallergic subjects.

## 4. Discussion and Future Work

Here, we conducted an experimental trial, where birch pollen allergic subjects and nonallergic control subjects had topical nasal challenge with birch pollen extract. We monitored both the immediate nasal reaction and simultaneous autonomic nervous system function by recording continuous nasal airflow resistance and by analyzing heart rate variability, respectively. We found that in allergic subjects the nasal airflow resistance increased and concomitantly the LF energy and LF/HF ratio decreased after allergen challenge indicating sympathetic withdrawal. In addition, the change in HF energy or the heart rate signal itself did not show similar dynamics. The sympathetic stimulus in the nose is known to cause vasoconstriction and thus increased nasal patency. Thus, our findings indicate that in allergic subjects the nasal

obstruction following topical nasal exposure to allergen is at least partially due to the dysfunction of the autonomic nervous system. The LF energy and LF/HF ratio were strong parameters that differentiated the allergy group from the nonallergy group. Additionally, we found out that there are differences in timing between the length of increase in nasal airflow resistance and the length of trend in LF energy and LF/HF ratio signals. This finding was only possible with our proposed technique to estimate continuous nasal airflow resistance and HRV parameters. To our knowledge, this is the first time this kind of differences is found out. Study of meaning and importance of this phenomenon remains as future work.

Our findings are in accordance with those of Pichon et al. who followed subjects with lower respiratory symptoms after diagnostic methacholine bronchial challenge using heart rate variability analysis and found that the hyperresponsive subjects had altered autonomic balance [24]. However, Pichon et al. found that the hyperresponsive subjects had higher parasympathetic tone (HF component) than those without airway responsiveness, both at baseline and after the challenge, whereas we found the decrease of sympathetic tone (LF component) to be responsible for the altered autonomic reaction in the allergic subjects after topical nasal challenge. Our findings are also in accordance with studies by Lan et al. [16], Taşcilar et al. [17], and Yokusoglu et al. [18], who concluded that autonomic dysfunction may play a role in allergic rhinitis.

Measuring nasal reactions after topical nasal challenge is difficult in clinical work. The measurement inevitably affects the delicate nose and easily causes a false reaction. For example, the weighing of nasal secretion after the challenge is done by a suctioning device which irritates the nose and can itself cause nasal obstruction and secretion. Similarly, the measurement of nasal breathing with conventional rhinomanometry or acoustic rhinometry involves occlusion of one nostril that interferes with the normal nasal breathing. These disadvantages can be totally avoided if nasal allergy can be measured from the heart rate without touching the nose at all, like our present results indicate.

The work included a number of limitations. Firstly, the study included only ten birch pollen allergic and ten nonallergic subjects. Still, the sample enabled us to find significant associations between the HRV results and the resistance values and allergy status. The study should be repeated with a larger data set in order to draw more general conclusions. Secondly, it was observed that the timing of ANS response to provocation was not the same as with nasal airflow resistance. We selected signal segments manually for the line fitting procedure. Automating the segment selection would be highly beneficial for practical applications and is left for future work. Thirdly, the window size for HRV analysis was chosen as 3 min for the following reasons. Our data contained strong dynamics after the challenge of birch pollen allergic subjects. Traditional 5 min window was too long for our purposes because the rise of nasal airflow resistance was shorter than 5 min for some allergic subjects. However, due to the dynamics, 1 min window produced very unstable data. The choice of 3 min window was an experimental compromise. However, robustness to dynamic variation and, indeed, analysis of the variation itself still remains as future work.

## 5. Conclusion

We presented a method to assess simultaneous dynamic changes in nasal airflow resistance and autonomic nervous system function during a provocation test. The continuous nasal airflow resistance was estimated with a method that applies LMS filtering technique to the nasal pressure signals and calibrated rib cage and abdominal effort belt signals to update adaptively an extended Broms model. LF and HF components of heart rate were quantified with bandpass FIR filter in 3 min 90% overlapping windows.

Quantitative results of nasal airflow resistance, LF, HF, and LF/HF ratio changes were presented for birch pollen allergic and nonallergic subjects. The main finding was that when the nasal airflow resistance of birch pollen allergic

subjects increases after the provocation, the LF energy and LF/HF ratio decrease with a clear trend. This could imply gradual sympathetic withdrawal in allergic patients after the provocation with allergen. Our findings further imply that the allergic and nonallergic subjects could be differentiated by following HRV after the provocation. We also found out that there are differences in timing between the length of increase in nasal airflow resistance and the length of trend in LF energy and LF/HF ratio signals. This finding was only possible with our proposed technique to estimate continuous nasal airflow resistance and HRV parameters. The proposed method opens entirely new opportunities to research accurately concomitant changes in nonstationary nasal breathing function and autonomic nervous system in provocation tests.

## Conflict of Interests

The authors declare that there is no potential conflict of interests.

## Acknowledgments

Allergy Research Foundation, Tauno Tönning Research Foundation, Seppo Säynäjäkangas Science Foundation, and International Doctoral Programme in Biomedical Engineering and Medical Physics (iBioMEP) are gratefully acknowledged for financial support.

## References

[1] J. Bousquet, P. Van Cauwenberge, N. Khaltaev, and WHO, "Allergic rhinitis and its impact on asthma," *Journal of Allergy and Clinical Immunology*, vol. 108, no. 5, supplement, pp. S147–S334, 2001.

[2] P. Van Cauwenberge, J. B. Watelet, T. Van Zele, J. Bousquet, P. Burney, and T. Zuberbier, "Spreading excellence in allergy and asthma: the GA2LEN (Global Allergy and Asthma European Network) project," *Allergy*, vol. 60, no. 7, pp. 858–864, 2005.

[3] J. Bousquet, R. Dahl, and N. Khaltaev, "Global alliance against chronic respiratory diseases," *Allergy*, vol. 62, no. 3, pp. 216–223, 2007.

[4] J. Bousquet, N. Khaltaev, A. A. Cruz et al., "Allergic rhinitis and its impact on asthma (ARIA) 2008," *Allergy*, vol. 63, supplement 86, pp. 8–160, 2008.

[5] L. Klimek, A. S. Hammerbacher, P. W. Helling et al., "The influence of European legislation on the use of diagnostic test allergens for nasal allergen provocation in routine care of patients with allergic rhinitis," *Rhinology*, vol. 53, no. 3, pp. 260–269, 2015.

[6] R. Starling-Schwanz, H. L. Peake, C. M. Salome et al., "Repeatability of peak nasal inspiratory flow measurements and utility for assessing the severity of rhinitis," *Allergy*, vol. 60, no. 6, pp. 795–800, 2005.

[7] P. A. R. Clement and F. Gordts, "Consensus report on acoustic rhinometry and rhinomanometry," *Rhinology*, vol. 43, no. 3, pp. 169–179, 2005.

[8] M. Chaaban and J. P. Corey, "Assessing nasal air flow: options and utility," *Proceedings of the American Thoracic Society*, vol. 8, no. 1, pp. 70–78, 2011.

# 12

# Kids' Perceptions toward Children's Ward Healing Environments: A Case Study of Taiwan University Children's Hospital

**Jeng-Chung Woo[1] and Yi-Ling Lin[2]**

[1]*Department of Product Design, Sanming University, Sanming City, Fujian, China*
[2]*Department of Arts and Plastic Design, Taipei University of Education, Taipei City, Taiwan*

Correspondence should be addressed to Jeng-Chung Woo; wu.jc2000@msa.hinet.net

Academic Editor: Jesus Favela

This paper summarizes the opinions of experts who participated in designing the environment of a children's hospital and reports the results of a questionnaire survey conducted among hospital users. The grounded theory method was adopted to analyze 292 concepts, 79 open codes, 25 axial codes, and 4 selective codes; in addition, confirmatory factor analysis and reliability analysis were performed to identify elements for designing a healing environment in a children's hospital, and 21 elements from 4 dimensions, namely, emotions, space design, interpersonal interaction, and pleasant surroundings, were determined. Subsequently, this study examined the perceptions of 401 children at National Taiwan University Children's Hospital. The results revealed that, regarding the children's responses to the four dimensions and their overall perception, younger children accepted the healing environment to a significantly higher degree than did older children. The sex effect was significant for the space design dimension, and it was not significant for the other dimensions.

## 1. Introduction

In the 1990s, "healing environments" became a crucial concept in designing and planning medical facilities. Healthcare operators consider their medical institutions to be healing environments, regardless of whether they can provide a definition for the term "healing environment" [1]. Currently, healing and treatment should be considered simultaneously in the establishment of a new healthcare model [2].

Wetton [3] stated that emotional design provides pleasure to viewers or users, a notion that has been widely accepted and applied in healthcare to satisfy patients' psychological needs. For example, a toy baby seal (Paro) was designed for nursing homes and hospitals in Japan and Europe [4]. Toys and games are the focus of children's lives, and they enable people to communicate with children and help doctors in establishing a relationship with children [5]. In nursing homes, elderly people who care for plants and participate in activities are physically and psychologically active and feel happy [6]. Healing design is widely accepted and involves using various types of software and hardware to heal patients.

A healing environment can be defined as a holistic environment that facilitates patient rehabilitation. In contrast to medical treatment, healing is a psychological concept of health [7]. Evidence-based design has become a theoretical concept in the creation of healing environments [8, 9]; healthcare providers prefer using evidence-based information to make decisions. Children and adolescents are often neglected in fields such as architectural and urban planning, although they are typically more sensitive to environments compared with adults [10]. Scanlon and Bauer [11] emphasized that because young children are more dynamic than adults are, more considerations should be included in healthcare for children. Therefore, developing an evidence-based method for designing a healing environment for a children's hospital is an appealing topic that warrants further research. Planning for National Taiwan University Children's Hospital (NTUCH) began in 1994, and the facility officially opened in December 2008. NTUCH was the first children's hospital in Taiwan to adopt a healing environment design. However, whether the design conforms with users' perception of a healing environment and whether it achieves the objective of such an environment must be evaluated. In addition, previous studies on hospital environments have primarily examined user satisfaction [12–14] and special tasks; however, only few studies have provided useful insights into the design-related interaction between users and their environments [15]. Therefore, the objectives of this study were twofold:

(1) Identify an evidence-based method for designing and establishing a healing environment that meets the requirements of children's hospitals.

(2) Determine whether the atmosphere created by the NTUCH healing environment design conforms with users' perception of a healing environment and whether it achieves the objectives of such an environment.

## 2. Literature Review

The "patient-centered" care concept poses a challenge to many healthcare service provision practices [16]. In 1978, Planetree, a nonprofit organization, was founded. Planetree emphasizes the importance of a patient-centered healing environment. The Society of Arts in Healthcare, founded in the United Kingdom in 1991, integrates art and healthcare facilities in its endeavor to provide an excellent healing environment for patients by reducing their stress, enhancing their sense of security, and improving their physical and mental health [17]. In 1993, the Center for Health Design in the United States was founded to advocate for a secure and healthy healthcare environment. This organization has facilitated the study of healing environment designs, and it launched the Pebble project to promote healing environments worldwide.

Biley [29] stated that rich and diverse visual (e.g., gardens, pictures, and colors) and auditory (e.g., relaxing music and natural sounds) environments facilitate the creation of a healing environment. The enjoyment derived from nature can distract patients from their ailments, thus alleviating their pain [30]. Ulrich [31] demonstrated that nature, green plants, and an extensive space can effectively reduce stress, alleviate pain, improve body immunity, and enhance human resilience. Improving healthcare environments can facilitate patients' recovery, enable patients to relax, and reduce the stress of healthcare staff, thereby indirectly improving doctor-patient relationships, enhancing healthcare quality, and reducing healthcare costs. The National Association of Children's Hospitals and Related Institutions (NACHRI) [32] indicated that active distraction strategies such as providing opportunities for patients to engage in art and music can reduce stress and anxiety and that natural sunlight can alleviate depression. Hence, exploring these topics related to designing a healing environment for children and adolescents is worthwhile.

Creating healing environments in children's hospitals is a current trend [33]. Psychologists have indicated that physical environments can influence treatment processes and results [34]. Moreover, environmental health is considered in healthcare engineering [35]. A physical environment can be divided into two categories: indoor and outdoor environments. Previous studies have reported that factors that influence a healing environment are safety, sound [29], color [2], artwork [36, 37], interactive art [38], lighting [39], outdoor view [40], furnishing [41], and atmosphere [42]. Moore [43] also indicated that playing outdoors positively influences the interaction between children and the society. Nature and gardens can effectively improve the emotions of children and adolescents, alleviate their pain, and produce a healing effect [18, 32]. The design features of healing environments should be able to provide users with multisensory experience as well as positive healing effects [37]. Ozcan [10] also revealed that face-to-face social interaction can enhance healing. In addition, Altimier [12] indicated that an outdoor view, natural sunlight, pastel colors, therapeutic sounds, and interaction with family members can facilitate healing; Altimier reported that these elements must be balanced with staff members' requirements in the design of essential care environments.

Evidence-based design is a theoretical concept applied for creating healing environments [8, 9]. In healing processes, actual environments are related to the well-being of patients, their family members, and healthcare staff [8, 13]; however, the perspectives of these people regarding healthcare design are often neglected during decision-making [9]. A study reported that nursing staff members' self-care was negatively correlated with their compassion fatigue and burnout [44]. Caring can strongly influence the efficiency of healing environments, such as patients' interaction with their caregivers. One of the goals of a healing environment is to restore wholeness through helpful design features that address the thoughts and emotions of patients and care providers. Moreover, Planetree advocates the concept of healthy healthcare service providers [38]. Incorporating a healing environment into healthcare also optimizes clinical care and outcomes as well as employee satisfaction and morale in addition to patient satisfaction [12].

The patient-centered concept entails enhancing patient well-being related to an aesthetic, comfortable, safe, and pleasant atmosphere; encouraging patients to interact with their family members, caregivers, and other patients; and providing a homelike environment [38, 45]. The designs of numerous hospitals have been based on experts' perspectives and have prioritized cost efficiency and clinical functionality; specifically, only the perspectives of management staff, architects, and policymakers have been considered in such designs [46]. Therefore, evidence-based healthcare design should consider hospital users' perception of a care unit [9].

As mentioned, a healing environment can be defined as a holistic environment (physical and nonphysical) that facilitates patient rehabilitation. In contrast to treatment, healing is a psychological concept of health [7]. However, children are generally neglected in architectural planning, despite them being typically more sensitive to environments than adults are [10]. Scanlon and Bauer [11] emphasized that young children are more dynamic than adults are and that various considerations should be included in children's healthcare because children's requirements differ from those of adults. Developing an evidence-based method for designing a healing environment for children's hospitals is an appealing topic that warrants further research.

# 3. Method and Design

*3.1. Questionnaire Development.* The ethics committee of the National Taiwan University Hospital approved this study. Moreover, all participants provided informed consent and agreed to participate voluntarily. The questionnaire development involved six stages:

(1) To obtain background knowledge for interviews, a literature review was conducted according to the connotations of a healing environment in a children's hospital.

(2) The interview topic was related to the design of a healing environment in a children's hospital. On the basis of the literature review, a questionnaire for in-depth semistructured interviews was developed (Supplementary Material A, in the Supplementary Material available online at http://dx.doi.org/10.1155/2016/8184653), and the interviewees expressed their opinions according to their expertise and experience. The interviews were audio-recorded with the interviewees' consent. The interviewees were a pediatrician (A), chief nurse executive from the pediatrics department of a hospital (B), hospital manager (C), medical manager from the pediatrics department of a hospital (D), architect (E), and art therapist (F).

(3) Transcripts of the interviews (a total of 65,395 Chinese characters) were analyzed and decoded using the grounded theory method. Strauss and Corbin [47] stated that a data analysis process includes open, axial, and selective coding procedures. Open coding involves decomposing, examining, comparing, conceptualizing, and categorizing data. Overall, 99, 47, 37, 47, 71, and 80 concepts were extracted from interviewees A, B, C, D, E, and F, respectively. After similar concepts were combined, 292 concepts remained. Moreover, after a decoding process, 79 open codes, 25 axial codes, and 4 selective codes (i.e., emotions, space design, interpersonal interaction, and pleasant surroundings) were obtained (Supplementary Material C). The "emotional preferences" axial code in the "emotions" dimension, which was a selective code, was used as an example to explain the coding processes. As shown in Supplementary Material D, emotional preferences included open codes such as personal preferences, self-healing, and moving people emotionally. These personal preferences comprised concepts C9, E40, and E43 (C9, the ninth concept extracted from the transcript of the interview with hospital manager C, posits that art appreciation varies among people; E40 and E43, the 40th and 43rd concepts extracted from the transcript of the interview with architect E, are personalized space and

TABLE 1: Demographic information on the pilot questionnaire subjects.

| Aged 7–18 | 7 | 8 | 9 | 10 | 11 | 12 | 13 | 14 | 15 | 16 | 17 | 18 | Sum |
|---|---|---|---|---|---|---|---|---|---|---|---|---|---|
| Girls | 7 | 7 | 7 | 10 | 10 | 9 | 3 | 3 | 3 | 6 | 5 | 6 | 76 |
| Boys | 7 | 6 | 6 | 7 | 6 | 7 | 3 | 2 | 2 | 2 | 2 | 2 | 52 |
| Children | 14 | 13 | 13 | 17 | 16 | 16 | 6 | 5 | 5 | 8 | 7 | 8 | 128 |

differences in art preferences, resp.). Supplementary Material D details the opening coding processes for self-healing and moving people emotionally.

(4) As shown in Supplementary Material E, 25 axial codes were transformed into a pilot questionnaire comprising 25 question items.

(5) Pilot data were collected from May 20 to May 31, 2013. The second author of this study conducted a pilot questionnaire survey among users aged 7–18 (including inpatients, outpatients, and visitors). Before distributing the questionnaire to a participant, the researcher introduced herself and informed the participant of the purposes of the study. Because all participants had not fully experienced the entire NTUCH environment, a 5-minute, 28-second video (https://youtu.be/I4fMCC9Ca1Q) was produced to introduce the hospital environment and associated activities to the subjects. Parents assisted the younger children in completing the questionnaire. Gorsuch suggested that, for factor analysis, the ratio of the number of question items to sample size should be approximately 1 : 5 and that the total number of subjects should be more than 100 [48]. In this study, the pilot questionnaire comprised 25 questions. A total of 140 questionnaires were distributed; 128 valid questionnaires were returned. Demographics are shown in Table 1.

(6) Confirmatory factor analysis and reliability analysis were conducted to determine the question items for each dimension of the final version of the questionnaire. Supplementary Material F presents a summary of the analysis process. The principal components method with varimax orthogonal rotation was used to perform factor analysis; this analysis included question items whose factor loadings were greater than .4 in the questionnaire. First, items q8 and q19 were removed according to the confirmatory factor analysis results. Subsequently, q12 and q18 were removed according to the reliability analysis results. Item q17 was next moved from the space design dimension to the interpersonal interaction dimension according to the confirmatory factor analysis results. The final version of the questionnaire comprised the 4 dimensions and 21 question items (Table 2). The four dimensions explained 59.538% of the score variance. According to the reliability analysis, the Cronbach $\alpha$ value for the four dimensions (emotions, space design, interpersonal interaction, and pleasant surroundings) and the overall value were 0.774, 0.873, 0.744, 0.8, and

TABLE 2: Resulting questionnaire items after grounded theory analysis versus those after factor and reliability analyses.

| Dimension | Emotions | Space design | Interpersonal interaction | Pleasant surroundings |
|---|---|---|---|---|
| Resulting question items for the pilot questionnaire after grounded theory analysis | q1, q2, q3, q4, q5, q6 | q7, q8, q9, q10, q11, q12, q13, q14, q15, q16, q17, q18 | q19, q20, q21 | q22, q23, q24, q25 |
| Resulting question items according to factor analysis and reliability analysis (question items for the formal questionnaire) | q1, q2, q3, q4, q5, q6 (01, 02, 03, 04, 05, 06) | q7, q9, q10, q11, q13, q14, q15, q16 (07, 08, 09, 10, 11, 12, 13, 14) | q17, q20, q21 (15, 16, 17) | q22, q23, q24, q25 (18, 19, 20, 21) |

*Note.* q8, q12, q18, and q19 were removed from the pilot questionnaire, and q17 was moved from the space design dimension to the interpersonal interaction dimension.

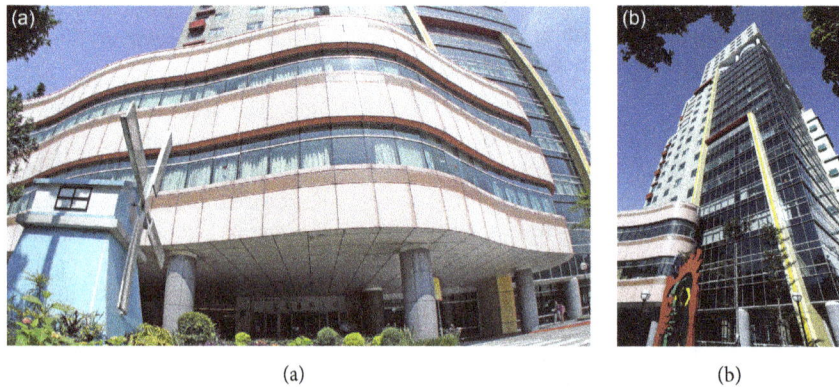

FIGURE 1: (a) Exterior of NTUCH (front view) and (b) exterior of NTUCH (side view).

0.918, respectively (Supplementary Material F). The criterion was the confirmed suitability of the questionnaire for factor analysis. Kaiser and Rice indicated that the Kaiser-Meyer-Olkin measure should not be less than 0.5. In this study, the measure was 0.875 (Supplementary Material F), indicating that it was suitable for factor analysis [49]. Internal consistency reliability was assessed using Cronbach's coefficient $\alpha$ [50]. For the questionnaire, Cronbach's $\alpha > 0.70$ was applied as the recommended value, with $\alpha > 0.9$ indicative of high reliability [51, 52]. As mentioned, this study exhibited construct validity and reliability.

As suggested by the results, a healing environment in a children's hospital should accommodate children's emotional preferences, be a homelike and reassuring environment that can be emotionally accepted by children, and encourage interpersonal interaction among children and between children and healthcare staff. In addition, the space design should be a visually aesthetic and child-friendly design that can provide a multifunctional and comfortable space for children. Moreover, in a children's hospital, pleasant surroundings should be created for children through both dynamic activities and static indoor and outdoor scenery.

For the formal questionnaire survey, participants were required to rate each question on a 5-point scale with anchors ranging from 1 (*strongly disagree*) to 5 (*strongly agree*). Each participant was required to provide demographic information.

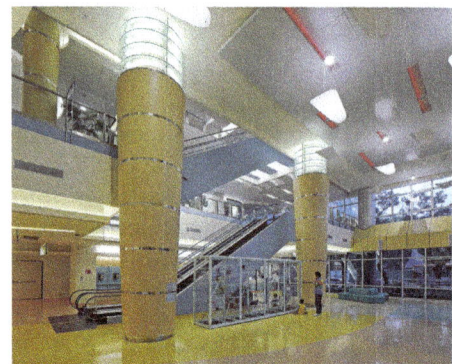

FIGURE 2: NTUCH lobby.

### 3.2. NTUCH and Study Participants

*3.2.1. NTUCH.* National Taiwan University Hospital is the oldest hospital in Taiwan, having provided healthcare services since 1895. The affiliated NTUCH was the first children's hospital in Taiwan to adopt a healing environment design. The NTUCH building has a glass curtain wall design (Figure 1), enabling a substantial amount of natural sunlight to enter the building through the windows. Colorful and uniquely shaped artworks including those suspending from the ceiling are installed in the hallways (Figure 2). The characteristics of the hospital's healing environment design are described in Supplementary Material B, and nonpharmacological intervention measures during children's medical

TABLE 3: Nonpharmacological intervention measures during children's medical procedures versus elements of the healing environment in the NTUCH.

| Intervention elements | Aim | Objective | Elements of the healing environment |
| --- | --- | --- | --- |
| Healing garden [18] | Anxiety, sadness, anger, worry, fatigue, and pain | Child (2–12 years old), adolescent (13–18 years old), and adult | Hanging garden |
| Playful activities [19] | Anxiety | 5 to 12 years old | Game room (colorful sky cave, touching republic, toy room, and youth blog), toy building bricks, craft activities, and balloons of various shapes activities |
| Music [20] | Anxiety and pain | 2–12 years old | Regular concerts |
| Electronic game [21] | Child distress | 3 to 7 years old | None |
| Clown [22, 23] | Anxiety/anxiety | 3–8 years old/5–12 years old | Clown and magic shows and theatres |
| Virtual reality [24, 25] | Anxiety and pain/anxiety and pain | 7–14 years old/6–14 years old | None |
| Cartoon movie [26] | Distress, restraint, and pain | 4 to 6 years old | Cartoon movies shown in waiting areas |
| Computer game [27] | Anxiety, symptom, and emotion | 10–16 years old | None |
| Instructional therapeutic toy [28] | Pain | 3–10 years old | Seeds-of-hope hospital activities |

procedures versus elements of the healing environment in the NTUCH are shown in Table 3.

*3.2.2. Study Participants.* Children who visited NTUCH were invited to participate in this study. According to the United Nations Convention on the Rights of the Child, "children" refers to people under 18 years old. On the basis of the requirement that respondents could express themselves clearly or read, children aged 7–18 who were outpatients or inpatients or accompanied their family members to the hospital were recruited to participate in this study.

*3.3. Data Collection.* The data were collected from June 3 to June 28, 2013. Informed consent was obtained from each participant. The data collection procedure was the same as that of the pilot data sampling. The sample size $n$ was determined as follows [53]:

$$n \geq \left(\frac{k}{\alpha}\right)^2 p\left(1 - p\right). \tag{1}$$

The value of $p$ is typically set at .5. In social and behavioral science research, the value of $\alpha$ (i.e., the significance level) is typically set at .05; therefore, the value of $k$ is 1.96. Under these conditions, the sample size $n$ should be equal to or greater than 384. In this study, the sample size was 430, and the number of valid questionnaires was 401. Hence, the return rate was 93.26%. Demographics are shown in Table 4.

*3.4. Limitations.* According to Piaget [54], children progress through four stages of cognitive development: sensorimotor (0–2 years old), preoperational (2–7 years old), concrete operational (7–11 years old), and formal operational (above 11 years old). Piaget noted that, during the preoperational stage of

TABLE 4: Study subjects demographic information.

| Aged 7–18 | 7 | 8 | 9 | 10 | 11 | 12 | 13 | 14 | 15 | 16 | 17 | 18 | Sum |
| --- | --- | --- | --- | --- | --- | --- | --- | --- | --- | --- | --- | --- | --- |
| Girls | | 18 | 18 | 12 | 24 | 22 | 18 | 20 | 18 | 15 | 18 | 18 | 14 | 215 |
| Boys | | 20 | 18 | 16 | 22 | 20 | 22 | 15 | 14 | 12 | 10 | 9 | 8 | 186 |
| Children | 38 | 36 | 28 | 46 | 42 | 40 | 35 | 32 | 27 | 28 | 27 | 22 | 401 |

cognitive development, children do not yet understand concrete logic and cannot mentally manipulate information. The concrete operational stage is characterized by an appropriate use of logic, and the formal operational stage is demonstrated through the logical use of symbols related to abstract concepts. Because children's abilities to express themselves and read are limited, the participants recruited for this study were children aged 7–18. A limitation of this study was that all participants had not fully experienced the entire environment of the hospital and its associated activities. Therefore, although the participants had experienced the hospital environment, they were shown a video introducing the hospital healing environment to ensure that they understood the entire healing environment. This study aimed to identify an evidence-based method for designing and establishing a healing environment. It did not include the comparison of kids' perceptions of a healing environment with those of a regular hospital environment.

## 4. Results and Discussion

The researchers used SPSS 20 software for data analysis, and they calculated the means and standard deviations of participant perception of the healing environment according to the four dimensions and overall perception. Two-way analysis of variance (ANOVA) was performed to examine the effects of age and sex on the perception of the healing environment in each dimension and on the overall perception.

*4.1. Descriptive Statistics for Children's Perceptions of the NTUCH Healing Environment.* As shown in Table 5, the average scores of all the children's responses to the four dimensions (emotions, space design, interpersonal interaction, and pleasant surroundings) and the average overall perception score were 4.21, 4.41, 4.09, 4.17, and 4.26, respectively. The average overall perception scores of the girls and boys were 4.29 and 4.23, respectively. The trends of the average scores for the four dimensions were consistent between the boys and the girls; specifically, for both the boys and the girls, the average scores for space design were the highest, followed by those for emotions, pleasant surroundings, and interpersonal interaction. Across all age levels, the children were most satisfied with the space design dimension and least satisfied with the interpersonal interaction dimension. The trends of the average scores for the four dimensions were consistent among the children at all age levels. All the average scores for each dimension also exceeded 3.90, signifying that all the age groups positively accepted the NTUCH healing environment. Moreover, the younger age groups accepted the healing environment to a greater extent than did the older age groups; the mean perception scores for the groups aged 7–9, 10–12, 13–15, and 16–18 years were 4.39, 4.32, 4.18, and 4.10, respectively (Table 5). In all groups, boys aged 16–18 also demonstrated the lowest average scores for the four dimensions and overall perception (4.02, 3.64, 3.73, 3.87, and 3.89, resp.; Table 5).

*4.2. Effects of Sex and Age on Children's Perception of the NTUCH Healing Environment.* As shown in Table 6, the interaction effects of sex and age on emotions, space design, interpersonal interaction, pleasant surroundings, and overall perception were nonsignificant.

Regarding the emotions dimension, the main effect of sex was nonsignificant ($F = .832$, $p > .05$) and that of age was significant ($F = 4.054$, $p = .007$). Fisher's least significant difference (LSD) post hoc test revealed that the average score of children aged 7–9 for the emotions dimension was significantly higher than those of children aged 13–15 and 16–18.

For the space design dimension, the main effects of sex ($F = 4.626$, $p = .032$) and age ($F = 3.482$, $p = .016$) were significant. The average score of girls was significantly higher than that of boys. Fisher's LSD post hoc test showed that the average score of children aged 7–9 for this dimension was significantly higher than that of children aged 16–18.

Regarding the interpersonal interaction dimension, the main effect of sex was nonsignificant ($F = 1.991$, $p > .05$), whereas that of age was significant ($F = 5.690$, $p = .001$). Fisher's LSD post hoc test indicated that the average scores of children aged 7–9 and 10–12 for this dimension were significantly higher than those of children aged 13–15 and 16–18.

For the pleasant surroundings dimension, the main effect of sex was nonsignificant ($F = 2.893$, $p > .05$), whereas that of

age was significant ($F = 14.764$, $p = .000$). Fisher's LSD post hoc test revealed that the average scores of children aged 7–9 and 10–12 for this dimension were significantly higher than those of children aged 13–15 and 16–18.

Concerning the overall perception dimension, the main effect of sex was nonsignificant ($F = 3.276$, $p > .05$), whereas that of age was significant ($F = 7.034$, $p = .000$). Fisher's LSD post hoc test indicated that, regarding the overall perception, the average score of children aged 7–9 was significantly higher than those of children aged 13–15 and 16–18, and that of children aged 10–12 was significantly higher than that of those aged 16–18.

*4.3. Discussion.* The statistical analysis conducted on the effect of age on children's perception of the healing environment according to the four dimensions (i.e., emotions, space design, interpersonal interaction, and pleasant surroundings) reveals that the average scores of younger children were significantly higher than those of older children. According to previous studies (Table 3), applying nonpharmacological intervention measures to manage stress, anxiety, and pain has become a widely recognized method. This type of intervention includes attention distraction strategies, such as using healing gardens [18], games [51], music [20], electronic game devices [21], clown doctors [22, 23], virtual reality [24, 25], and cartoons [26], or game-based cognitive learning tools, such as computer games and educational healing toys [27, 28]. These intervention measures target children aged 2–18. At NTUCH, most of these intervention strategies were used with children under 12 years old. Healing gardens, virtual reality, and computer games were also used with children above 12 years old (Table 3). Landreth [5] indicated that toys and games are at the center of children's lives and that using toys and games to communicate with children is a natural method that can facilitate establishing a relationship between children and healthcare staff. Children use digital toys and games that help them to pursue dominant values [55].

Because younger children typically spend considerable time playing games, nonpharmacological intervention measures can be effectively applied among them. Previous studies have also demonstrated that younger children exhibit stronger anxiety and pain responses during diagnosis and treatment processes than do older children [24, 56], signifying that more attention should be paid to younger children during healthcare processes. The results of previous studies are mainly applicable to younger children. In addition to virtual reality and computer games, other healing elements have been applied in the NTUCH healing environment (Table 3), and this may explain why the younger children accepted the healing environment to a higher degree in each of the four dimensions compared with the older children.

The sex variable significantly affected children's perception of space design, and the average score of the girls was significantly higher than that of the boys. The results are consistent with those reported by Mourshed and Zhao [15], who studied healthcare providers' perceptions toward hospital environment design factors and determined that females are more sensitive to healthcare environments than

TABLE 5: Descriptive statistics for the perceptions of children toward the NTUCH healing environment.

| Sex | Age (~years old) | Mean | | | | | Standard deviation | | | | | Frequency |
|---|---|---|---|---|---|---|---|---|---|---|---|---|
| | | Emotions | Space design | Interpersonal interaction | Pleasant surroundings | Overall | Emotions | Space design | Interpersonal interaction | Pleasant surroundings | Overall | |
| Girls | 7–9 | 4.35 | 4.51 | 4.23 | 4.44 | 4.41 | .565 | .595 | .845 | .695 | .545 | 48 |
| | 10–12 | 4.26 | 4.48 | 4.27 | 4.37 | 4.37 | .624 | .545 | .637 | .632 | .547 | 64 |
| | 13–15 | 4.08 | 4.38 | 3.89 | 3.92 | 4.14 | .540 | .555 | .640 | .552 | .479 | 53 |
| | 16–18 | 4.18 | 4.44 | 4.04 | 4.01 | 4.22 | .575 | .561 | .721 | .610 | .531 | 50 |
| | Average | 4.22 | 4.45 | 4.11 | 4.19 | 4.29 | .584 | .561 | .720 | .657 | .534 | 215 |
| Boys | 7–9 | 4.31 | 4.49 | 4.22 | 4.35 | 4.37 | .532 | .472 | .700 | .708 | .494 | 54 |
| | 10–12 | 4.22 | 4.39 | 4.09 | 4.23 | 4.27 | .586 | .540 | .711 | .594 | .530 | 64 |
| | 13–15 | 4.24 | 4.41 | 4.07 | 3.98 | 4.23 | .584 | .521 | .633 | .654 | .518 | 41 |
| | 16–18 | 3.89 | 4.02 | 3.64 | 3.73 | 3.87 | .632 | .738 | .745 | .707 | .614 | 27 |
| | Average | 4.20 | 4.37 | 4.06 | 4.14 | 4.23 | .589 | .567 | .715 | .687 | .549 | 186 |
| All children | 7–9 | 4.33 | 4.50 | 4.23 | 4.39 | 4.39 | .545 | .531 | .768 | .700 | .516 | 102 |
| | 10–12 | 4.24 | 4.44 | 4.18 | 4.30 | 4.32 | .603 | .542 | .678 | .615 | .538 | 128 |
| | 13–15 | 4.15 | 4.39 | 3.97 | 3.94 | 4.18 | .562 | .538 | .639 | .596 | .496 | 94 |
| | 16–18 | 4.08 | 4.29 | 3.90 | 3.91 | 4.10 | .608 | .655 | .749 | .655 | .583 | 77 |
| | Average | 4.21 | 4.41 | 4.09 | 4.17 | 4.26 | .585 | .564 | .717 | .671 | .541 | 401 |

TABLE 6: Summary of two-way analysis of variance results regarding the effects of sex and age on children's perception of the NTUCH healing environment.

| Dependent variable (dimension) | Source | Type III sum of squares | df | Mean square error | F | p | Eta-squared | Post hoc comparisons |
|---|---|---|---|---|---|---|---|---|
| Emotions | Sex | .278 | 1 | .278 | .832 | .362 | .002 | |
| | Age | 4.070 | 3 | 1.357 | 4.054* | .007 | .030 | 7–9 > 13–15 years old 7–9 > 16–18 years old |
| | Sex × age | 1.976 | 3 | .659 | 1.968 | .118 | .015 | |
| Space design | Sex | 1.436 | 1 | 1.436 | 4.626* | .032 | .012 | Girls > boys |
| | Age | 3.243 | 3 | 1.081 | 3.482* | .016 | .026 | 7–9 > 16–18 years old |
| | Sex × age | 2.302 | 3 | .767 | 2.472 | .061 | .019 | |
| Interpersonal interaction | Sex | .984 | 1 | .984 | 1.991 | .159 | .005 | |
| | Age | 8.437 | 3 | 2.812 | 5.690* | .001 | .042 | 7–9 > 13–15 years old 7–9 > 16–18 years old 10–12 > 13–15 years old 10–12 > 16–18 years old |
| | Sex × age | 3.668 | 3 | 1.223 | 2.474 | .061 | .019 | |
| Pleasant surroundings | Sex | 1.183 | 1 | 1.183 | 2.893 | .090 | .007 | |
| | Age | 18.121 | 3 | 6.040 | 14.764* | .000 | .101 | 7–9 > 13–15 years old 7–9 > 16–18 years old 10–12 > 13–15 years old 10–12 > 16–18 years old |
| | Sex × age | 1.163 | 3 | .388 | .948 | .417 | .007 | |
| Overall perception | Sex | .914 | 1 | .914 | 3.276 | .071 | .008 | |
| | Age | 5.889 | 3 | 1.963 | 7.034* | .000 | .051 | 7–9 > 13–15 years old 7–9 > 16–18 years old 10–12 > 16–18 years old |
| | Sex × age | 2.013 | 3 | .671 | 2.404 | .067 | .018 | |

$^*p < .05.$

males. Moir and Jessel [57] (pp. 17-18) reported that females see larger images than males do, and this is because females have wider peripheral vision and their retina contains more cone and rod cells for receiving visual information.

According to the preceding results, children aged 7–18 positively accepted the NTUCH healing environment; in addition, they were most satisfied with space design and least satisfied with interpersonal interaction. Poor outdoor playground design reduces the frequency of children's interaction with the opposite sex [58]. NTUCH should thus improve its interpersonal interaction design to enhance healing effects. Prensky [59] reported that playing with others is fun and helps a player become involved in a community. Space design can be considered a component of hardware facilities. As presented in Supplementary Material B, game rooms (e.g., the toy room, colorful sky cave, touching republic, and youth blog), the hanging garden, family resource center, and waiting areas (e.g., fantastic journey, fantastic forest, Buddi's adventure, and animal carnival) were the healing elements that attracted children. The elements of space design were installed in the open space of NTUCH and were readily available to children in the hospital. This space design is in accordance with the suggestions proposed by Turner et al. [60] regarding a hospital's physical environment. This may be

the reason why the children were most satisfied with space design.

## 5. Conclusion and Recommendation

An evidence-based healthcare design should be based on the evaluation of the perceptions of hospital care unit users [9]; this design strategy was used in the current study, and the results are as follows:

(1) This study proposed qualitative and quantitative analyses and systematically summarized essential factors for designing and evaluating a healing environment in a children's hospital. Questionnaires about the design of a healing environment in a children's hospital were collected and analyzed, and related elements are summarized in this paper (Table 2 and Supplementary Material E). These elements include 4 dimensions, namely, emotions, space design, interpersonal interaction, and pleasant surroundings, and 21 elements.

(2) Children aged 7–18 positively accepted the NTUCH healing environment, and they were most satisfied with space design and least satisfied with interpersonal interaction. Two-way ANOVA was performed

to investigate the effects of sex and age on children's perception of the healing environment. The results indicate that the average score of girls was significantly higher than that of boys for space design, whereas the effect on the other dimensions and overall perception was nonsignificant. The main effect of age on the four dimensions and overall perception was significant; specifically, younger children accepted the healing environment to a higher degree than did older children.

This study proposes a method for evaluating the perceptions of users of children's ward healing environments, and the proposed method is applicable to children aged 7–18. Future studies should include children aged 2–6. Nevertheless, children at these ages are limited in their ability to express themselves and read; therefore, other evaluation methods should be considered. In addition, further research is necessary to examine the comparison of kids' perceptions of a healing environment with those of a regular hospital environment.

## Competing Interests

The authors declare that there are no competing interests.

## References

[1] B. J. Huelat, *Healing Environments: Design for the Body, Mind and Spirit*, Medzyne Press, Alexandria, Va, USA, 2003.

[2] S. Ananth, "The natural next step," *Explore*, vol. 4, no. 4, pp. 273–274, 2008.

[3] B. Wetton, *Robots: Blood-A Methodology*, Kolding School of Design, Kolding, Denmark, 2007.

[4] J. Fehrenbacher and Y. Yoneda, *PARO: Therapeutic Baby Seal Robot!*, 2009, http://www.inhabitots.com/paro-therapeutic-baby-seal-robot/.

[5] G. L. Landreth, *Play Therapy: The Art of the Relationship*, Brunner-Routledge, New York, NY, USA, 2nd edition, 2002.

[6] E. J. Langer and J. Rodin, "The effects of choice and enhanced personal responsibility for the aged: a field experiment in an institutional setting," *Journal of Personality and Social Psychology*, vol. 34, no. 2, pp. 191–198, 1976.

[7] R. Ghazali and M. Y. Abbas, "Assessment of healing environment in paediatric wards," *Procedia—Social and Behavioral Sciences*, vol. 38, pp. 149–159, 2012.

[8] E. R. C. M. Huisman, E. Morales, J. van Hoof, and H. S. M. Kort, "Healing environment: a review of the impact of physical environmental factors on users," *Building and Environment*, vol. 58, pp. 70–80, 2012.

[9] N. Watkins and A. Keller, "Lost in translation: bridging gaps between design and evidence-based design," *Health Environments Research & Design Journal*, vol. 1, no. 2, pp. 39–46, 2008.

[10] H. Ozcan, *Healing design: A holistic approach to social interaction in pediatric intensive care units in the United States and Turkey [Ph.D. thesis]*, Texas A&M University, College Station, Tex, USA, 2006.

[11] M. C. Scanlon and P. Bauer, "Human factors and ergonomics in pediatrics," in *Handbook of Human Factors and Ergonomics in Health Care and Patient Safety*, P. Carayon, Ed., pp. 865–882, CRC Press, Boca Raton, Fla, USA, 2007.

[12] L. B. Altimier, "Healing environments: for patients and providers," *Newborn and Infant Nursing Reviews*, vol. 4, no. 2, pp. 89–92, 2004.

[13] C. Andrade, M. L. Lima, F. Fornara, and M. Bonaiuto, "Users' views of hospital environmental quality: validation of the perceived hospital environment quality indicators (PHEQIs)," *Journal of Environmental Psychology*, vol. 32, no. 2, pp. 97–111, 2012.

[14] R. Crow, H. Gage, S. Hampson et al., "The measurement of satisfaction with healthcare: implications for practice from a systematic review of the literature," *Health Technology Assessment*, vol. 6, no. 32, pp. 1–244, 2002.

[15] M. Mourshed and Y. Zhao, "Healthcare providers' perception of design factors related to physical environments in hospitals," *Journal of Environmental Psychology*, vol. 32, no. 4, pp. 362–370, 2012.

[16] L. Sun, M. Yamin, C. Mushi, K. Liu, M. Alsaigh, and F. Chen, "Information analytics for healthcare service discovery," *Journal of Healthcare Engineering*, vol. 5, no. 4, pp. 457–478, 2014.

[17] M. Miles, *Art, Space and the City: Public Art and Urban Futures*, Routledge, New York, NY, USA, 1997.

[18] S. A. Sherman, J. W. Varni, R. S. Ulrich, and V. L. Malcarne, "Post-occupancy evaluation of healing gardens in a pediatric cancer center," *Landscape and Urban Planning*, vol. 73, no. 2-3, pp. 167–183, 2005.

[19] F. S. Weber, "The influence of playful activities on children's anxiety during the preoperative period at the outpatient surgical center," *Jornal de Pediatria*, vol. 86, no. 3, pp. 209–214, 2010.

[20] H. Yu, Y. Liu, S. Li, and X. Ma, "Effects of music on anxiety and pain in children with cerebral palsy receiving acupuncture: a randomized controlled trial," *International Journal of Nursing Studies*, vol. 46, no. 11, pp. 1423–1430, 2009.

[21] B. Pringle, L. Hilley, K. Gelfand et al., "Decreasing child distress during needle sticks and maintaining treatment gains over time," *Journal of Clinical Psychology in Medical Settings*, vol. 8, no. 2, pp. 119–130, 2001.

[22] G. Golan, P. Tighe, N. Dobija, A. Perel, and I. Keidan, "Clowns for the prevention of preoperative anxiety in children: a randomized controlled trial," *Paediatric Anaesthesia*, vol. 19, no. 3, pp. 262–266, 2009.

[23] L. Vagnoli, S. Caprilli, A. Robiglio, and A. Messeri, "Clown doctors as a treatment for preoperative anxiety in children: a randomized, prospective study," *Pediatrics*, vol. 116, no. 4, pp. e563–e567, 2005.

[24] L. M. Dahlquist, K. E. Weiss, L. D. Clendaniel, E. F. Law, C. S. Ackerman, and K. D. McKenna, "Effects of videogame distraction using a virtual reality type head-mounted display helmet on cold pressor pain in children," *Journal of Pediatric Psychology*, vol. 34, no. 5, pp. 574–584, 2009.

[25] K. Wolitzky, R. Fivush, E. Zimand, L. Hodges, and B. O. Rothbaum, "Effectiveness of virtual reality distraction during a painful medical procedure in pediatric oncology patients," *Psychology and Health*, vol. 20, no. 6, pp. 817–824, 2005.

[26] L. L. Cohen, R. L. Blount, and G. Panopoulos, "Nurse coaching and cartoon distraction: an effective and practical intervention to reduce child, parent, and nurse distress during immunizations," *Journal of Pediatric Psychology*, vol. 22, no. 3, pp. 355–370, 1997.

[27] J. E. Beck, T. A. Lipani, K. F. Baber et al., "Attentional bias to pain and social threat in pediatric patients with functional abdominal pain and pain-free youth before and after performance evaluation," *Pain*, vol. 152, no. 5, pp. 1061–1067, 2011.

[28] M. T. Kiche and F. D. Almeida, "Therapeutic toy: strategy for pain management and tension relief during dressing change in children," *Acta Paulista de Enfermagem*, vol. 22, no. 2, pp. 125–130, 2009.

[29] F. C. Biley, "Hospitals: healing environments?" *Complementary Therapies in Nursing and Midwifery*, vol. 2, no. 4, pp. 110–115, 1996.

[30] R. S. Ulrich and R. Parsons, "Influences of passive experiences with plants on individual well-being and health," in *The Role of Horticulture in Human Well-Being and Social Development*, D. Relf, Ed., pp. 93–105, Timber Press, Portland, Ore, USA, 1992.

[31] R. S. Ulrich, "Effects of gardens on health outcomes: theory and research," in *Healing Gardens: Therapeutic Benefits and Design Recommendations*, C. Cooper-Marcus and M. Barnes, Eds., pp. 27–86, John Wiley, New York, NY, USA, 1999.

[32] NACHRI, *Evidence for Innovation, National Association of Children's Hospitals and Related Institutions (NACHRI) Issue*, 2008, http://www.premiersafetyinstitute.org/wp-content/uploads/evidenceforinnovation-execsum-small.pdf.

[33] M. Y. Abbas and R. Ghazali, "Healing environment: paediatric wards-status and design trend," *Procedia—Social and Behavioral Sciences*, vol. 49, pp. 28–38, 2012.

[34] R. Gross, Y. Sasson, M. Zarhy, and J. Zohar, "Healing environment in Psychiatric Hospital design," *General Hospital Psychiatry*, vol. 20, no. 2, pp. 108–114, 1998.

[35] M.-C. Chyu, T. Austin, F. Calisir et al., "Healthcare engineering defined: a white paper," *Journal of Healthcare Engineering*, vol. 6, no. 4, pp. 635–648, 2015.

[36] N. Daykin, E. Byrne, T. Soteriou, and S. O'Connor, "The impact of art, design and environment in mental healthcare: a systematic review of the literature," *Journal of the Royal Society for the Promotion of Health*, vol. 128, no. 2, pp. 85–94, 2008.

[37] S. Whitehouse, J. W. Varni, M. Seid et al., "Evaluating a children's hospital garden environment: utilization and consumer satisfaction," *Journal of Environmental Psychology*, vol. 21, no. 3, pp. 301–314, 2001.

[38] J. F. Stichler, "Healing by design," *Journal of Nursing Administration*, vol. 38, no. 12, pp. 505–509, 2008.

[39] K. M. Beauchemin and P. Hays, "Sunny hospital rooms expedite recovery from severe and refractory depressions," *Journal of Affective Disorders*, vol. 40, no. 1-2, pp. 49–51, 1996.

[40] R. S. Ulrich, "View through a window may influence recovery from surgery," *Science*, vol. 224, no. 4647, pp. 420–421, 1984.

[41] S. Baldwin, "Effects of furniture rearrangement on the atmosphere of wards in a maximum-security hospital," *Hospital & Community Psychiatry*, vol. 36, no. 5, pp. 525–528, 1985.

[42] T. Moran, "Hospital Hotel Crain's Detroit Business," *Detroit*, vol. 9, no. 18, p. 11, 1993.

[43] R. Moore, "Healing gardens for children," in *Healing Gardens: Therapeutic Benefits and Design Recommendations*, C. Cooper-Marcus and M. Barnes, Eds., pp. 323–384, John Wiley & Sons, New York, NY, USA, 1999.

[44] K. A. Richards and J. Nelson, "Overcoming obstacles to create the optimal healing environment," *Nurse Leader*, vol. 9, no. 2, pp. 37–57, 2011.

[45] D. P. Martin, P. Diehr, D. A. Conrad, J. Hunt Davis, R. Leickly, and E. B. Perrin, "Randomized trial of a patient-centered hospital unit," *Patient Education and Counseling*, vol. 34, no. 2, pp. 125–133, 1998.

[46] W. Gesler, M. Bell, S. Curtis, P. Hubbard, and S. Francis, "Therapy by design: evaluating the UK hospital building program," *Health & Place*, vol. 10, no. 2, pp. 117–128, 2004.

[47] A. Strauss and J. Corbin, *Basics of Qualitative Research. Grounded Theory Procedures and Techniques*, Sage, Newbury Park, Calif, USA, 1990.

[48] R. L. Gorsuch, *Factor Analysis*, Lawrence Erlbaum Associates, Hillsdale, NJ, USA, 2nd edition, 1983.

[49] H. F. Kaiser and J. Rice, "Little Jiffy, Mark Iv," *Educational and Psychological Measurement*, vol. 34, no. 1, pp. 111–117, 1974.

[50] L. J. Cronbach, "Coefficient alpha and the internal structure of tests," *Psychometrika*, vol. 16, no. 3, pp. 297–334, 1951.

[51] R. F. DeVells, *Scale Development Theory and Applications*, Sage, London, UK, 1991.

[52] J. C. Nunnally, *Psychometric Theory*, McGraw-Hill, New York, NY, USA, 2nd edition, 1978.

[53] D. P. Doane and L. W. Seward, *Essential Statistics in Business and Economics*, McGraw-Hill, New York, NY, USA, 2010.

[54] J. Piaget, *The Psychology of Intelligence*, Littlefield, Totowa, NJ, USA, 1972.

[55] M. Ruckenstein, "Toying with the world: children, virtual pets and the value of mobility," *Childhood*, vol. 17, no. 4, pp. 500–513, 2010.

[56] C. Kleiber and D. C. Harper, "Effects of distraction on children's pain and distress during medical procedures: a meta-analysis," *Nursing Research*, vol. 48, no. 1, pp. 44–49, 1999.

[57] A. Moir and D. Jessel, *Brain Sex: The Real Difference between Men and Women*, Carol, New York, NY, USA, 1991.

[58] L. Karsten, "Children's use of public space: the gendered world of the playground," *Childhood*, vol. 10, no. 4, pp. 457–473, 2003.

[59] M. Prensky, *Digital Game-Based Learning*, McGraw-Hill, New York, NY, USA, 2007.

[60] J. Turner, J. Fralic, K. Newman-Bennett, and L. Skinner, "Everybody needs a break! Responses to a playgarden survey," *Pediatric Nursing*, vol. 35, no. 1, pp. 27–34, 2009.

# 13

# An Overview of the 2009 A(H1N1) Pandemic in Europe: Efficiency of the Vaccination and Healthcare Strategies

**Funda Samanlioglu and Ayse Humeyra Bilge**

*Faculty of Engineering and Natural Sciences, Kadir Has University, 34083 Istanbul, Turkey*

Correspondence should be addressed to Funda Samanlioglu; fsamanlioglu@khas.edu.tr

Academic Editor: Mohamad Sawan

2009 A(H1N1) data for 13 European countries obtained from the weekly influenza surveillance overview (WISO) reports of European Centre for Disease Prevention and Control (ECDC) in the form of weekly cumulative fatalities are analyzed. The variability of relative fatalities is explained by the health index of analyzed countries. Vaccination and healthcare practices as reported in the literature are used to explain the departures from this model. The timing of the vaccination with respect to the peak of the epidemic and its role in the efficiency of the vaccination is discussed. Simulations are used to show that on-time vaccination reduces considerably the final value of $R(t)$, $R_f$, but it has little effect on the shape of normalized curve $R(t)/R_f$.

## 1. Introduction

The 2009 A(H1N1) pandemic was a major influenza pandemic that caused global alert. It was a variant of 1918 influenza that caused millions of fatalities. All countries applied some type of intervention and vaccines were developed but it turned out that the pandemic was not as deadly as anticipated and vaccination campaigns were not as effective as planned in most of the countries. As summarized in Section 2.1, a large number of research papers addressed various aspects of the pandemic: basic parameters were measured from clinical information and review articles on the healthcare measures and on epidemiological research were published for various countries.

In this paper, we study the 2009 A(H1N1) pandemic in 13 European countries, based on weekly influenza surveillance overview (WISO) reports published by European Centre for Disease Prevention and Control (ECDC) [1]. The official pandemic period for A(H1N1) is from week 18 of 2009 to week 35 of 2010 and the formal end is declared as week 32 of 2010 [2]. Here we study the fatality data for the so-called second wave (or autumn/winter wave), from week 36 of 2009 to week 15 of 2010. In the following, for practical purposes, we will count weeks from the beginning of 2009, hence our data will cover the period from week 36 to week 68.

The aim of the present work is to study the inference of the epidemic parameters from fatality data only, as discussed in our previous work [3]. We show that the scatter in relative fatalities can be explained by the healthcare measures and we use pulse vaccination simulations for the Susceptible-Infected-Removed (SIR) model to measure the effects of timing of vaccinations.

## 2. Preliminaries

*2.1. Literature Survey.* In the literature there are a number of papers devoted to the study of 2009 A(H1N1) pandemic in a single country such as Turkey [4], Denmark [5], Canada [6], Iran [7], Morocco [8], and Mexico [9] or to a comparative study [10–14]. Several others focus on the transmission dynamics of the pandemic, providing estimates of "basic reproduction number," "incubation period (latent period)," "generation time," and "serial interval" as below.

The "basic reproduction number" ($R_0$) is the average number of secondary cases generated from a single infected case in a population with no immunity to the disease and in the absence of interventions to control the infection. The "incubation period" is defined as the time between infection and symptom onset while the "latent period" is defined as the time of being infected and becoming infectious. The latent period is the notion that is relevant in epidemiological dynamics but for influenza type diseases the latent period and incubation period are used synonymously. The "generation time (interval)" is the average delay between the time of infection of a case and the time of infection of secondary cases infected by that case; and the "serial interval" is defined as the difference between the onset of symptoms of the primary and secondary cases [15, 16]. The serial interval is more easily observable than the generation time; however generation time is more relevant in the epidemic spread. For influenza type diseases, the distinction is not crucial. For A(H1N1), the mean incubation period is estimated as 1.4 days (95% confidence interval (CI), 1.0–1.8); the mean generation time of the pandemic is estimated as 2.5 to 3 days, and the serial interval is estimated as 2.2 to 2.3 days [11, 17]. Since $R_0$ depends on the contact rate which may differ from country to country, the estimate of $R_0$ has certain spread. For example, it is estimated as 1.1–1.4 in United Kingdom [12], 1.8 (95% CI, 1.5–2.2) in United States [17], 1.3–1.4 in Brazil [12], 1.4–1.6 in Mexico [18], 1.2–1.6 in Peru [19], 1.8–2.1 in Thailand [20], 1.2–1.5 in Australia [12], and 1.2–1.4 in Chili [12]. A review of studies presenting estimates of transmission parameters of the 2009 A(H1N1) pandemic is given in Boëlle et al.'s [13] work, where they show that the mean generation time of 2009 A(H1N1) pandemic was lower than the median for 1889, 1918, 1957, and 1968 influenza pandemics; and the median reproduction number was similar to 1968 pandemic and slightly smaller than 1889, 1918, and 1957 pandemics.

*2.2. Preprocessing of the Data.* Data collected for the European Union and European Economic Area (EU/EEA) WISO includes sentinel syndromic surveillance of influenza-like illness (ILI) and acute respiratory infection (ARI) and virological surveillance data, hospital-based sentinel surveillance of severe acute respiratory infection (SARI) data, and qualitative reporting data as well as influenza deaths. Data related to weakly influenza deaths includes case based deaths resulting from severe acute respiratory infection (SARI) and weakly aggregated influenza deaths reported by countries, which is also complemented by active monitoring of official websites for deaths [2, 21]. The first WISO report, published on 15.09.2009, includes the data of week 36 of 2009. Our study covers the period from week 36 of 2009 to week 15 of 2010 (or from week 36 to week 68 counted cumulatively for practical purposes) called the "second wave." In Table 1, we present 33 weeks of cumulative fatality data, from September 2009 to May 2010, of 13 different European countries, obtained from WISO reports.

Fatality data related to weeks 44, 45, and 52 were not available in WISO reports; linear interpolation was used to fill the missing values. It has been reported that the weekly mortality reports might be unreliable due to reporting delays [2].

The time series for fatalities for the analyzed countries are presented in Figure 1. From this figure we can see that the epidemic starts earlier in Netherlands, Ireland, Norway, and Sweden and later in Czech Republic, Estonia, France,

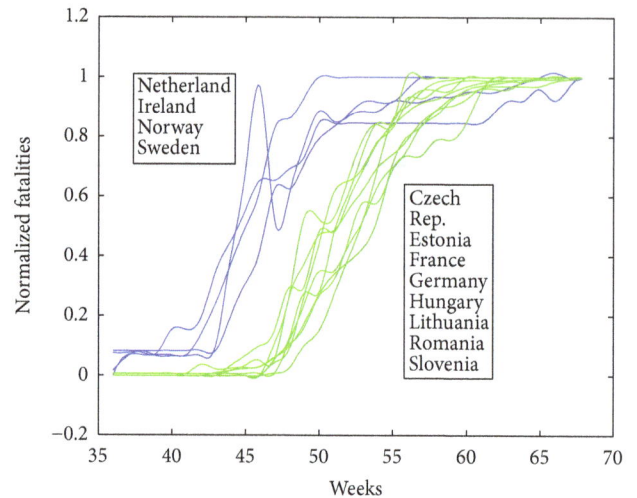

FIGURE 1: Normalized fatalities for analyzed European countries.

Germany, Hungary, Lithuania, Romania, and Slovenia. The reason of this early start-up may be the early start of the influenza season due to climate in Northern countries.

*2.3. Demographic Structure and Healthcare Measures.* Geographic and demographic information of various European countries is presented in Table 2 [22]. This piece of information is used to normalize and compare the number of fatalities in different countries. The age structure of the population is also a key issue since the 2009 A(H1N1) pandemic is characterized with low infection rate among people over the age of 60 presumably due to their prior exposure to antigenically related influenza viruses, resulting in the development of cross-protective antibodies [2, 23]. As opposed to seasonal influenza, during the 2009 A(H1N1) pandemic, 80% of fatalities were within the age group under 65, and about 25%–30% of fatalities were among healthy adults that were not considered as part of risk groups [2]. It is reported by several studies [14, 24, 25] that during the 2009 A(H1N1) pandemic, the proportion of fatalities among the young increased in comparison to seasonal influenza deaths. In fact, Van Kerkhove et al. [26] reported that globally the median age was 46 among fatalities. We have included information on age structure for the countries we analyzed in Table 2; however since their age structure was more or less homogeneous we overlooked this information and decided to use total figures. In this table, Human Development Index (HDI) and health index (HI) of countries are also presented along with average latitudes. The census data and average latitudes are obtained from CIA (*The World Factbook*) [22] and *Eurostat Yearbook* [27]; HDI and HI values are acquired from Human Development Reports [28]. HI published in the framework of the United Nations Development Program [28] is one of the objective measures of the efficiency of the healthcare system. HDI that includes HI as a component can also be considered as an alternative [28]. HDI is a measure of human development, and it has three basic dimensions: a long and healthy life (health index), access to knowledge (education index), and a decent standard of living (income index).

TABLE 1: Cumulative weekly fatalities due to A(H1N1) pandemic in Europe.

| Week | 1st day | Czech R. | Estonia | France | Germany | Greece | Hungary | Ireland | Lithuania | Netherlands | Norway | Romania | Slovenia | Sweden |
|---|---|---|---|---|---|---|---|---|---|---|---|---|---|---|
| 36 (36/09) | 30.08.2009 | 0 | 0 | 0 | 0 | 1 | 1 | 2 | 0 | 1 | 0 | 0 | 0 | 2 |
| 37 (37/09) | 07.09.2009 | 0 | 0 | 0 | 0 | 1 | 1 | 2 | 0 | 4 | 2 | 0 | 0 | 2 |
| 38 (38/09) | 14.09.2009 | 0 | 0 | 0 | 0 | 1 | 1 | 2 | 0 | 5 | 2 | 0 | 0 | 2 |
| 39 (39/09) | 21.09.2009 | 0 | 0 | 0 | 0 | 1 | 1 | 2 | 0 | 4 | 2 | 0 | 0 | 2 |
| 40 (40/09) | 28.09.2009 | 0 | 0 | 0 | 0 | 1 | 1 | 4 | 0 | 4 | 2 | 0 | 0 | 2 |
| 41 (41/09) | 05.10.2009 | 0 | 0 | 0 | 0 | 1 | 1 | 4 | 0 | 4 | 2 | 0 | 0 | 2 |
| 42 (42/09) | 12.10.2009 | 0 | 0 | 0 | 0 | 1 | 5 | 5 | 0 | 4 | 4 | 0 | 0 | 2 |
| 43 (43/09) | 19.10.2009 | 1 | 0 | 0 | 0 | 1 | 3 | 9 | 0 | 6 | 7 | 0 | 0 | 2 |
| 44 (44/09) | 26.10.2009 | 1.6 | 0 | 10.3 | 4.3 | 1 | 3.3 | 11.6 | 0 | 23.6 | 10.6 | 0 | 0 | 4.6 |
| 45 (45/09) | 02.11.2009 | 2.3 | 0 | 20.6 | 8.6 | 1 | 3.6 | 14.3 | 0 | 41.3 | 14.3 | 0 | 0 | 7.3 |
| 46 (46/09) | 09.11.2009 | 3 | 0 | 31 | 13 | 1 | 4 | 17 | 0 | 59 | 18 | 0 | 0 | 10 |
| 47 (47/09) | 16.11.2009 | 6 | 1 | 46 | 13 | 1 | 8 | 17 | 1 | 32 | 24 | 1 | 2 | 15 |
| 48 (48/09) | 23.11.2009 | 12 | 2 | 92 | 66 | 16 | 13 | 18 | 2 | 37 | 25 | 3 | 5 | 15 |
| 49 (49/09) | 30.11.2009 | 27 | 3 | 92 | 94 | 33 | 23 | 19 | 6 | 47 | 27 | 12 | 10 | 17 |
| 50 (50/09) | 07.12.2009 | 27 | 5 | 150 | 119 | 49 | 36 | 22 | 10 | 54 | 29 | 18 | 10 | 19 |
| 51 (51/09) | 14.12.2009 | 46 | 6 | 150 | 123 | 49 | 45 | 22 | 14 | 52 | 29 | 32 | 10 | 20 |
| 52 (52/09) | 21.12.2009 | 59.5 | 8.5 | 182 | 140 | 61 | 51 | 22 | 15 | 53 | 29 | 47.5 | 12.5 | 21 |
| 53 (53/09) | 28.12.2009 | 73 | 11 | 214 | 157 | 73 | 57 | 22 | 16 | 54 | 29 | 63 | 15 | 22 |
| 54 (01/10) | 04.01.2010 | 83 | 11 | 243 | 176 | 89 | 70 | 22 | 18 | 54 | 29 | 84 | 16 | 22 |
| 55 (02/10) | 11.01.2010 | 83 | 13 | 261 | 187 | 98 | 94 | 22 | 19 | 56 | 29 | 104 | 16 | 22 |
| 56 (03/10) | 18.01.2010 | 91 | 14 | 275 | 199 | 106 | 107 | 22 | 21 | 56 | 29 | 110 | 19 | 23 |
| 57 (04/10) | 25.01.2010 | 91 | 14 | 285 | 215 | 118 | 112 | 22 | 22 | 56 | 29 | 116 | 19 | 24 |
| 58 (05/10) | 01.02.2010 | 94 | 15 | 289 | 225 | 123 | 119 | 22 | 22 | 57 | 29 | 120 | 19 | 24 |
| 59 (06/10) | 08.02.2010 | 96 | 15 | 296 | 235 | 130 | 121 | 22 | 22 | 57 | 29 | 121 | 19 | 24 |
| 60 (07/10) | 15.02.2010 | 97 | 16 | 302 | 239 | 135 | 124 | 22 | 23 | 58 | 29 | 122 | 19 | 24 |
| 61 (08/10) | 22.02.2010 | 97 | 18 | 306 | 243 | 137 | 129 | 22 | 23 | 58 | 29 | 122 | 19 | 24 |
| 62 (09/10) | 01.03.2010 | 97 | 19 | 308 | 243 | 138 | 130 | 23 | 23 | 58 | 29 | 122 | 19 | 24 |
| 63 (10/10) | 08.03.2010 | 98 | 19 | 309 | 243 | 139 | 130 | 24 | 23 | 59 | 29 | 122 | 19 | 24 |
| 64 (11/10) | 13.03.2010 | 98 | 19 | 310 | 250 | 139 | 130 | 24 | 23 | 60 | 29 | 122 | 19 | 24 |
| 65 (12/10) | 22.03.2010 | 98 | 19 | 311 | 252 | 140 | 130 | 25 | 23 | 61 | 29 | 122 | 19 | 24 |
| 66 (13/10) | 29.03.2010 | 98 | 19 | 312 | 254 | 140 | 132 | 24 | 23 | 62 | 29 | 122 | 19 | 24 |
| 67 (14/10) | 05.04.2010 | 98 | 19 | 312 | 253 | 141 | 133 | 25 | 23 | 61 | 29 | 122 | 19 | 24 |
| 68 (15/10) | 12.04.2010 | 98 | 19 | 312 | 253 | 141 | 134 | 26 | 23 | 61 | 29 | 122 | 19 | 24 |

TABLE 2: Demographic information.

| Country | $D_f$ | $N$ | $A$ | $d = N/A$ | $N < 65$ (%) | $(D_f/N)10^3$ | HDI | HI | $\lambda$ |
|---|---|---|---|---|---|---|---|---|---|
| Czech Rep. | 98 | 10 467 | 78 866 | 132.7 | 85.1 | 9.4 | 0.841 | 0.901 | 49.45 |
| Estonia | 19 | 1 340 | 45 226 | 29.63 | 82.9 | 14 | 0.812 | 0.851 | 59.00 |
| France | 312 | 64 367 | 643 548 | 100.0 | 83.3 | 4.9 | 0.872 | 0.976 | 46.00 |
| Germany | 253 | 82 002 | 357 021 | 229.7 | 79.6 | 3.1 | 0.885 | 0.953 | 51.00 |
| Greece | 141 | 11 260 | 131 940 | 85.34 | 81.3 | 13 | 0.855 | 0.945 | 39.00 |
| Hungary | 134 | 10 031 | 93 030 | 107.8 | 83.6 | 13 | 0.805 | 0.853 | 47.00 |
| Ireland | 26 | 4 450 | 70 280 | 63.32 | 88.9 | 5.8 | 0.895 | 0.955 | 53.00 |
| Lithuania | 23 | 3 349 | 65 200 | 51.37 | 84.0 | 6.9 | 0.783 | 0.824 | 56.00 |
| Netherlands | 61 | 16 485 | 41 526 | 397.0 | 85.0 | 3.7 | 0.890 | 0.955 | 52.30 |
| Norway | 29 | 4 799 | 385 252 | 12.46 | 85.3 | 6.0 | 0.938 | 0.966 | 62.00 |
| Romania | 122 | 21 498 | 238 391 | 90.18 | 85.1 | 5.7 | 0.767 | 0.842 | 46.00 |
| Slovenia | 19 | 2 032 | 20 253 | 100.3 | 83.6 | 9.4 | 0.828 | 0.931 | 46.00 |
| Sweden | 24 | 9 256 | 449 964 | 20.57 | 82.2 | 2.6 | 0.885 | 0.970 | 62.00 |

Note: $D_f$: total fatality; $N$: population in thousands; $A$: area (km$^2$); $d$: population density (thousand/km$^2$); $N < 65$ (%): percentage of 0–64 years; $(D_f/N)10^3$: relative fatalities; HDI: Human Development Index; HI: health index; $\lambda$: average latitude degree north.

The HDI value is calculated as the geometric mean of normalized indices measuring achievements in each dimension.

During the 2009 A(H1N1) pandemic, several pharmaceutical (antivirals, vaccination) and nonpharmaceutical (school closures, travel restrictions, limiting public gatherings, etc.) measures were recommended across communities [29, 30]. All countries agreed on EU Health Security Committee (HSC) recommendations to immunize risk and target groups such as healthcare workers, pregnant women, and those older than six months with chronic ill health; however some countries even targeted children or entire population [2, 10]. Hungary was the first EU country able to start vaccination (during week 40), and other countries followed afterwards. In EU/EEA, at least 46.2 million (9% of the population) was vaccinated as of mid-July 2010 [2].

Vaccination coverage of various European countries is presented in Table 3 based on Mereckiene et al.'s [10] study. The vaccination coverage data for Lithuania was not available and presented data related to Germany corresponds to the vaccinated people above the age of 14.

In this table, $t_i$ and $t_e$ denote, respectively, the onset and the end of the epidemic wave which are estimated as the week before the first fatality and the week after the last fatality, $t_e$ being counted from the beginning of 2009. The values $t_1$ and $t_2$ denote the weeks at which vaccination starts and ends, as reported in [10], $t_2$ being counted cumulatively. Latest reported time is week 86 corresponding to the end of the survey. The duration of the epidemic wave, $\Delta T$, is defined as $\Delta T = t_e - t_i$, with $t_i$ and $t_e$ estimated in Table 3. The time span between the onset of the epidemic pulse and the starting of the pulse vaccination $\Delta V$ is defined as $\Delta V = t_1 - t_i$. $QV = \Delta V / \Delta T$ is the relative timing of the vaccination campaign within the epidemic pulse and a negative or small positive value indicates on-time vaccination campaign. $QV$ together with the total vaccination percentage $V_f$ will be considered as a measure of the efficiency of the vaccination strategy. In many countries, vaccination timing goes beyond

TABLE 3: Vaccination coverage.

| Country | $t_i$ | $t_1$ | $t_e$ | $t_2$ | $\Delta T$ | $\Delta V$ | $QV$ | $V_f$ |
|---|---|---|---|---|---|---|---|---|
| Czech Rep. | 41 | 48 | 64 | 76 | 23 | 7 | 0.30 | 0.6 |
| Estonia | 45 | 51 | 63 | 86 | 18 | 6 | 0.33 | 3 |
| France | 42 | 43 | 67 | 86 | 25 | 1 | 0.04 | 8 |
| Germany | 42 | 44 | 67 | 85 | 25 | 2 | 0.08 | 8 |
| Greece | 46 | 47 | 68 | 86 | 22 | 1 | 0.04 | 3 |
| Hungary | 40 | 40 | 63 | 86 | 23 | 0 | 0.00 | 27 |
| Ireland | 38 | 43 | 51 | 86 | 13 | 5 | 0.38 | 23 |
| Lithuania | 45 | 53 | 61 | 86 | 16 | 8 | 0.50 | — |
| Netherlands | 41 | 44 | 61 | 56 | 20 | 3 | 0.15 | 30 |
| Norway | 40 | 43 | 51 | 66 | 11 | 3 | 0.27 | 45 |
| Romania | 45 | 48 | 61 | 77 | 16 | 3 | 0.19 | 9 |
| Slovenia | 45 | 44 | 57 | 58 | 12 | −1 | −0.08 | 5 |
| Sweden | 42 | 42 | 58 | 86 | 16 | 0 | 0.00 | 59 |

Note: $t_i$: the onset of the epidemic wave estimated as the week before the first fatality; $t_1$: the first week of vaccination; $t_e$: the end of the epidemic wave estimated as the week after the last fatality; $t_2$: the last week of vaccination (counted from the beginning of 2009); $\Delta T$: the duration of the epidemic wave, $\Delta T = t_e - t_i$; $\Delta V$: the time span between the onset of the epidemic pulse and the starting of the pulse vaccination, $\Delta V = t_1 - t_i$; $QV = \Delta V / \Delta T$: the relative timing of the vaccination campaign within the epidemic pulse (a negative or small positive value indicated on time vaccination campaign); $V_f$: total vaccination percentage.

the end of the epidemic but presumably the vaccination rate drops towards the end of the epidemic and the vaccination percentage saturates. Thus we will assume that vaccination is practically terminated at the end of the epidemic as if pulse vaccination was applied.

*2.4. SIR and SEIR Epidemic Models with Vaccination.* Compartmental models in epidemiology are based on the subdivision of the individuals in a society into distinct groups with respect to their status regarding the disease. The basic compartmental models are the Susceptible-Infected-Removed (SIR) and the Susceptible-Exposed-Infected-Removed (SEIR) models that represent quite adequately the spread of an epidemic in a society where the total population is constant, the characteristics of the disease are time independent, and no vaccination policy is in force. In these models, it is further assumed that immunity, once acquired, cannot be lost; hence the passage among the compartments is one-directional. This situation fits well with the spread of seasonal epidemics in a homogeneous closed society.

The standard Susceptible-Infected-Removed (SIR) and Susceptible-Exposed-Infected-Removed (SEIR) models [31, 32] consist of differential equations governing the dynamics of a population where the individuals can be "Susceptible" $(S)$, "Exposed" $(E)$, "Infected" $(I)$, and "Removed" $(R)$. Vaccination is incorporated in the model by adding the group of "Vaccinated" $(V)$ individuals who gain immunity without going through an infectious period. We reserved the term "Removed" to the group of individuals who gain immunity after going through an infectious period.

The resulting differential equations for the SIR and the SEIR system with vaccination are given as

$$\frac{dS}{dt} = \beta SI - \nu S(t),$$

$$\frac{dI}{dt} = \beta SI - \eta I,$$

$$\frac{dR}{dt} = \eta I,$$

$$\frac{dV}{dt} = \nu S(t), \tag{1}$$

$$\frac{dE}{dt} = \beta SI - \varepsilon E,$$

$$\frac{dI}{dt} = \varepsilon E - \eta I.$$

In these equations, the parameters $\beta$, $\varepsilon$, $\eta$, and $\nu$ are constants. In the SIR and SEIR models, the ratio of the parameters $\beta/\eta$ turns out to be equal to the basic reproduction number $R_0$, when a first-order approximation is used for $I(t)$ [33, 34].

The reciprocals of the parameters $\eta$ and $\varepsilon$ are, respectively, the infection period and the incubation period (latent period), respectively. The parameter $\nu$ is the vaccination rate; hence models without vaccination are obtained by putting $\nu = 0$. Since the total population is assumed to be constant, the normalization conditions are $S + I + R + V = 1$ and $S + E + I + R + V = 1$.

*2.5. Exact Solutions for Pulse Vaccination.* The differential equations for the SIR system with or without vaccination are solved implicitly for $I$ and $S$ as

$$(I - I_i) + (S - S_i) + \left(\frac{\nu}{\beta}\right)\ln\left(\frac{I}{I_i}\right) - \left(\frac{\eta}{\beta}\right)\ln\left(\frac{S}{S_i}\right) = 0, \tag{2}$$

where $S_i$ and $I_i \neq 0$ are the initial values of $S$ and $I$, respectively. For the SEIR system without vaccination we have a similar relation:

$$(E + I) - (E_i + I_i) + (S - S_i) - \left(\frac{\eta}{\beta}\right)\ln\left(\frac{S}{S_i}\right) = 0, \tag{3}$$

where $E_i$ is the initial value of $E$. The SEIR system with vaccination is an essentially third-order system that could not be integrated as in the case of the SIR system with vaccination.

In the following we assume that vaccination starts at $t = t_1$ and stops at $t = t_2$. The conditions as $t \rightarrow -\infty$ are characterized by $S \rightarrow 1$, $I \rightarrow 0$, $E \rightarrow 0$, and $R \rightarrow 0$; hence the initial conditions should be specified according to $I_i + E_i + S_i - (\eta/\beta)\ln(S_i) = 1$. It follows that at the initial stage prior to vaccination the implicit relations for the SIR and the SEIR models are, respectively,

$$I + S - \left(\frac{\eta}{\beta}\right)\ln(S) = 1,$$

$$E + I + S - \left(\frac{\eta}{\beta}\right)\ln(S) = 1, \tag{4}$$

regardless of the initial conditions. Let $S_f$, $R_f$, and $V_f$ be the final proportions of Susceptible, Removed, and Vaccinated individuals, respectively. Since the final state is characterized by $I = E = 0$, for both models the implicit relations are reduced to

$$S_f - \left(\frac{\eta}{\beta}\right)\ln(S_f) = 1. \tag{5}$$

It follows that the basic reproduction number $R_0 = \beta/\eta$ is expressed in terms of $S_f$ as

$$R_0 = \frac{\beta}{\eta} = -\frac{\ln(1 - R_f - V_f)}{(R_f + V_f)} = -\frac{\ln(S_f)}{1 - S_f}, \tag{6}$$

regardless of the vaccination coverage. If vaccination has never been applied, $S_f = 1 - R_f$, while if pulse vaccination has been in effect, $S_f = 1 - R_f - V_f$. Thus in the case of pulse vaccination, $R_0$ can be obtained by knowing the total percentage of Removed and Vaccinated individuals.

## 3. The Effects of Healthcare Quality of Countries

The basic parameter of the epidemic $R_0$ and the final proportion of the Removed individuals $R_f$ in the SIR and SEIR models are related by a one-to-one nonlinear relationship. Thus the basic reproduction number that can be measured from clinical studies at the early phases of an epidemic can also be found from the total proportion of Removed individuals at the postepidemic phase. The difficulty here lies in the fact that the final proportion of Removed individuals is hard to estimate. Nevertheless, the total number of fatalities can be considered as a measure of the individuals affected by the disease. The proportion of individuals who die from

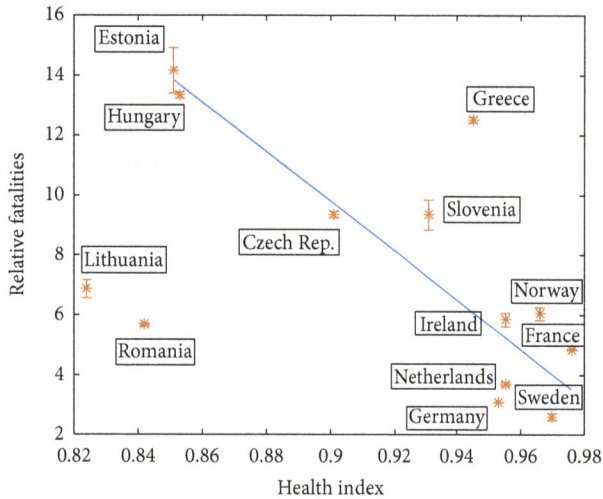

FIGURE 2: Relative fatalities versus the health index.

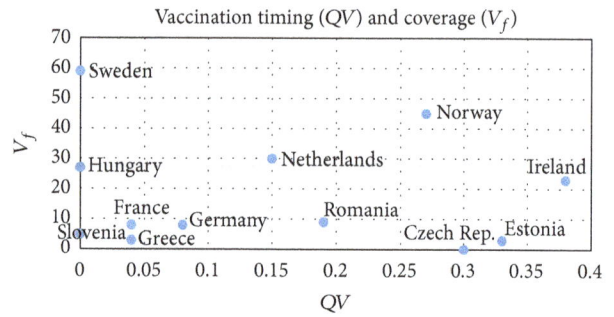

FIGURE 3: Vaccination timing versus vaccination coverage.

a disease is known as the case fatality rate (CFR). In the case of an influenza-like illness, the case fatality rate possibly depends on the quality of healthcare. The purpose of this section is to study the effects of healthcare, specifically, the relation between the relative fatalities and the healthcare indices for the countries that we study.

In order to examine the correlations between the relative fatalities and HDI and HI values, associated correlation coefficients are calculated. Weak negative correlations are found based on correlation coefficients of −0.4386 and −0.4834, respectively. Relative fatalities $(D_f/N)10^3$ versus the health index (HI) are shown in Figure 2, which displays roughly this negative correlation, despite numerous exceptions that will be discussed. In preliminary work, we have studied the effect of both indices and we have seen that for the countries under consideration they are closely correlated and we decided to work with HI values of the countries.

In this figure, the linear fit is obtained by minimizing the number of outliers with trial and error method. The countries that lie well off the linear fit are Lithuania and Romania with lower than expected relative fatalities and Greece with higher than expected relative fatalities. These countries are considered as outliers with the minimum error of 2.9%.

At the right lower part of the graph, corresponding to high HI, we observe that the relative fatalities are lower for Germany compared to France and lower for Sweden compared to Norway. Furthermore, the relative fatalities of Netherlands are also well below the regression line. In the next subsections, we discuss these relations.

### 3.1. Discussion of the Results for Netherlands.

The time evolution of the data has excessive fluctuations but we may consider the total number of fatalities data reliable. From Table 3, we can see that vaccination timing was appropriate and the coverage was as high as 30%. This may explain the low relative fatalities but we should also take into account the fact that Netherlands is the most densely populated country among the ones analyzed and the dependency of the parameter $\beta$ on the population density may have a saturation effect.

### 3.2. Comparison of the Results for Germany and France.

Merler et al. [35] reported that the peak of the pandemic was delayed in France due to timing of the school holidays (weeks 44 and 45) and the peak was predicted to happen on average at week 43.6 but actually happened at week 49. We can see that although Germany and France have similar demographic structures and vaccination policies and even though France has higher HI, the relative fatalities of France were higher than Germany. Detailed vaccination policies and strategies followed by France are presented in Schwarzinger et al.'s [36] study. The difference can be explained by epidemic-specific precautions and healthcare procedures applied in Germany as reported in [37]. Wilking et al. [37] suggested that mortality in Germany due to 2009 A(H1N1) pandemic seems to have been one of the lowest fatality ratios in Europe and early treatment might have had an impact on overall mortality.

### 3.3. Comparison of the Results for Norway and Sweden.

Norway and Sweden have similar geographic, demographic, and social characteristics. The difference between Sweden and Norway can be explained by their vaccination strategies. From Table 3, we can see that although vaccination started almost at the same time in both countries, for Norway it was almost 1/3 of the epidemic pulse, but for Sweden it was right at the beginning. It has actually been reported that in Norway vaccination campaign started too late to be effective [38] although probably above 40% of the Norwegian population got vaccinated [39]. In the study of de Blasio et al. [38], the effect of vaccination timing and sales of antivirals in Norway is analyzed with an age-structured SEIR model, and it is indicated that the countermeasures only prevented 11-12% of the potential cases relative to an unmitigated pandemic, and if the vaccination campaign would have started 6 weeks earlier, rather than week 43/2009, it is estimated that the vaccination alone might have reduced the clinical attack rate by 50%.

### 3.4. Vaccination Timing and Coverage of Analyzed Countries.

In Figure 3, vaccination timing ($QV$) versus vaccination coverage percentage ($V_f$) are shown for each analyzed country.

In this figure, lower right corner corresponds to late vaccination campaigns with low percentage coverage. The ones at the upper right correspond to late vaccination and high coverage so these are relatively inefficient campaigns.

(a)

(b)

(c)

(d)

(e)

(f)

(g)

(h)

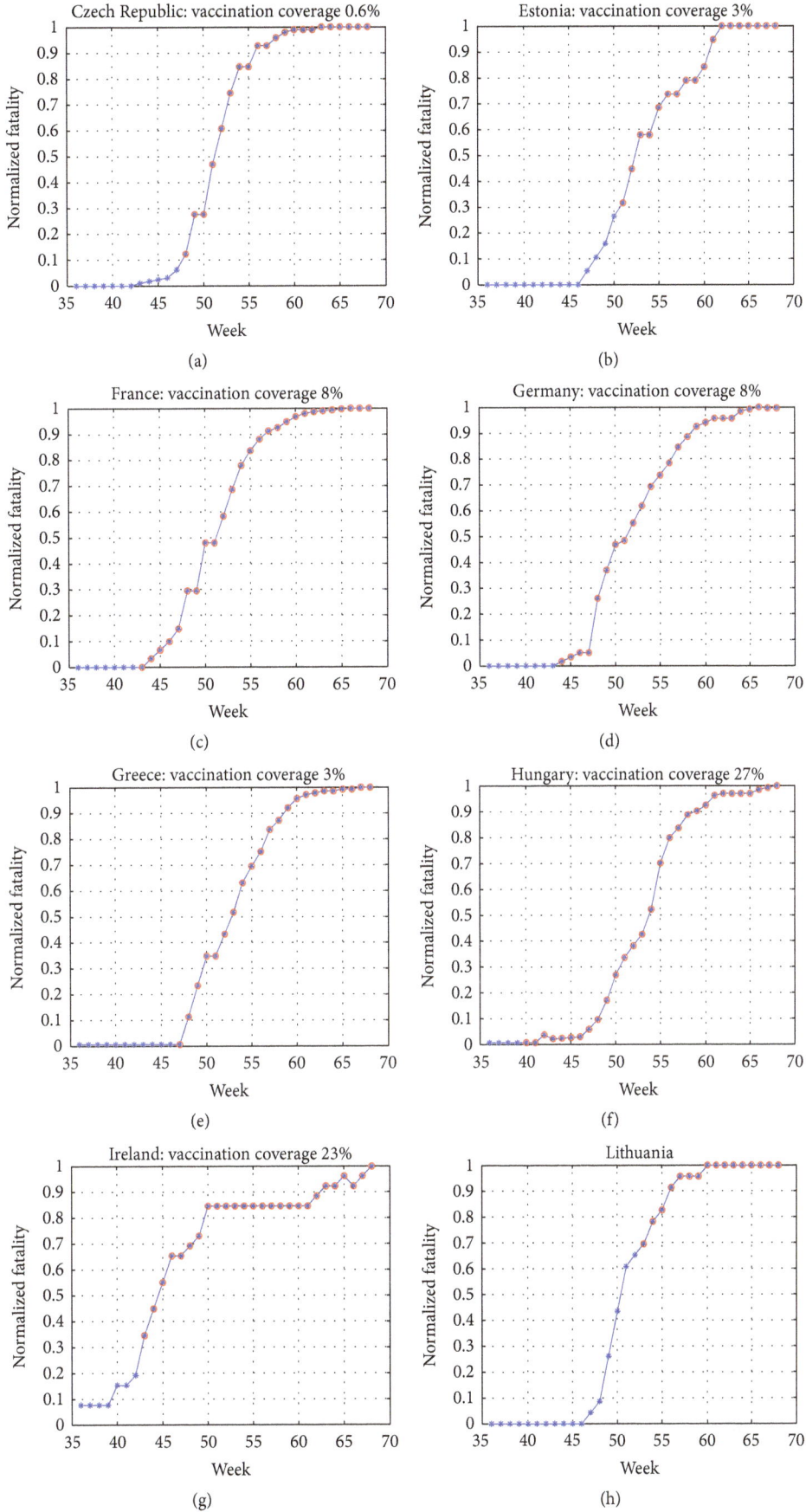

FIGURE 4: Continued.

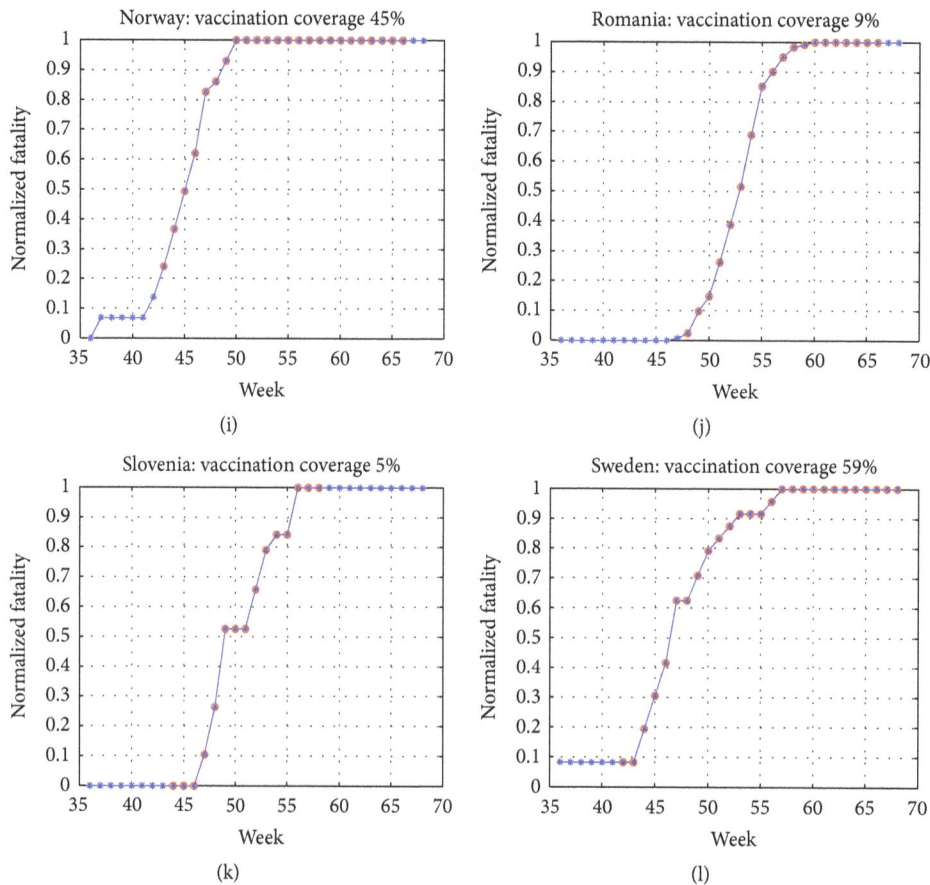

FIGURE 4: The normalized fatality data and the vaccination timings.

The ones at the upper left are the most efficient with on-time vaccination campaigns and high coverage. This figure explains the difference between Sweden and Norway. Both countries have similar HI, and their geographic and demographic properties are similar, the absolute timing difference for starting vaccination is just 1 week but the relative difference is large, and this reflects to the burden of the epidemic.

In Figures 4(a)–4(l), we present the data for each country and the vaccination timings, based on the vaccination information given in Table 3. Many countries claim having continued vaccination past the epidemic wave but the number of vaccinated people as a function of time is not given. It is reasonable to assume that the majority of the people have been vaccinated during the epidemic wave and vaccination continues only for specific target groups.

The timing of the vaccination should be measured by its location in the epidemic wave, as indicated in Table 3. For an efficient vaccination campaign, the ratio $QV$ should be small, even negative. We see that in many countries the ratio $QV$ is too high to be effective. From Table 3, we see that vaccination campaigns should have been most effective in Hungary, Sweden, and Netherlands. In Figures 4(a)–4(l), we can see this effect clearly for Sweden and Netherlands but not for Hungary.

## 4. Simulations for Pulse Vaccination Strategies

In this section, we present simulations for vaccination coverage and timing to conclude that on-time vaccinations have a considerable impact in reducing the final value $R_f$, but vaccination effects are practically unobservable in normalized time evolution curves $R(t)/R_f$.

In Table 3, the latest reported week is 86, corresponding to the end of the survey, but our study stops at week 68. The temporal distribution of vaccination rates is not given in these reports. However, it is reasonable that mass vaccination campaigns would be discontinued after the stabilization of the number of fatalities which signals the end of epidemic. In fact, the vaccination rates for France [10] confirm this. We thus assumed that total vaccination ratios are achieved by the end of week 68. Even if vaccination goes beyond the stabilization of $R(t)$, it does not change $R_f$; it simply decreases $S_f$ to zero.

*4.1. The Effect of Very Low Vaccination Coverage.* The total vaccination coverage given in Table 3 shows that total percentage of Vaccinated individuals was as low as 3% except for Hungary, Ireland, Netherlands, Norway, and Sweden. A comparison of the no vaccination and 3% vaccination for the SIR model is shown in Figures 5(a)-5(b).

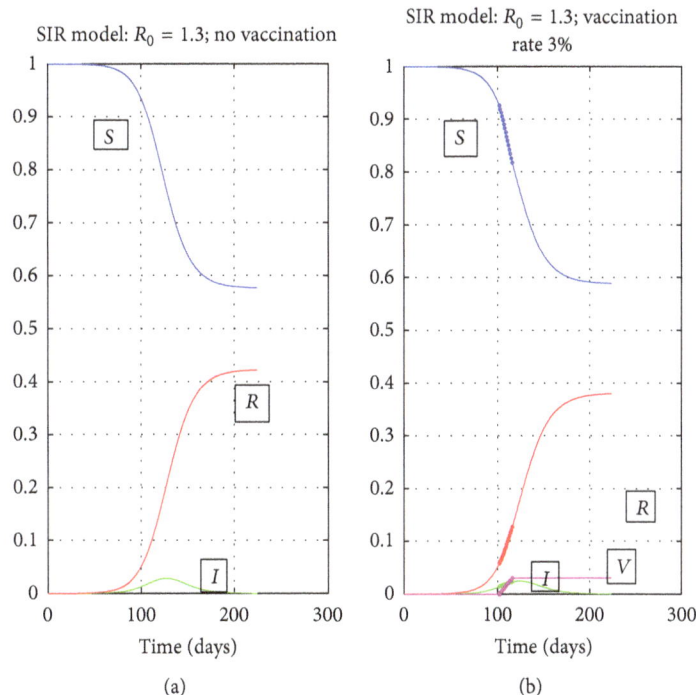

FIGURE 5: Comparison of no vaccination (a) and 3% vaccination (b) for the SIR model.

In this simulation, vaccination starts when $I(t)$ reaches half of its peak value and it is applied for 14 days. The final value of $S(t)$ is more or less the same, but the final value of $R(t)$ is lower. This issue is discussed in some detail in [40], where it is shown that the predicted number of cases of infections decreases linearly with vaccination coverage. Based on this, we considered vaccination to be effective on $R_f$ only for Hungary, Ireland, Netherlands, Norway, and Sweden, where the coverage was above 20%.

*4.2. The Effect of Vaccination Timing.* It is well known that the timing of pulse vaccination is crucial in controlling the spread of the infection. It is reported that the progression of the epidemic is from west to east, as seen from Figure 1 where we present the timing of the epidemic. We also note that it started earlier in Norway compared to Sweden and this had a crucial effect on the efficiency of vaccination [2]. In Table 3, the onset of the epidemic wave is considered as the week before the first fatality and the end of the epidemic as the week after the stabilization of $R(t)$. We thus measure "early" or "late" vaccination by the location of the starting time of the vaccination within this epidemic wave period.

In Figures 6(a)-6(b) we present a simulation of 30% vaccination, starting "early" and "late." The terms early and late refer to the timing of the vaccination with respect to the time $t_m$ where $I(t)$ for the no vaccination model reaches its maximum value. In our simulations, we used early and late pulse vaccinations as the ones starting one week earlier or later than $t_m$. The reductions in $R_f$ for each case show the importance of the vaccination timing.

Here we see that vaccination that starts late has little effect in reducing the number of Removed individuals. Vaccination

that continues beyond the stabilization of $R(t)$ is useless for influenza type epidemics. The simulations also show that even 2-week or 4-week campaigns may be sufficient.

*4.3. The Effect of Vaccination on Normalized Curves.* Although the efficiency of the vaccination on reducing the burden of the epidemic is unquestionable, it was a surprise to see that it had little effect on the shape of the time evolution curve, $R(t)$. In Figures 7(a)-7(b), we present the actual and normalized time evolution curves $R(t)$ and $R(t)/R_f$ for various vaccination coverage percentages, ranging from no vaccination (top and right) to 50% vaccination. From Figure 7(b), we see that the effect of high vaccination coverage on the normalized curves is a back-shift in time, rather than a distinguishable change in the shape. From these figures, we see that vaccination at low rates is practically unobservable in normalized curves. Even at high rates, it appears as a shift and a reduction in the curvature of the first turn if it is applied early and a reduction of the curvature of the second turn, if it is applied late.

*4.4. The Efficiency of Vaccination Campaigns.* In order to compare the efficiency of various vaccination campaigns, we ran a pulse vaccination simulation using SIR model. The simulation runs over 3 parameters, the duration of the vaccination campaign, the onset of the campaign, and the percentage of Vaccinated individuals. For each of these cases, we ran the SIR model with pulse vaccination using representative parameters $R_0$ = 1.5, $\eta$ = 1/4 and we computed the final percentage of Removed individuals $R_f$ as a function of these 3 parameters.

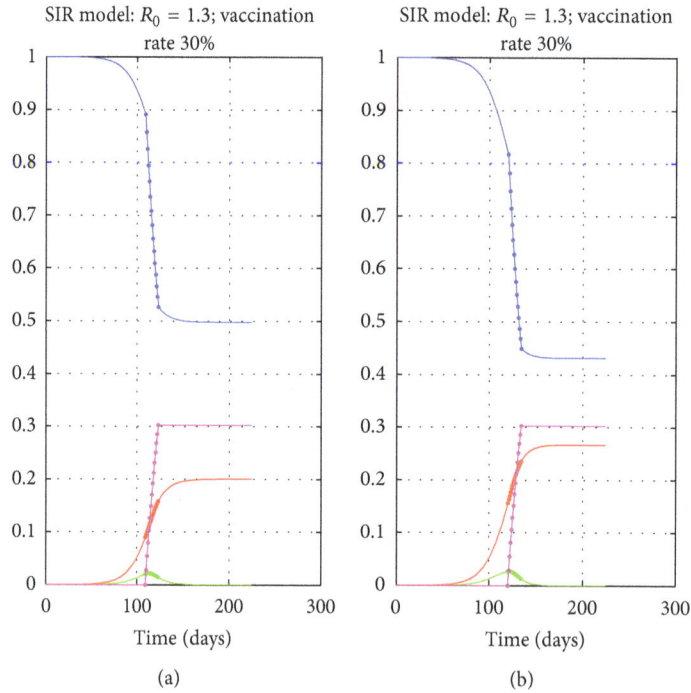

FIGURE 6: Comparison of early (a) and late (b) timings for 30% vaccination for the SIR model.

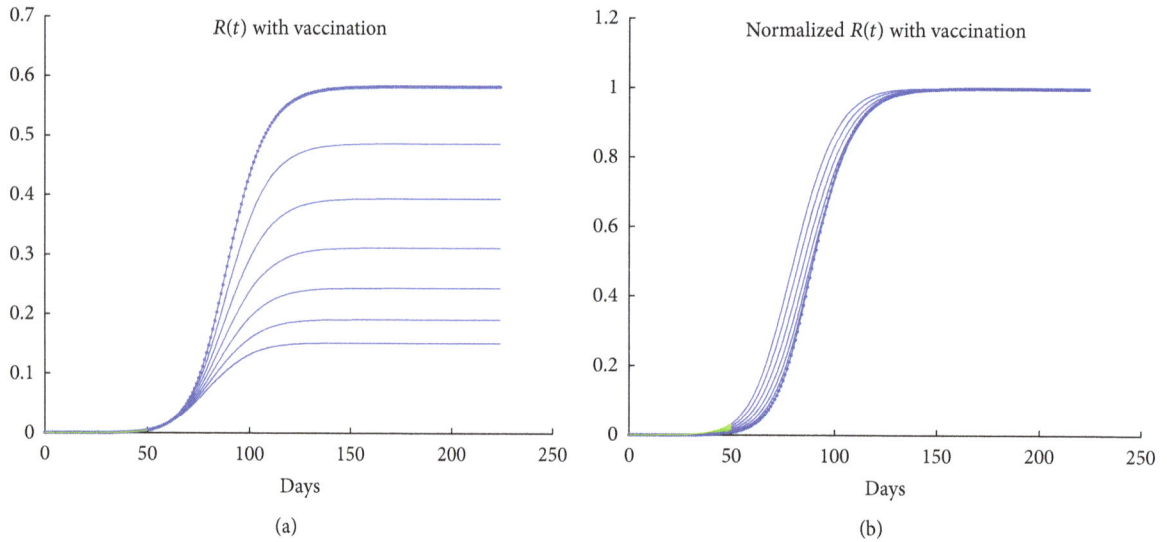

FIGURE 7: The effect of vaccination on actual (a) and normalized (b) $R(t)$.

We have chosen the duration of the pulse vaccinations as $k$ = 14, 28, 70, and 140 days, as presented, respectively, in Figures 8(a)–8(d). In these figures, the curves from top to down correspond to vaccination ratios ranging from 10% to 50% in steps of 5%, respectively. Points of these curves are the ratio of the final percentage of Removed individuals with pulse vaccination ($R_f$) and without pulse vaccination ($R_{f0}$). The horizontal axis is day $j$ of the onset of the vaccination campaign and the time origin is chosen at the peak $I(t)$ without vaccination. As an example, the top curve in Figure 8(a) corresponds to a 14-day campaign

with 10% vaccination ratio and one can see that a campaign that starts about 40 days before the expected peak of the epidemic reduces the final percentage of individuals affected by the epidemic to approximately 60% of this value when no vaccination is applied.

These figures can be useful in decisions related to vaccination strategies. For example, a short ($k$ = 14) but early ($j$ = −80) campaign with low coverage (15%) is as efficient as a long ($k$ = 70) but relatively late ($j$ = −40) campaign with higher (20%) coverage, both leading to approximately 30% improvement. On the other hand, campaigns with duration

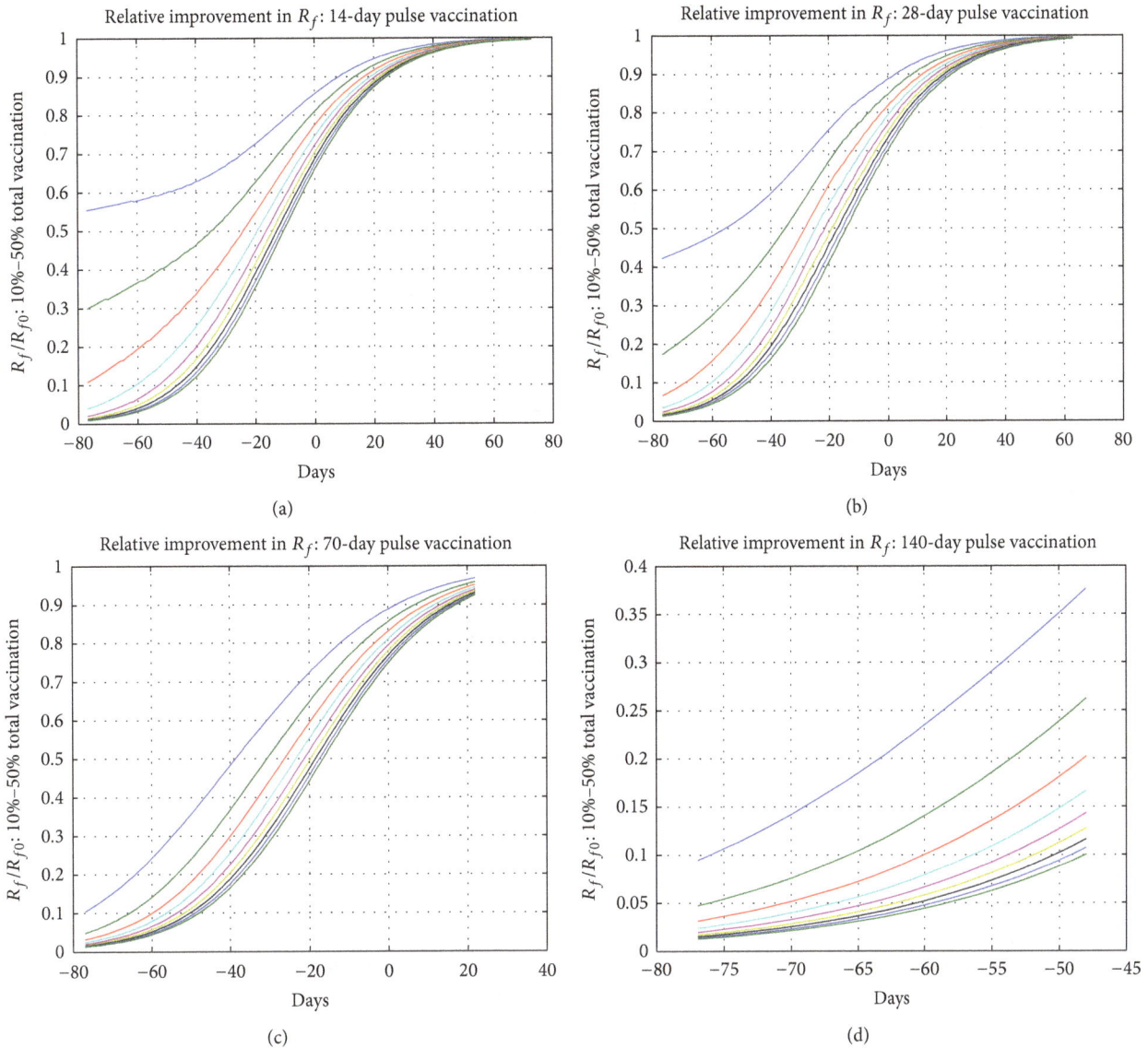

FIGURE 8: The improvement in $R_f$ for total vaccination ratios ranging from 10% (top curves) to 50% in steps of 5% for the SIR model. Time origin is chosen as the peak of $I(t)$ with no vaccination. Pulse vaccination starts at day $j$ (horizontal axis) and lasts for 14 days (a), 28 days (b), 70 days (c), and 140 days (d).

$k = 70$ that start later than day $j = -30$ can never reach this improvement level. Thus, vaccination campaigns should start as early as possible *with respect to the expected peak of the epidemic* and one should be aware that longer campaigns that start late would have limited efficiency despite their higher coverages.

## 5. Discussion

We have studied the relation between the HI and the relative fatalities of countries and obtained a linear fit by minimizing the outliers with trial and error method. We realized a roughly negative correlation and Lithuania, Romania, and Greece were considered outliers. Netherlands had lower relative

fatalities than expected and this may be due to appropriate timing, high coverage of vaccination, and the saturation effect of the parameter $\beta$ on the high population density of Netherlands. The relative fatalities in France were higher than in Germany although they have similar demographic structures and vaccination policies and the difference may be explained by epidemic-specific precautions and healthcare procedures applied by Germany. Norway had higher relative fatalities than Sweden although they are demographically and HI-wise similar, and this can be explained by vaccination strategies, specifically by the timing of the vaccination and vaccination coverage percentage. Even though vaccination started almost at the same time in both countries, in Norway it was too late to be effective since the relative timing of the starting time of the vaccination, its location in the epidemic wave, is significant. For an efficient vaccination campaign the ratio $QV$ should be small and even negative and in many countries the $QV$ ratio was too high to be effective.

We presented simulations for vaccination coverage and the timing of the vaccination with respect to the peak of the epidemic to study their role in vaccination efficiency. We realized that on-time vaccinations considerably reduce the final value of $R_f$, but these effects are practically too little to be observed on the shape of the normalized curve $R(t)/R_f$. To study the effect of percentage of vaccination coverage, we compared no vaccination policy and 3% vaccination for the SIR model and realized that $R_f$ is lower in 3% strategy than no vaccination policy even though final value of $S(t)$ is more or less the same. Hungary, Ireland, Netherlands, Norway, and Sweden have vaccination coverage percentages above 20%, so in these countries vaccinations were considered to be effective on $R_f$. To study the effect of the timing of pulse vaccination, we presented SIR model results of 30% vaccination coverage percentage starting early and late, one week earlier or later than the time $t_m$, where $I(t)$ for the no vaccination model reaches its maximum value. Based on these results, we see that vaccinations that start late have little effect on reductions of $R_f$, and also even 2–4-week campaigns may be sufficient and campaigns that continue beyond the stabilization of $R(t)$ are not effective for influenza type epidemics. To study the effect of vaccination coverage percentages on actual and normalized curves, we presented $R(t)$ and $R(t)/R_f$ curves for different vaccination coverage percentages and realized that percentage of vaccination had little effect on the shape of $R(t)$. Low rates were practically unobservable in $R(t)/R_f$ curves but at high vaccination percentage rates the effect on $R(t)/R_f$ was a shift and a reduction in the curvature of the first turn for early vaccination timing and a reduction of the curvature of the second turn for late vaccination timing. Finally, SIR model simulations were used to show the relative improvements in $R_f$ when different pulse vaccination strategies are used.

## 6. Conclusions

We have seen that healthcare practices and HI of countries as well as vaccination campaigns explain the variations among relative fatalities. On-time vaccinations have a considerable effect on reducing the ratio of individuals that are Removed after going through an infections cycle, $R_f$; however, this effect is not practically observable in normalized time evolution curves $R(t)/R_f$, especially at low vaccination rates. An efficient vaccination campaign should start early in the phases of the epidemic but does not need to continue over the peak of the epidemic. We recall that $R_0$ can be estimated at the beginning of an epidemic; hence the peak of $I(t)$ can be estimated without the vaccine intervention. Based on this pieces of information, the timing and the coverage percentage of the vaccination can be planned effectively.

As a tool for controlling the epidemic, the timing of the pulse vaccination is crucial. The simulations show the importance of the timing of the vaccination and show that vaccinations that start late have little effect in reducing $R_f$. In order to be effective, vaccination should start in the early

phases of the epidemic but does not need to continue over the peak of the epidemic. The comparison of the vaccination timings for Norway and Sweden is a good example for this situation. The simulation results presented in Section 4.4 support the importance of the timing in vaccination campaigns.

Our study is limited to what can be inferred from publicly available data; we used WISO reports of ECDC and restricted our investigation to European countries. These countries display relatively small variations in their demographic structures and healthcare systems; hence our conclusions should not be generalized worldwide.

## Conflict of Interests

The authors declare that there is no conflict of interests regarding the publication of this paper.

## References

[1] ECDC surveillance reports 2009-2010, July 2015, http://www.ecdc.europa.eu/en/publications/surveillance_reports/influenza/Pages/influenza.aspx.

[2] European Centre for Disease Prevention and Control, *The 2009 A (H1N1) Pandemic in Europe*, ECDC, Stockholm, Sweden, 2010.

[3] A. H. Bilge, F. Samanlioglu, and O. Ergonul, "On the uniqueness of epidemic models fitting a normalized curve of removed individuals," *Journal of Mathematical Biology*, vol. 71, no. 4, pp. 767–794, 2015.

[4] Ö. Ergönül, S. Alan, Ö. Ak et al., "Predictors of fatality in pandemic influenza A (H1N1) virus infection among adults," *BMC Infectious Diseases*, vol. 14, no. 1, article 317, 2014.

[5] Writing Committee of the WHO Consultation on Clinical Aspects of Pandemic (H1N1) 2009 Influenza, "Clinical aspects of pandemic 2009 influenza A (H1N1) virus infection," *The New England Journal of Medicine*, vol. 362, no. 18, pp. 1708–1719, 2010.

[6] A. R. Tuite, A. L. Greer, M. Whelan et al., "Estimated epidemiologic parameters and morbidity associated with pandemic H1N1 influenza," *Canadian Medical Association Journal*, vol. 182, no. 2, pp. 131–136, 2010.

[7] A. A. Haghdoost, M. M. Gooya, and M. R. Baneshi, "Modelling of H1N1 flu in Iran," *Archives of Iranian Medicine*, vol. 12, no. 6, pp. 533–541, 2009.

[8] A. Barakat, H. Ihazmad, F. El Falaki, S. Tempia, I. Cherkaoui, and R. El Aouad, "2009 pandemic influenza a virus subtype H1N1 in Morocco, 2009-2010: epidemiology, transmissibility, and factors associated with fatal cases," *Journal of Infectious Diseases*, vol. 206, no. 1, pp. S94–S100, 2012.

[9] E. Navarro-Robles, L. Martínez-Matsushita, R. López-Molina, J. Fritz-Hernández, B. A. Flores-Aldana, and J. C. Mendoza-Pérez, "Model to estimate epidemic patterns of influenza A (H1N1) in Mexico," *Revista Panamericana de Salud Pública*, vol. 31, no. 4, pp. 269–274, 2012.

[10] J. Mereckiene, S. Cotter, J. T. Weber et al., "Influenza A(H1N1)pdm09 vaccination policies and coverage in Europe," *Eurosurveillance*, vol. 17, no. 4, 2012.

[11] World Health Organization, "Mathematical modelling of the pandemic H1N1 2009," The Weekly Epidemiological Record (WER), 21 August 2009, 84th Year, No. 34, 2009, 84, 341–352, http://www.who.int/wer.

[12] World Health Organization, "Transmission dynamics and impact of pandemic influenza A (H1N1) 2009 virus, Weekly epidemiological record," November 2009, 84th Year, no. 46, 2009, http://www.who.int/wer.

[13] P.-Y. Boëlle, S. Ansart, A. Cori, and A.-J. Valleron, "Transmission parameters of the A/H1N1 (2009) influenza virus pandemic: a review," *Influenza and Other Respiratory Viruses*, vol. 5, no. 5, pp. 306–316, 2011.

[14] L. Simonsen, P. Spreeuwenberg, R. Lustig et al., "Global mortality estimates for the 2009 influenza pandemic from the GLaMOR project: a modeling study," *PLoS Medicine*, vol. 10, no. 11, Article ID e1001558, 2013.

[15] G. Scalia Tomba, A. Svensson, T. Asikainen, and J. Giesecke, "Some model based considerations on observing generation times for communicable diseases," *Mathematical Biosciences*, vol. 223, no. 1, pp. 24–31, 2010.

[16] E. Kenah, M. Lipsitch, and J. M. Robins, "Generation interval contraction and epidemic data analysis," *Mathematical Biosciences*, vol. 213, no. 1, pp. 71–79, 2008.

[17] L. F. White, J. Wallinga, L. Finelli et al., "Estimation of the reproductive number and the serial interval in early phase of the 2009 influenza A/H1N1 pandemic in the USA," *Influenza and Other Respiratory Viruses*, vol. 3, no. 6, pp. 267–276, 2009.

[18] C. Fraser, C. A. Donnelly, S. Cauchemez et al., "Pandemic potential of a strain of influenza A (H1N1): early findings," *Science*, vol. 324, no. 5934, pp. 1557–1561, 2009.

[19] C. Munayco V, J. Gomez, V. A. Laguna-Torres et al., "Epidemiological and transmissibility analysis of influenza A(H1N1)v in a southern hemisphere setting: Peru," *Eurosurveillance*, vol. 14, no. 13, pp. 1–5, 2009.

[20] U. C. de Silva, J. Warachit, S. Waicharoen, and M. Chittaganpitch, "A preliminary analysis of the epidemiology of influenza A(H1N1)v virus infection in Thailand from early outbreak data, June-July 2009," *Euro Surveillance*, vol. 14, no. 31, pp. 1–3, 2009.

[21] European Centre for Disease Prevention and Control (ECDC), "Overview of surveillance of Influenza 2009/2010 in the EU/EEA," http://ecdc.europa.eu/en/publications/Publications/0909_TED_Overview_of_Surveillance_of_Influenza_2009-2010_in_EU-EEA.pdf.

[22] Central Intelligence Agency of United States of America (CIA), "The World Factbook," https://www.cia.gov/library/publications/the-world-factbook/.

[23] Writing Committee of the WHO Consultation on Clinical Aspects of Pandemic (H1N1) 2009 Influenza, "Clinical aspects of pandemic 2009 influenza A (H1N1) virus infection," *The New England Journal of Medicine*, vol. 362, no. 18, pp. 1708–1719, 2010.

[24] M. Lemaitre, F. Carrat, G. Rey, M. Miller, L. Simonsen, and C. Viboud, "Mortality Burden of the 2009 A/H1N1 influenza pandemic in France: comparison to seasonal influenza and the A/H3N2 pandemic," *PLoS ONE*, vol. 7, no. 9, Article ID e45051, 2012.

[25] C. C. van den Wijngaard, L. van Asten, M. P. G. Koopmans et al., "Comparing pandemic to seasonal influenza mortality: moderate impact overall but high mortality in young children," *PLoS ONE*, vol. 7, no. 2, Article ID e31197, 2012.

[26] M. D. Van Kerkhove, K. A. H. Vandemaele, V. Shinde et al., "Risk factors for severe outcomes following 2009 influenza A (H1N1) infection: a global pooled analysis," *PLoS Medicine*, vol. 8, no. 7, Article ID e1001053, 2011.

[27] Europe in Figures, Eurostat yearbook 2011, Eurostat Statistical Books, http://ec.europa.eu/eurostat.

[28] Human Development Reports 2010, 2015, http://hdr.undp.org/en/.

[29] J. K. Kelso, N. Halder, and G. J. Milne, "Vaccination strategies for future influenza pandemics: a severity-based cost effectiveness analysis," *BMC Infectious Diseases*, vol. 13, article 81, 2013.

[30] S. Cauchemez, M. D. Van Kerkhove, B. N. Archer et al., "School closures during the 2009 influenza pandemic: national and local experiences," *BMC Infectious Diseases*, vol. 14, no. 207, pp. 1–11, 2014.

[31] W. O. Kermack and A. G. McKendrick, "A contribution to the mathematical theory of epidemics," *Proceedings of the Royal Society of London Series A: Mathematical, Physical and Engineering Sciences*, vol. 115, no. 772, pp. 700–721, 1927.

[32] R. M. Anderson and R. M. May, "Population biology of infectious diseases: part I," *Nature*, vol. 280, no. 5721, pp. 361–367, 1979.

[33] C. Castillo-Chavez, Z. L. Feng, and W. Z. Huang, "On the computation of $R_0$ and its role on global stability," in *Proceedings of the Workshop on Emerging and Reemerging Diseases*, C. Castillo Chavez, S. Blower, P. VandenDriessche et al., Eds., University of Minnesota, Institute of Mathematics and Its Applications, Minneapolis, Minn, USA, May 1999.

[34] C. Castillo-Chavez, S. Blower, P. van den Driessche, D. Kirschner, and A.-A. Yakubu, Eds., *Mathematical Approaches for Emerging and Reemerging Infectious Diseases: An Introduction*, vol. 125 of *IMA Volumes in Mathematics and Its Applications*, Springer, 2002.

[35] S. Merler, M. Ajelli, A. Pugliese, and N. M. Ferguson, "Determinants of the spatiotemporal dynamics of the 2009 h1n1 pandemic in Europe: implications for real-time modelling," *PLoS Computational Biology*, vol. 7, no. 9, Article ID e1002205, 2011.

[36] M. Schwarzinger, R. Flicoteaux, S. Cortarenoda, Y. Obadia, and J.-P. Moatti, "Low acceptability of A/H1N1 pandemic vaccination in french adult population: did public health policy fuel public dissonance?" *PLoS ONE*, vol. 5, no. 4, Article ID e10199, 2010.

[37] H. Wilking, S. Buda, E. von der Lippe et al., "Mortality of 2009 pandemic influenza A(H1N1) in Germany," *Eurosurveillance*, vol. 15, no. 49, p. 19741, 2010.

[38] B. F. de Blasio, B. G. Iversen, and G. S. Tomba, "Effect of vaccines and antivirals during the major 2009 A(H1N1) pandemic wave in Norway—and the influence of vaccination timing," *PLoS ONE*, vol. 7, no. 1, Article ID e30018, 2012.

[39] K. Waalen, A. Kilander, S. G. Dudman, G. H. Krogh, T. Aune, and O. Hungnes, "High prevalence of antibodies to the 2009 pandemic influenza A(H1N1) virus in the Norwegian population following a major epidemic and a large vaccination campaign in autumn," *Eurosurveillance*, vol. 15, no. 31, p. 19633, 2009.

[40] M. Keeling, M. Tildesley, T. House, and L. Danon, "The mathematics of vaccination," *Mathematics Today*, no. 4, pp. 40–43, 2013.

# 14

# Challenges of Identifying Clinically Actionable Genetic Variants for Precision Medicine

**Tonia C. Carter[1] and Max M. He[1,2,3]**

[1]Center for Human Genetics, Marshfield Clinic Research Foundation, Marshfield, WI 54449, USA
[2]Biomedical Informatics Research Center, Marshfield Clinic Research Foundation, Marshfield, WI 54449, USA
[3]Computation and Informatics in Biology and Medicine, University of Wisconsin-Madison, Madison, WI 53706, USA

Correspondence should be addressed to Max M. He; he.max@mcrf.mfldclin.edu

Academic Editor: Saverio Affatato

Advances in genomic medicine have the potential to change the way we treat human disease, but translating these advances into reality for improving healthcare outcomes depends essentially on our ability to discover disease- and/or drug-associated clinically actionable genetic mutations. Integration and manipulation of diverse genomic data and comprehensive electronic health records (EHRs) on a big data infrastructure can provide an efficient and effective way to identify clinically actionable genetic variants for personalized treatments and reduce healthcare costs. We review bioinformatics processing of next-generation sequencing (NGS) data, bioinformatics infrastructures for implementing precision medicine, and bioinformatics approaches for identifying clinically actionable genetic variants using high-throughput NGS data and EHRs.

## 1. Introduction

High-throughput genomics technology has made possible the era of precision medicine, an approach to healthcare that involves integrating a patient's genetic, lifestyle, and environmental data and then comparing these data to similar data collected for thousands of other individuals to predict illness and determine the best treatments. Precision medicine aims to tailor healthcare to patients by using clinically actionable genomic mutations to guide preventive interventions and clinical decision making [1]. In the past 25 years, more than 4,000 Mendelian disorders have been studied at the genetic level [2]. In addition, more than 80 million genetic variants have been uncovered in the human genome [3, 4]. Clinical pharmacology research using electronic health record (EHR) systems has recently become feasible as EHRs have been implemented more widely [5]. Also, studies such as the Electronic Medical Records and Genomics-Pharmacogenomics (eMERGE-PGx) project [6], GANI_MED project [7], SCAN-B initiative [8], and Cancer 2015 study [9] have been designed to assess the value of next-generation sequencing (NGS) in healthcare.

Combining the functional characterization of identified genomic mutations with comprehensive clinical data available in EHRs has the potential to provide compelling evidence to implicate novel disease- and/or drug-associated mutations in phenotypically well-characterized patients. NGS is increasingly used in biomedical research and clinical practice. NGS technological advances in clinical genome sequencing and adoption of EHRs will pave the way to create patient-centered precision medicine in clinical practice. NGS technology is an essential component supporting genomic medicine but the volume and complexity of the data pose challenges for its use in clinical practice [10]. Sequencing a single human genome generates megabytes of data; therefore, investment in a bioinformatics infrastructure is required to implement NGS in clinical practice.

The term "big data" is defined differently by different people [11]. Gartner defines big data as "high-volume, high-velocity, and/or high-variety information assets that demand cost-effective, innovative forms of information processing that enable enhanced insight, decision making, and process automation" (http://www.gartner.com/it-glossary/big-data/) while others define it as the 5 Vs, which are Volume, Velocity,

TABLE 1: Sequencing assays.

| Characteristic | DNA sequencing | | | RNA-seq | |
| --- | --- | --- | --- | --- | --- |
| | Targeted genomic regions | Whole exome | Whole genome | Targeted | Transcriptome profiling |
| Capture method[*] | Amplicon-based targeting; hybrid capture; in-solution capture | Hybrid capture; in-solution capture | None | Hybridization only; hybridization and extension; multiplexed PCR | None |
| Amount of genome/transcriptome sequenced | ~150 bp–62 Mb (≤2% of genome) | ~30–60 Mb (1-2% of genome) | ~3 Gb (≥95% of genome) | Variable: transcripts of ~10–1000 genes | Entire transcriptome |
| Amplification | Yes | Yes | Not required | Yes | Required for low-quantity RNA samples |
| Sequencing depth | 100–1000x[Ü] | 80–100x[Ü] | 30–50x[Ü] | 0.3–25 million reads[‡] | 15–200 million reads[‡] |
| Amount of sequence data generated per sample | ~0.3–5 Gb | ~4-5 Gb | ~90 Gb | ~0.5–3 Gb | ~5-6 Gb |

bp, base pairs; Mb, megabases; Gb, gigabases; PCR, polymerase chain reaction.
[*]Method used to select genomic regions for sequencing.
[Ü]Number of times a single base is read during a sequencing run.
[‡]A greater number of reads are needed to detect rare transcripts.

Variety, Verification/Veracity, and Value [12]. In this review, we describe how one source of big data, in the form of genomic data generated by NGS, is processed and being used to improve healthcare and clinical research. We give an overview of NGS technologies, bioinformatics processing of NGS data, bioinformatics approaches for identifying clinically actionable variants in sequence data, guidelines for maintaining high standards when generating genomic data for clinical use, bioinformatics infrastructures of studies aimed at implementing precision medicine, and methods for ensuring the security of genomic data. We also discuss the need for the efficient integration of genomic information into EHRs.

## 2. Genomic Data Generation

*2.1. Approaches to Sequencing.* NGS includes DNA sequencing and RNA sequencing (RNA-seq) (Table 1). DNA sequencing approaches include (1) whole-genome sequencing (WGS), (2) whole exome sequencing (WES) of the coding regions of all known genes, and (3) targeted sequencing of genomic regions or genes implicated in a disease [13]. In addition, RNA-seq is used in transcriptome profiling to sequence all RNA transcripts (the transcriptome) in cells at a given time point to measure gene expression, targeted sequencing for measuring the expression of transcripts encoded by a specific genomic region, and sequencing of small RNAs. Targeted DNA sequencing is already being applied in some areas of clinical practice such as pharmacogenomics (e.g., the eMERGE-PGx project [6]), while WGS, and particularly WES, is emerging into the clinic for the evaluation of developmental brain disorders such as intellectual disability [14], autism [15], and seizures [16]. With continuing decreases in the costs of sequencing, it is expected that the use of WES/WGS and RNA sequencing in healthcare will become more common.

*2.2. Read Depth.* NGS involves breaking DNA into fragments and determining the order of the nucleotide bases in each fragment. The sequence of each fragment is called a "read." Because the distribution of reads across the genome is uneven (due to biases in sample preparation, sequencing-platform chemistry, and bioinformatics methods for genomic alignment and assembly of the reads) [17, 18], some bases are present in more reads and others in fewer reads. Read depth refers to the number of reads that contain a base; for example, a 10x read depth means that each base was present in an average of 10 reads. For RNA-seq, read depth is more often stated in terms of the number of millions of reads. Variant calling is more reliable with increasing read depth, and a greater depth is advantageous for detecting rare genetic variants with confidence. The read depth needed can depend on multiple factors including guidelines from the scientific community, the presence of repetitive genomic regions (these are more difficult to sequence), the error rate of the sequencing platform, the algorithm used for assembling reads into a genomic sequence, and gene expression level (for RNA-seq). Read depth recommendations from the scientific literature include 100x for heterozygous single nucleotide variant detection by WES [19], 35x for genotype detection by WGS [20], 60x for detecting insertions/deletions (INDELs) by WGS [21], 10–25 million reads for differential gene expression profiling by RNA-seq [22], and 50–100 million reads for allele-specific gene expression by RNA-seq [23].

### 2.3. Sequencing Technologies

*2.3.1. Description of Technologies.* Commercially available sequencing platforms use a variety of methods to generate sequence data (Table 2). Sequencing-by-synthesis (MiSeq and HiSeq 4000 platforms) is the enzymatic synthesis of a DNA strand complementary to a template DNA strand. For

TABLE 2: Comparison of sequencing instruments.

| Characteristic | MiSeq | PacBio RS II | Ion S5 | HiSeq 4000 | 454 GS FLX Titanium XL+ | SOLiD 5500xl W | Sanger Genetic Analyzer 3500xL |
|---|---|---|---|---|---|---|---|
| Instrument price | ~$125 K | ~$695 K | ~$65 K | ~$900 K | ~$500 K | ~$595 K | ~$173 K |
| Sequencing mechanism | Sequencing-by-synthesis | Single-molecule, real-time sequencing | Semiconductor sequencing | Sequencing-by-synthesis | Pyrosequencing | Oligonucleotide ligation | Dideoxynucleotide chain termination |
| Sequencing application | Targeted | Targeted; transcriptome profiling | Targeted; whole exome; transcriptome profiling | Whole exome/genome; transcriptome profiling | Whole exome/genome; transcriptome profiling | Whole exome/genome; transcriptome profiling | Next-generation sequencing validation, targeted sequencing of mutations or small insertions/deletions |
| Maximum read length | 300 bp PE | 10,000 bp | 200 bp | 150 bp PE | 700 bp | 75 bp SE, 50 bp mate-paired | 850 bp |
| Reads per run | 15 million | 55–900 K | 60–80 million | 2.5–5 billion | ~1 million | 100 million–4.8 billion | Not applicable |
| Output data per run | 0.5–15 Gb | 0.5–16 Gb | ~44 Gb | 125–1500 Gb | ~0.7 Gb | 160–320 Gb | 2–100 Kb |
| Run time | 4–55 hours | 6 hours | 1–2 days | <1–3.5 days | 23 hours | 2–7 days | 0.5–3 hours |
| Advantages | Low error rate; short run time | Long read length; short run time | Short run time; low start-up cost | Low error rate; high throughput | Long read length | Low error rate | Low error rate; long read length |
| Disadvantages | Higher cost per base compared to HiSeq instruments | Medium/high cost per base | High error rate for homopolymer tracts and insertions/deletions | Short read length | High error rate for homopolymer tracts | Short read length; long run time | High cost per base; low throughput |

bp, base pairs; Gb, gigabases; K, thousand; Kb, kilobases; PE, paired-end; SE, single-end.

NGS, the procedure involves DNA fragmentation, creation of a DNA library by attaching adaptors to each fragment, amplification of the fragments on a solid surface, synthesis of a DNA strand complementary to each template DNA fragment (using DNA polymerase), and fluorescence imaging to identify each newly incorporated nucleotide on the synthesized DNA strands [24]. Single-molecule, real-time sequencing (PacBio RS II platform) is a modification of sequencing-by-synthesis [25]. In this approach, each DNA polymerase molecule is immobilized at the bottom of a nanoscale well called a zero-mode waveguide. A laser light illuminates the well from below and emits a pulse of light when a fluorescent-labelled nucleotide is added to the nascent DNA strand by DNA polymerase (bound to a template DNA fragment), allowing detection of the incorporated nucleotide. Semiconductor sequencing (Ion S5 platform) is another modification of sequencing-by-synthesis that uses a semiconductor-sensing device to detect the addition of unmodified nucleotides during DNA synthesis [26]. Pyrosequencing (454 GS FLX Titanium XL+ platform) is a technique that couples sequencing-by-synthesis to a chemiluminescent enzyme (luciferase) reaction that generates visible light allowing detection of nucleotide incorporation during DNA synthesis [27]. Oligonucleotide ligation (SOLiD 5500xl W platform) involves ligating oligonucleotide probes to template DNA strands to determine the sequence of the template [28]. Sequencing by dideoxynucleotide (ddNTP) chain termination (Sanger Genetic Analyzer 3500xL platform), often called Sanger sequencing, involves incorporation of ddNTPs by DNA polymerase during DNA synthesis [29]. Fluorescence labelling allows identification of each of the ddNTPs added to the synthesized DNA strands.

*2.3.2. Comparison of Sequencers.* The MiSeq, PacBio RSII, and Ion S5 sequencers were designed for targeted sequencing and sequencing small genomes (e.g., the genomes of microorganisms) whereas the HiSeq 4000, 454 GS FLX Titanium XL+, and SOLiD 5500xl W can be used for WES and WGS of human genomes (Table 2). The instruments most often used in precision medicine programs performing WES/WGS of the human genome in clinical care settings are the HiSeq sequencers [30] that have the advantages of a relatively high sample throughput and a low sequencing error rate. However, all of the NGS technologies are being applied to health research [31–36]. The single-molecule, real-time sequencing technology generates the longest reads (Table 2), making the PacBio RS II instrument well suited for de novo sequencing (by assembly of reads into long contiguous sequences) of the genomes of organisms that do not have a reference genome (e.g., many microbial genomes) [37].

The sequencers that cost the least are the bench-top Ion S5 and MiSeq instruments (Table 2), and for many laboratories it would be feasible to buy more than one of these instruments. While they can be used to perform WES of the human genome, the sequencing cost per base would be much higher compared with WES on the HiSeq instrument. The HiSeq 4000, 454 GS FLX Titanium XL+, and SOLiD 5500xl W instruments are more expensive, costing between $500,000 and $900,000 each, but they are capable of sequencing

several human genomes or exomes within a few days to one week. Large laboratories that expect to assay many samples routinely by WES/WGS might consider it cost-efficient to buy more than one of these sequencers to meet assay demand. All six next-generation sequencers in Table 2 produce at least 0.5 gigabases per run and most output several gigabases per run, giving an idea of the volume of data that needs to be considered when planning for the data storage and processing capabilities of bioinformatics pipelines to be used in clinical laboratories that perform NGS assays.

*2.3.3. Sequencing Accuracy.* With continued refinement in technology, many NGS platforms have demonstrated a low rate of errors in variant detection (1/1000 to 1/50 bases depending on the instrument and read depth) [38, 39]. Previous reports have compared sequencing accuracy among the technologies presented in Table 2. In a comparison of the HiSeq 2000 and SOLiD 5500xl platforms for WGS of human DNA samples, the HiSeq 2000 had higher sensitivity for calling single nucleotide variants but the SOLiD 5500xl had a lower false positive rate [40]. When the Ion PGM, MiSeq, and PacBio RS sequencers were compared by sequencing four microbial genomes, the PacBio RS had the highest sequencing error rate, and Ion PGM data had slightly more variant calls and a higher false positive rate than MiSeq data [41]. Compared with other technologies, the 454 and PacBio RS platforms have demonstrated the most unbiased read distribution in genomic regions with a high GC content [41, 42], an important factor affecting the probability of calling a variant in these regions. However, the 454 platform has a tendency to assess the length of homopolymer tracts incorrectly, resulting in false positive single nucleotide variant calls in these tracts [42].

In comparison with NGS technologies, Sanger sequencing is widely considered the most accurate sequencing method (error rate as low as 1 in 10,000 bases) [43] and remains the gold standard. Genetic variants detected using NGS should always be validated by an independent method if the variants are relevant to clinical care or are associated with health outcomes in research studies. Because of its high accuracy, Sanger sequencing is often used for validation. Other methods of validation, especially for common single nucleotide variants, INDELs, or structural variants, include polymerase chain reaction (PCR) and genotype/copy number variant arrays.

# 3. Genomic Data Processing and Quality Control

*3.1. Data Processing.* Data files generated by next-generation sequencers contain raw sequence reads, each with a unique identifier, and their quality scores. Sequence reads need to be evaluated for data quality and to exceed minimum quality thresholds, before being processed for read alignment [44], variant calling [45], and variant annotation [46, 47] in a bioinformatics pipeline (Figure 1). Read alignment involves aligning the sequence reads to a reference sequence [48, 49] of the human genome to allow comparison of sequence data from the patient sample with the reference sequence. Reads

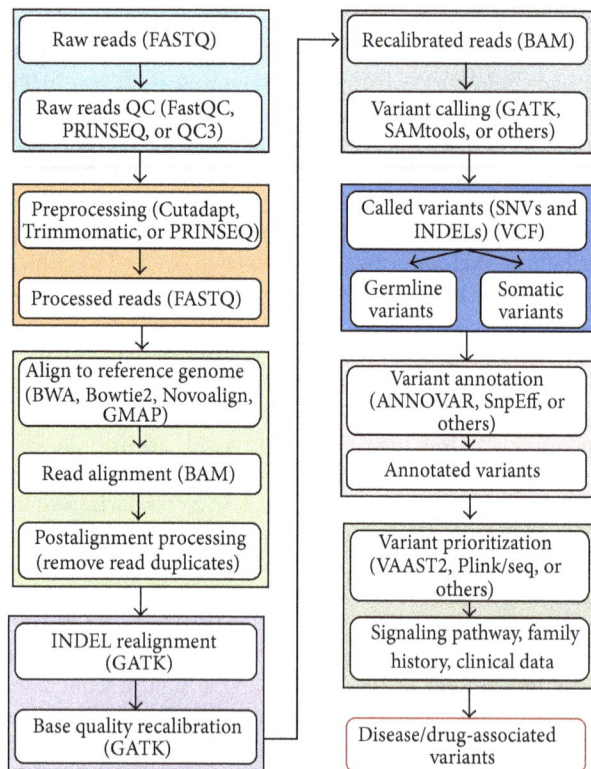

FIGURE 1: A flow chart of processing next-generation sequencing data.

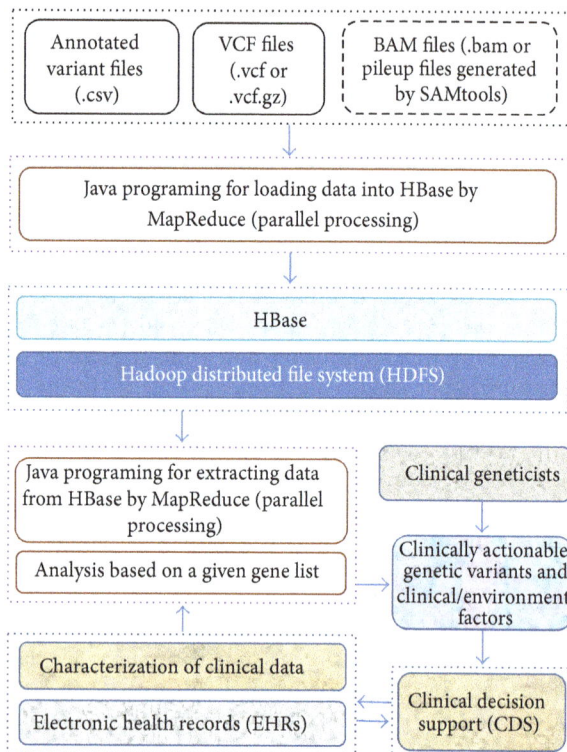

FIGURE 2: The basic framework of SeqHBase for detecting clinically actionable genetic variants.

with an uncertain alignment location need to be removed before further data processing. Alignment allows a number of quality control measures to be determined, for example, the percentage of all reads that align to a reference sequence, the percentage of unique reads that align to a reference sequence, and the number of reads that align at a specific locus (read depth). These measures influence the reliability of variant calling, the next step in a NGS bioinformatics pipeline. Variant calling tools, such as SAMtools [50], GATK [45], and others, are used to identify differences in sequence between the patient sample and a reference. These differences can include changes of one nucleotide (single nucleotide variants, SNVs), a few nucleotides (small INDELs), or larger regions, such as copy number variants (CNVs) and other structural variations (SVs). These software programs allow users to specify different parameters to adjust for minimizing false positive and false negative variant calls. Variant annotation depends on biological knowledge and provides information on the known or likely impact of variants on gene and protein function [46, 47]. To produce a patient report, annotated variants are interpreted in a disease-specific context and are often classified based on their known or expected clinical impact. For instance, the ClinVar [51] variant database, released on May 4, 2015 (http://www.ncbi.nlm.nih.gov/clinvar/), by the National Center for Biotechnology Information (NCBI), contained more than 110,000 unique genetic variants having clinical interpretations [52].

3.2. Clinically Actionable Variants. In clinical care, the American College of Medical Genetics and Genomics (ACMG) has recommended the identification and return of incidental findings (IFs) for clinically significant variants in a set of 56 "highly medically actionable" genes associated with 24 inherited conditions [53, 54]. Also, the National Heart, Lung, and Blood Institute (NHLBI) Exome Sequencing Project (ESP) has reported actionable exomic IFs from 112 genes in 6,503 participants [55]. The 112 genes included 52 ACMG genes and an additional 60 "actionable" genes. To infer biological insights from massive amounts of NGS data and comprehensive clinical data in a short period of time, we have developed an analysis pipeline within a software framework called SeqHBase [56] (Figure 2) to quickly identify disease- or drug-associated genetic variants. There were more than 27 million unique variants among 300 patients with WGS data that we analyzed using SeqHBase. In addition to identifying variants that are annotated as "pathogenic" or "likely pathogenic" by ClinVar [51], we compiled a list of low frequency or rare variants that are possibly damaging, and novel loss-of-function (LoF) variants that are absent in the ClinVar database, to allow clinical geneticists to review the potential pathogenicity of these variants further. As SeqHBase is a big data-based toolset, it takes only a few minutes to analyze WGS data for 300 individuals and to generate a candidate list of actionable genomic variants. More detailed discoveries from these WGS data will be described in future reports.

SeqHBase is one of several, freely accessible bioinformatics tools for prioritization of variants from WES/WGS data. Daneshjou et al. reported a web-based tool for identifying clinically actionable variants in the 56 ACMG genes [57], and Zhou et al. developed a variant characterization framework for targeted analysis of relevant reads from high-throughput sequencing data [58]. Other tools include PHIVE [59] which prioritizes variants in genes responsible for mouse model phenotypes that are similar to the phenotypes of patients being tested by WES and OVA [60] that performs prioritization by integrating data on human and model organism phenotypes, gene function, and known biological pathways.

Identifying clinically actionable variants remains a challenge despite the availability of variant prioritization tools. A workshop convened by the National Human Genome Research Institute and the Wellcome Trust identified limited evidence of the clinical significance of genetic variants and the lack of a comprehensive database of genetic variant-phenotype associations as barriers to the implementation of precision medicine [61]. It was noted that existing catalogs of clinically actionable variants are not standardized, are maintained by different entities (e.g., laboratories or government organizations), and are not designed to interact with EHRs. To speed the incorporation of genomic data into clinical care, the workshop advocated for a dynamic, centralized database that can be updated with available, reliable evidence on variant pathogenicity. The Clinical Genome Resource (ClinGen) program [52], developed in response to this recommendation, provides resources (e.g., ClinVar [51]) to aid the understanding of genetic variation and the use of genetic variation in clinical practice.

*3.3. Quality Control.* Best practices for quality control in the bioinformatics processing of NGS data have been reported in the scientific literature [45, 62]. Quality control metrics include total reads, ratio of unique reads to total reads, proportion of bases covered at a specified minimum read depth, mean read depth, raw sequence error rates, ratio of transitions (pyrimidine-to-pyrimidine or purine-to-purine mutation) to transversions (pyrimidine-to-purine mutation or vice versa), missingness (proportion of genomic sites at which a variant could not be called), homozygosity, heterozygosity, and distribution of known and novel variants relative to those contained in the dbSNP database. For targeted or exome sequencing, an additional metric is capture efficiency, the percentage of targeted bases that are covered by one or more reads.

These metrics can be calculated using the PLINK/SEQ (https://atgu.mgh.harvard.edu/plinkseq/) or VCFtools [63] software programs that can readily be incorporated into a bioinformatics pipeline, allowing assessment of NGS data quality in both clinical and research settings. Values for the first four metrics depend on the type of sequencing assay performed but, in general, higher values indicate better data quality. The raw sequence error rates and missingness should be as low as possible. The ratio of transitions to transversions (Ti/Tv ratio) is expected to be ~2.0–2.1 for WGS data overall, 2.10 for known variants in WGS data, 2.07 for new variants in WGS data, ~3.0–3.3 for WES data overall, 3.5 for known variants in WES data, and 3.0 for new variants in WES data [45]. Homozygosity and heterozygosity depend on the type of population: heterozygosity is expected to be more frequent in admixed populations and homozygosity to be more frequent in inbred populations. It is estimated that each person has ~200 novel SNPs not present in the dbSNP database [64]; therefore, a value that is much larger than 200 is indicative of a high false positive rate of single nucleotide variant calls. Capture efficiency is reported to range within ~50–75% [65].

There are no existing, quality control standards that relate to generating clinical interpretations for genetic variants. However, substantial efforts are being made to identify clinically actionable pharmacogenetics variants, and it is instructive to review the approach being used. The Coriell Personalized Medicine Collaborative [66], the Clinical Pharmacogenetics Implementation Consortium [67], the Pharmacogenetics Working Group established by the Royal Dutch Association for the Advancement of Pharmacy [68], and the Evaluation of Genomic Applications in Practice and Prevention initiative sponsored by the Centers for Disease Control and Prevention [69] have independently developed similar processes for selecting candidate drugs, reviewing the published literature to identify drug-gene associations, scoring the evidence supporting associations between genetic variants and drug response, and interpreting the evidence to provide treatment guidelines.

This approach involving review and interpretation of the scientific literature by an expert committee can be considered the gold standard for determining whether a variant is clinically relevant or actionable but also can be expensive and time-consuming. It will not be feasible for experts, either individually or in committees, to review the large number of genetic variants identified in NGS data. Tools such as POLYPHEN-2 [70], VEP [71], MutationAssessor [72], and SIFT [73] can be used to predict variant effects. However, because these tools are sometimes inaccurate [74] and often differ in their predictions for the same variant [75, 76], there will likely be many variants that have no clear predicted, clinical interpretation. Furthermore, an additional problem is that the predictions made by these tools are not specific to a given gene or class of genes. For example, many genes would tolerate the substitution of glycine for another amino acid, but, in a gene that encodes a collagen fibril, loss of a glycine would impair fiber assembly resulting in a significant phenotype [77]. New methods that are both accurate and efficient need to be developed for predicting the pathogenicity of genetic variants found by NGS.

A limitation of using the ClinVar database [51] to identify clinically actionable genomic mutations is that a genetic variant in ClinVar can be described as having a different potential for pathogenicity by different submitters. For example, of the 12,895 unique variants with multiple clinical interpretations that have been submitted by more than one laboratory, 2,229 (17%) were interpreted differently by different submitters, with one- or two-step differences between any of three major levels: "pathogenic or likely pathogenic," "uncertain significance," and "likely benign or benign" [52]. Differences in interpreting the pathogenicity of variants have also been reported by the Clinical Sequencing Exploratory Research

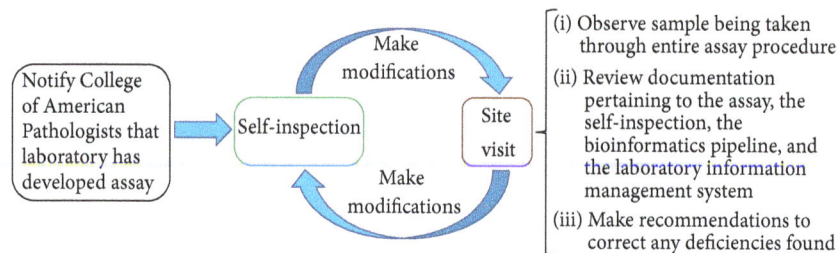

FIGURE 3: Overview of steps for a laboratory to obtain accreditation by the College of American Pathologists.

(CSER) program [30], an initiative designed to trial the use of WES/WGS data in clinical practice. The program compared CSER laboratories on their clinical interpretations of 98 variants and observed one-step differences in interpretation for 42% of variants and two-step or larger differences for 20% of variants [78]. To estimate and interpret the pathogenicity of new variants that are absent in the ClinVar database and to achieve some level of consensus on the clinical interpretations of variants, evaluations from experts, such as clinical geneticists, and/or further biological functional studies are needed.

## 4. Guidelines for Bioinformatics Processes

*4.1. Summary of Guidelines.* Bioinformatics pipelines are constituted of multiple databases and software programs to convert raw sequence reads to a list of clinically actionable or candidate variants. To promote the transparency of pipeline processes and data flow, the ACMG [79], the College of American Pathologists (CAP) [80], Weiss et al. [81], and Gargis et al. [82] have offered guidelines for NGS and the operation of bioinformatics pipelines in a clinical setting. The recommendations of these guidelines include thorough documentation of the pipeline and of deviations from pipeline standard operating procedures (e.g., software updates, changes in software settings, operator error, hardware failure, or other failures in the pipeline), validation of the pipeline, development of a pipeline quality management program, and implementation of policies to ensure secure data storage and data transfer.

The recommendations for written patient reports state that gene names should be provided according to HUGO Gene Nomenclature Committee nomenclature (http://www.genenames.org/) and genetic variants according to the nomenclature guidelines of the Human Genome Variation Society (http://www.hgvs.org/). Laboratories should follow the recommendations of the ACMG [53, 54] for interpreting the clinical significance of variants. Patient reports should also include the genome build and reference sequence used for variant detection, the genomic coordinates of identified variants, and mention of whether clinically significant variants were confirmed by an independent assay method [81]. Laboratories should also report genetic variant data (gene name, zygosity, cDNA nomenclature, protein nomenclatures, exon number, and clinical significance) in a structured format according to HL7 standards (HL7 version 2 Implementation Guide: Clinical Genomics,

http://www.hl7.org/implement/standards/). This is aimed at providing sufficient data to facilitate both clinical decision support and the display of genetic information in the EHR.

Challenges to implementing these guidelines include the constantly evolving nature of NGS technologies, bioinformatics tools (necessitating frequent updates of the bioinformatics pipeline), clinical interpretation (necessitating frequent updates of genetic variant annotation), the limited capacity of health care organizations/laboratories to store the voluminous data generated by NGS platforms (data storage options considered must ensure security of the stored genetic data), and the need for personnel trained in bioinformatics and statistics to develop a bioinformatics pipeline and to process and analyze NGS data. However, these challenges are not insurmountable, and it is likely that health care institutions that want to use NGS data in clinical care will attempt to overcome these hurdles and follow the guidelines.

*4.2. Accreditation from the College of American Pathologists (CAP).* Clinical laboratories that develop Clinical Laboratory Improvement Amendments- (CLIA-) certified NGS assays based on CAP standards [80] can seek accreditation from CAP, an agency that can provide accreditation on behalf of the CLIA program. The accreditation process involves a site visit inspection by a peer institution/laboratory once every two years and a self-inspection in alternate years (Figure 3). For the self-inspection, CAP sends the laboratory a list of items, specific to the NGS assay, that need to be checked by the laboratory. Completing the self-inspection for a NGS assay would allow the laboratory to determine how closely it adheres to the CAP standards for the assay. For the site visit, the inspectors would observe a sample being taken through the entire assay procedure. Any deficiencies found must be corrected, and CAP should be provided with a report describing the corrective measures within 30 days after the site visit. Through the mechanism of CAP accreditation, the laboratory would inform external entities that it provides a CLIA-certified assay that meets CAP standards for the assay.

## 5. Bioinformatics Infrastructure for Genomic Data

*5.1. Separate Databases for Different Types of Data.* Welch et al. have proposed an infrastructure comprised of independent, interacting databases for processing and storing genomic data in a clinical setting [83] (Figure 4). These

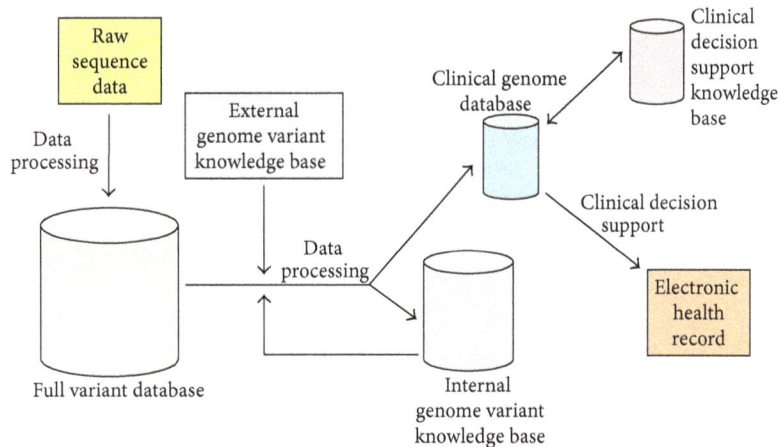

FIGURE 4: Elements of a proposed infrastructure for bioinformatics processing of sequencing data in clinical laboratories.

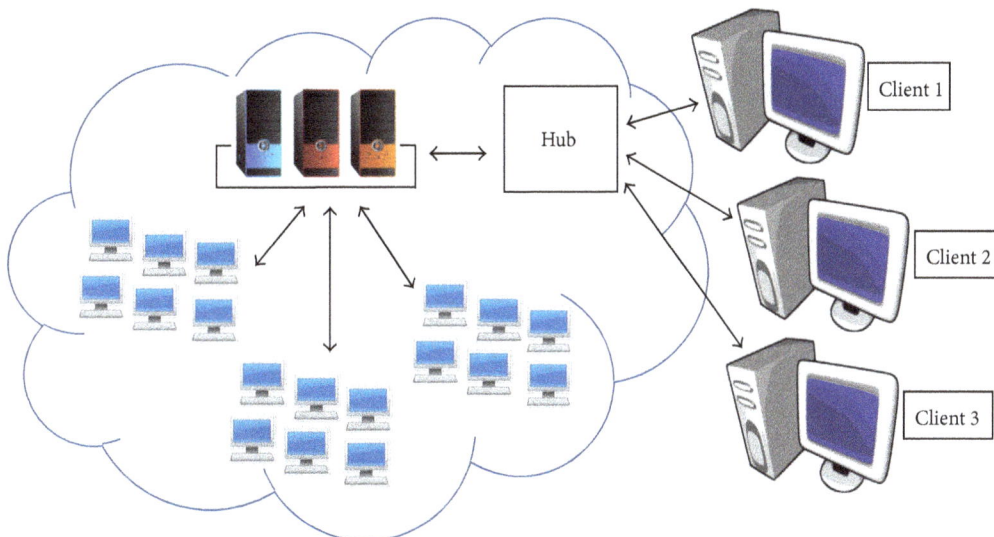

FIGURE 5: Cloud computing diagram.

databases include a "full variant database" to store all genetic variants for each patient, a clinical genome database to store only the clinically relevant variants for each patient, a clinical decision support knowledge base that integrates decision rules and guidelines for providing care (e.g., drug dosing rules) with genomic and clinical information, and a genome variant knowledge base to store known genetic variants and their clinical interpretations. ClinVar [51] is an example of a freely accessible genome variant knowledge base but clinical laboratories will likely also maintain their own internal genome variant knowledge bases (based on the genomic data of patients they test). The proposed infrastructure can potentially accommodate large amounts of genomic data because it involves warehousing the data external to EHRs. However, it would require investment in data storage capacity external to the EHR database system and the development and maintenance of interfaces between the genomic databases and the EHR database system [84].

5.2. Cloud Computing. Cloud computing, involving the use of remote servers to store and access data and software programs (Figure 5), has also been proposed for genomic data processing and storage. Cloud computing providers offer infrastructure, software, and programming platforms as services and incur the costs for developing and maintaining these services [85]. Because clients pay only for the services they use, cloud computing offers an economical approach to genomic data management compared with investment in the creation and maintenance of databases by healthcare entities to house genomic data. Hadoop is an open-source programming platform that is already being used to develop software for genomic data processing in a cloud computing environment [85]. Hadoop breaks data into small fragments, distributes the fragments over many computers, distributes computation to where the fragments are located so all fragments are processed in parallel, and aggregates the results at the end of computation [85]. The parallel processing of many small pieces of data greatly reduces computation time. Examples of open-source software developed on the Hadoop platform for processing genomic data are Crossbow [86], GATK [87], and Hadoop-BAM [88]. Challenges to the use of cloud computing for genomic data include the long data transfer times for uploading NGS data files to the cloud, the perceived lack of data security in the cloud computing environment, and the need for advanced programming skills in Java to develop software using Hadoop [85].

*5.3. Infrastructure for Data Sharing.* The separation of genomic and clinical data repositories facilitates the use of genomic data in research as well as clinical care. To engage in collaborative research, infrastructure for sharing genomic data with researchers internal and external to the institution that generated the data is required. The Global Alliance for Genomics and Health (GA4GH) [89], an international coalition of healthcare and academic centers that aims to advance the sharing of genomic and clinical data to improve health, has launched efforts to create such an infrastructure. The group has developed an application programming interface (API) to support the sharing of data on DNA sequences and genomic variants across organizations and bioinformatics pipelines [90]. GA4GH is also developing APIs for other types of genomics-related data including variant annotations, RNA-seq, and genotype-phenotype associations. These tools will allow genomic data from multiple organizations to be analyzed in aggregate, increasing statistical power to identify genetic variants that have a clinical effect.

*5.4. Security of Genomic Data.* Genomic data is protected health information; therefore, its privacy and confidentiality should be maintained similarly to other protected health information. Safeguards include the use of data encryption, password protected files, secure data transfer, audits of data transfer processes, and the implementation of institutional policies against data breeches and malicious use of the data [91]. The use of cloud computing presents added security concerns because data storage and/or processing services are provided by an entity external to the healthcare organization. Measures that the cloud service provider can take to address these concerns include logging access to the data, creating a role-based access system (level of access depends on the type of user), complying with third-party certifications for information security (e.g., the International Organization for Standardization/International Electrotechnical Commission 21001:2013 information security standard http://www.iso.org/iso/home/standards/management-standards/iso27001.htm/), protecting the security of the computer network, using notification alarms to track when changes are made to stored data, and guaranteeing the complete removal of data from its servers once the cloud storage service is no longer being used [92].

# 6. Examples of Implementing Genomic Data in Clinical Care

*6.1. Clinical Sequencing Exploratory Research Program.* A survey of six health centers participating in the CSER consortium

has described how the centers have integrated genomic data into the EHR [30]. Five centers performed sequencing at their own laboratories, and one site used an external laboratory but confirmed variants on-site using Sanger sequencing. Each center created a local bioinformatics pipeline for variant annotation, but all used multiple online catalogs of variants (e.g., ClinVar [51] and dbSNP) for annotation. Each site also built and maintained its own genome variant knowledge base (based on genetic variants ascertained in patients at the site) and created tools to use data from this internal database in variant annotation. Additionally, sites used manual or semiautomated methods to search the scientific literature or online gene-specific databases to determine the clinical significance of variants. EHR software was obtained from commercial providers at four centers and was locally developed at two centers. The laboratories at all six centers generated a human-readable PDF document, containing genetic results, that was designed to be incorporated into the EHR. The two sites with custom-built EHRs, and one site with commercial EHR software, also reported results in a structured, machine-readable format. Active clinical decision support (automated alerts through the EHR) for genetic variants was available at two of the centers. Only one center had an automated system for sending alerts to physicians when new genomic findings resulted in the reclassification of a genetic variant's clinical significance (e.g., a variant initially classified as being of unknown significance was subsequently discovered to have serious clinical consequences).

*6.2. eMERGE Network Pharmacogenetics Study.* Sites in the eMERGE network are also engaged in pilot efforts to incorporate genomic data, particularly data relevant to pharmacogenetics, into EHRs [6]. At one eMERGE site, separate data repositories were created for unprocessed sequence/genotype data and for variants of known pharmacogenetics relevance [93]. Software that applied approved pharmacogenetics-medication guidelines to patients' genetic data was used to determine a patient's pharmacogenetics phenotype (e.g., predicted poor metabolizer of a specific drug), and the phenotype data were stored as a laboratory result in the EHR. The site developed software that extended its existing, custom-built medication alert system, enabling the system to check for a relevant pharmacogenetics laboratory result when a physician prescribes a pharmacogenetics-related drug. If a patient has a pharmacogenetics phenotype, the system sends an alert to the physician and suggests alternative treatment. Another eMERGE site reported developing similar infrastructure that supported storage of all genetic variants separately from variants with pharmacogenetics relevance, the translation of genetic data into genotype-phenotype associations, and active clinical decision support for physicians prescribing pharmacogenetics-related drugs [94]. Changes in the clinical interpretation of genetic variants (based on new knowledge) that resulted in phenotype reassignment prompted the site to update its genotype-phenotype translation database to reflect the newly determined genotype-phenotype relationships. Because this database was linked to the site's clinical information system, pharmacogenetics data in the EHR was automatically updated.

*6.3. Lessons from CSER and eMERGE.* The CSER and eMERGE pharmacogenetics programs are in progress and have not yet reported on improvements in patient outcomes as a result of incorporating genomic data into clinical care. Each site in these programs had its own customized bioinformatics pipeline, laboratory information management system, clinical decision support capabilities, and electronic health records that would not be generalizable to other sites. This presents a challenge as a more uniform infrastructure for genomic data processing could be adopted more widely and easily. Based on their experiences, sites in both programs identified a number of factors that need to be addressed to facilitate the integration of genomic data into healthcare: (1) the requirement for active clinical decision support; (2) tools to examine and interpret sequence variants, especially new, undefined variants; (3) approaches to update changes in the clinical significance of sequence variants over time; (4) giving healthcare providers access to consultants trained in genetics; (5) infrastructure for secure and reliable delivery of results to external healthcare providers; and (6) methods for explaining genomic information to patients.

# 7. Discussion

The ideal, preventive model of patient care is to understand as much about a patient as possible, as early in his/her life as possible, to detect warning signs of serious but preventable illness at an early stage so that preemptive health interventions can be simpler and/or less expensive than treatment implemented at a later stage. Also, knowing a person's individual characteristics is often relevant for providing effective treatment against disease because patients can respond differently to the same treatment. By facilitating precision medicine, advances in genomics have the potential to change the way we prevent and treat diseases. However, the translation of these advances into reality for patient care depends mainly on our ability to discover disease- and/or drug-associated clinically actionable genetic mutations and on our understanding of the roles of these mutations in the disease process.

Healthcare centers that are conducting pilot studies of the integration of genomic data into clinical care have developed a bioinformatics infrastructure for processing NGS data that consists of a group of databases ancillary to the EHR [30, 93, 94]. The infrastructures were, for the most part, locally developed and proprietary, but this is because these centers are among the first healthcare providers to use genomic data in clinical care and there are no established infrastructures to meet their bioinformatics needs. The infrastructures were built along the same general plan: a bioinformatics pipeline for processing NGS data, a database for storing all genetic variants detected in patient samples, a genome variant knowledge base for storing known genetic variants and their clinical interpretation, a database for the subset of variants deemed to be clinically actionable (with variants linked to a specific clinical phenotype), links between databases allowing data transfer, and a method for reporting the results of clinically actionable variants in the EHR. Developing and maintaining a bioinformatics infrastructure for NGS data requires substantial investment in resources and personnel and can be too expensive for small clinical laboratories. However, because genetic variant databases are maintained separately from the EHR, it might be possible for multiple, small laboratories to pool resources to build and share a common bioinformatics infrastructure. The storage and bioinformatics processing of raw NGS data output by sequencing platforms might exceed the infrastructure capacity of even some large healthcare organizations. Therefore, healthcare providers might want to consider cooperatively establishing a cloud computing service designed to store and process genomic data securely for the healthcare community. Clinical laboratories must also consider the cost of sequencing instruments as part of infrastructure costs. Bench-top instruments used for targeted sequencing are less expensive and output less data than instruments that perform WES/WGS. For these reasons, more laboratories are likely to perform targeted sequencing before, or instead of, attempting to build infrastructure to support WES/WGS.

A major challenge to incorporating genomic data into clinical care is the lack of standards for generating NGS data, bioinformatics processing, data storage, and clinical decision support. Standards would promote consistency in data quality, and adherence to standards would facilitate the routine use of genomic data in clinical practice, but it is difficult to create standards when NGS technology and bioinformatics software are constantly evolving. Further, approaches to clinical decision support vary across healthcare institutions [30]. In a survey of 17 health centers participating in the CSER program or the eMERGE network, most centers did not have active clinical decision support for genetic data in the EHR although there were existing mechanisms for clinically actionable information to trigger alerts in the majority of the EHR systems [95]. Centers with active clinical decision support either built their own software locally or customized the clinical decision support capabilities of commercial EHR software [30]. Most centers reported that genetics results were available as a portable document format (PDF) file in the EHR and recommended the development of clinical decision support for disease-defining and pharmacogenetics variants and creation of a clinical decision support knowledge base to advise on appropriate clinical actions (e.g., a change in treatment).

Appropriately integrating EHRs with genomic data for the discovery of clinically actionable variants can generate new insights into disease mechanisms and provide better predictions about effective treatments, all leading to improved targeting of interventions to patients. To generate knowledge on the nature of disease from comprehensive EHR data, new methods such as machine learning, natural language processing, and other artificial intelligence methods are needed. However not all patients are likely to benefit from the use of big data in healthcare due to our current knowledge gaps on how to extract useful information from large-volume genomic and clinical data and how to interpret discovered genetic variants appropriately. At the same time, targeted therapies are not yet available for many important genes, and regulatory issues need to be resolved before some useful bioinformatics tools can be applied in a healthcare setting.

Finally, as EHRs are extremely personal, measures to protect patient data have to be put in place to make certain that patient information is only shared with those who need to see it. Despite this challenge, the potential advantages that genomic data can bring to healthcare far outweigh the potential disadvantages. The growing trend towards integration of genomic data and EHRs will cause concern, but as long as patient privacy and data security can be rigorously maintained, genomic data is certain to play an essential role in precision medicine.

## 8. Conclusion

To reach the goal of precision medicine, healthcare institutions need to invest in a bioinformatics infrastructure and in personnel trained in bioinformatics and genetics, to develop the capacity to process, store, and interpret genomic data and to link these data with EHRs. In addition, more efforts are needed to distinguish genetic variants that are truly clinically actionable; that is, the variants are useful for guiding clinical decisions regarding interventions to improve health outcomes. Clinical research studies of the implementation of genomic data in healthcare can provide valuable lessons about how genomic data should be managed, and patient privacy protected, when incorporating genomic data into clinical practice on a larger scale. These lessons can alert healthcare institutions to the scientific and technical challenges of using genomic data in precision medicine.

## Competing Interests

The authors indicated no potential competing interests.

## Acknowledgments

The authors would like to thank Dr. Rachel Stankowski in the Office of Scientific Writing and Publication at the Marshfield Clinic Research Foundation for assistance with editing of this paper. This work was supported by the Clinical and Translational Science Award program through a grant from the National Institutes of Health, National Center for Advancing Translational Sciences [UL1TR000427] and by the Marshfield Clinic Research Foundation.

## References

[1] J. L. Vassy, B. R. Korf, and R. C. Green, "How to know when physicians are ready for genomic medicine," *Science Translational Medicine*, vol. 7, no. 287, Article ID 287fs219, 2015.

[2] L. R. Brunham and M. R. Hayden, "Hunting human disease genes: lessons from the past, challenges for the future," *Human Genetics*, vol. 132, no. 6, pp. 603–617, 2013.

[3] G. R. Abecasis, D. Altshuler, A. Auton et al., "A map of human genome variation from population-scale sequencing," *Nature*, vol. 467, no. 7319, pp. 1061–1073, 2010.

[4] G. R. Abecasis, A. Auton, L. D. Brooks et al., "An integrated map of genetic variation from 1,092 human genomes," *Nature*, vol. 491, no. 7422, pp. 56–65, 2012.

[5] O. Gottesman, H. Kuivaniemi, G. Tromp et al., "The Electronic Medical Records and Genomics (eMERGE) Network: past, present, and future," *Genetics in Medicine*, vol. 15, no. 10, pp. 761–771, 2013.

[6] L. J. Rasmussen-Torvik, S. C. Stallings, A. S. Gordon et al., "Design and anticipated outcomes of the eMERGE-PGx project: a multicenter pilot for preemptive pharmacogenomics in electronic health record systems," *Clinical Pharmacology and Therapeutics*, vol. 96, no. 4, pp. 482–488, 2014.

[7] H. J. Grabe, H. Assel, T. Bahls et al., "Cohort profile: greifswald approach to individualized medicine (GANI_MED)," *Journal of Translational Medicine*, vol. 12, article 144, 2014.

[8] L. H. Saal, J. Vallon-Christersson, J. Häkkinen et al., "The Sweden Cancerome Analysis Network—breast (SCAN-B) Initiative: a large-scale multicenter infrastructure towards implementation of breast cancer genomic analyses in the clinical routine," *Genome Medicine*, vol. 7, no. 1, article 20, 2015.

[9] S. Q. Wong, A. Fellowes, K. Doig et al., "Assessing the clinical value of targeted massively parallel sequencing in a longitudinal, prospective population-based study of cancer patients," *British Journal of Cancer*, vol. 112, no. 8, pp. 1411–1420, 2015.

[10] R. R. Gullapalli, M. Lyons-Weiler, P. Petrosko, R. Dhir, M. J. Becich, and W. A. LaFramboise, "Clinical Integration of Next-Generation Sequencing Technology," *Clinics in Laboratory Medicine*, vol. 32, no. 4, pp. 585–599, 2012.

[11] E. Baro, S. Degoul, R. Beuscart, and E. Chazard, "Toward a literature-driven definition of big data in healthcare," *BioMed Research International*, vol. 2015, Article ID 639021, 9 pages, 2015.

[12] Q. Huang, S. Jing, J. Yi, and W. Zhen, *Innovative Testing and Measurement Solutions for Smart Grid*, John Wiley & Sons, Singapore, 2014.

[13] A. Sboner and O. Elemento, "A primer on precision medicine informatics," *Briefings in Bioinformatics*, vol. 17, no. 1, Article ID bbv032, pp. 145–153, 2016.

[14] C. Gilissen, J. Y. Hehir-Kwa, D. T. Thung et al., "Genome sequencing identifies major causes of severe intellectual disability," *Nature*, vol. 511, no. 7509, pp. 344–347, 2014.

[15] I. Iossifov, B. J. O'Roak, S. J. Sanders et al., "The contribution of de novo coding mutations to autism spectrum disorder," *Nature*, vol. 515, no. 7526, pp. 216–221, 2014.

[16] A. S. Allen, S. F. Berkovic, P. Cossette et al., "De novo mutations in epileptic encephalopathies," *Nature*, vol. 501, no. 7466, pp. 217–221, 2013.

[17] E. S. Lander and M. S. Waterman, "Genomic mapping by fingerprinting random clones: a mathematical analysis," *Genomics*, vol. 2, no. 3, pp. 231–239, 1988.

[18] D. Sims, I. Sudbery, N. E. Ilott, A. Heger, and C. P. Ponting, "Sequencing depth and coverage: key considerations in genomic analyses," *Nature Reviews Genetics*, vol. 15, no. 2, pp. 121–132, 2014.

[19] M. J. Clark, R. Chen, H. Y. K. Lam et al., "Performance comparison of exome DNA sequencing technologies," *Nature Biotechnology*, vol. 29, no. 10, pp. 908–916, 2011.

[20] S. S. Ajay, S. C. J. Parker, H. O. Abaan, K. V. Fuentes Fajardo, and E. H. Margulies, "Accurate and comprehensive sequencing of personal genomes," *Genome Research*, vol. 21, no. 9, pp. 1498–1505, 2011.

[21] H. Fang, Y. Wu, G. Narzisi et al., "Reducing INDEL calling errors in whole genome and exome sequencing data," *Genome Medicine*, vol. 6, no. 10, article 89, 2014.

[22] Y. Liu, J. Zhou, and K. P. White, "RNA-seq differential expression studies: more sequence or more replication?" *Bioinformatics*, vol. 30, no. 3, pp. 301–304, 2014.

[23] Y. Liu, J. F. Ferguson, C. Xue et al., "Evaluating the impact of sequencing depth on transcriptome profiling in human adipose," *PLoS ONE*, vol. 8, no. 6, Article ID e66883, 2013.

[24] C. W. Fuller, L. R. Middendorf, S. A. Benner et al., "The challenges of sequencing by synthesis," *Nature Biotechnology*, vol. 27, no. 11, pp. 1013–1023, 2009.

[25] J. Eid, A. Fehr, J. Gray et al., "Real-time DNA sequencing from single polymerase molecules," *Science*, vol. 323, no. 5910, pp. 133–138, 2009.

[26] J. M. Rothberg, W. Hinz, T. M. Rearick et al., "An integrated semiconductor device enabling non-optical genome sequencing," *Nature*, vol. 475, no. 7356, pp. 348–352, 2011.

[27] S. Balzer, K. Malde, A. Lanzén, A. Sharma, and I. Jonassen, "Characteristics of 454 pyrosequencing data—enabling realistic simulation with flowsim," *Bioinformatics*, vol. 26, no. 18, pp. i420–i425, 2010.

[28] A. Valouev, J. Ichikawa, T. Tonthat et al., "A high-resolution, nucleosome position map of *C. elegans* reveals a lack of universal sequence-dictated positioning," *Genome Research*, vol. 18, no. 7, pp. 1051–1063, 2008.

[29] F. Sanger, S. Nicklen, and A. R. Coulson, "DNA sequencing with chain-terminating inhibitors," *Proceedings of the National Academy of Sciences of the United States of America*, vol. 74, no. 12, pp. 5463–5467, 1977.

[30] P. Tarczy-Hornoch, L. Amendola, S. J. Aronson et al., "A survey of informatics approaches to whole-exome and whole-genome clinical reporting in the electronic health record," *Genetics in Medicine*, vol. 15, no. 10, pp. 824–832, 2013.

[31] K. S. Poon, K. M. Tan, and E. S. Koay, "Targeted next-generation sequencing of the ATP7B gene for molecular diagnosis of Wilson disease," *Clinical Biochemistry*, vol. 49, no. 1-2, pp. 166–171, 2016.

[32] V. Rehvathy, M. H. Tan, S. P. Gunaletchumy et al., "Multiple genome sequences of *Helicobacter pylori* strains of diverse disease and antibiotic resistance backgrounds from malaysia," *Genome Announcements*, vol. 1, no. 5, Article ID e00687, 2013.

[33] I. Vanni, S. Coco, A. Truini et al., "Next-generation sequencing workflow for NSCLC critical samples using a targeted sequencing approach by ion torrent PGM platform," *International Journal of Molecular Sciences*, vol. 16, no. 12, pp. 28765–28782, 2015.

[34] M. A. Choudhury, W. B. Lott, S. Banu et al., "Nature and extent of genetic diversity of dengue viruses determined by 454 pyrosequencing," *PLOS ONE*, vol. 10, no. 11, Article ID e0142473, 2015.

[35] B. Maranhao, P. Biswas, A. D. H. Gottsch et al., "Investigating the molecular basis of retinal degeneration in a familial cohort of Pakistani decent by exome sequencing," *PLoS ONE*, vol. 10, no. 9, Article ID e0136561, 2015.

[36] A. Webb, A. C. Papp, A. Curtis et al., "RNA sequencing of transcriptomes in human brain regions: protein-coding and noncoding RNAs, isoforms and alleles," *BMC Genomics*, vol. 16, no. 1, article 990, 2015.

[37] A. Shiroma, Y. Terabayashi, K. Nakano et al., "First complete genome sequences of *Staphylococcus aureus* subsp. *aureus* Rosenbach 1884 (DSM 20231T), determined by PacBio single-molecule real-time technology," *Genome Announcements*, vol. 3, no. 4, Article ID e00800, 2015.

[38] O. Harismendy, P. C. Ng, R. L. Strausberg et al., "Evaluation of next generation sequencing platforms for population targeted sequencing studies," *Genome Biology*, vol. 10, no. 3, article R32, 2009.

[39] L. Liu, Y. Li, S. Li et al., "Comparison of next-generation sequencing systems," *Journal of Biomedicine and Biotechnology*, vol. 2012, Article ID 251364, 11 pages, 2012.

[40] N. Rieber, M. Zapatka, B. Lasitschka et al., "Coverage bias and sensitivity of variant calling for four whole-genome sequencing technologies," *PLoS ONE*, vol. 8, no. 6, Article ID e66621, 2013.

[41] M. A. Quail, M. Smith, P. Coupland et al., "A tale of three next generation sequencing platforms: comparison of Ion Torrent, Pacific Biosciences and Illumina MiSeq sequencers," *BMC Genomics*, vol. 13, article 341, 2012.

[42] A. Ratan, W. Miller, J. Guillory, J. Stinson, S. Seshagiri, and S. C. Schuster, "Comparison of sequencing platforms for single nucleotide variant calls in a human sample," *PLoS ONE*, vol. 8, no. 2, Article ID e55089, 2013.

[43] B. Ewing and P. Green, "Base-calling of automated sequencer traces using phred. II. Error probabilities," *Genome Research*, vol. 8, no. 3, pp. 186–194, 1998.

[44] H. Li and R. Durbin, "Fast and accurate short read alignment with Burrows-Wheeler transform," *Bioinformatics*, vol. 25, no. 14, pp. 1754–1760, 2009.

[45] M. A. Depristo, E. Banks, R. Poplin et al., "A framework for variation discovery and genotyping using next-generation DNA sequencing data," *Nature Genetics*, vol. 43, no. 5, pp. 491–501, 2011.

[46] K. Wang, M. Li, and H. Hakonarson, "ANNOVAR: functional annotation of genetic variants from high-throughput sequencing data," *Nucleic Acids Research*, vol. 38, no. 16, article e164, 2010.

[47] P. Cingolani, A. Platts, L. L. Wang et al., "A program for annotating and predicting the effects of single nucleotide polymorphisms, SnpEff: SNPs in the genome of *Drosophila melanogaster* strain w1118; iso-2; iso-3," *Fly*, vol. 6, no. 2, pp. 80–92, 2012.

[48] E. S. Lander, L. M. Linton, B. Birren et al., "Initial sequencing and analysis of the human genome," *Nature*, vol. 409, no. 6822, pp. 860–921, 2001.

[49] D. M. Church, V. A. Schneider, K. M. Steinberg et al., "Extending reference assembly models," *Genome Biology*, vol. 16, article 13, 2015.

[50] H. Li, B. Handsaker, A. Wysoker et al., "The Sequence Alignment/Map format and SAMtools," *Bioinformatics*, vol. 25, no. 16, pp. 2078–2079, 2009.

[51] M. J. Landrum, J. M. Lee, G. R. Riley et al., "ClinVar: public archive of relationships among sequence variation and human phenotype," *Nucleic Acids Research*, vol. 42, no. 1, pp. D980–D985, 2014.

[52] H. L. Rehm, J. S. Berg, L. D. Brooks et al., "ClinGen—the clinical genome resource," *The New England Journal of Medicine*, vol. 372, no. 23, pp. 2235–2242, 2015.

[53] R. C. Green, J. S. Berg, W. W. Grody et al., "ACMG recommendations for reporting of incidental findings in clinical exome and genome sequencing," *Genetics in Medicine*, vol. 15, no. 7, pp. 565–574, 2013.

[54] H. Hampel, R. L. Bennett, A. Buchanan, R. Pearlman, and G. L. Wiesner, "A practice guideline from the American College of Medical Genetics and Genomics and the National Society of Genetic Counselors: referral indications for cancer predisposition assessment," *Genetics in Medicine*, vol. 17, no. 1, pp. 70–87, 2015.

[55] L. M. Amendola, M. O. Dorschner, P. D. Robertson et al., "Actionable exomic incidental findings in 6503 participants: challenges of variant classification," *Genome Research*, vol. 25, no. 3, pp. 305–315, 2015.

[56] M. He, T. N. Person, S. J. Hebbring et al., "SeqHBase: a big data toolset for family based sequencing data analysis," *Journal of Medical Genetics*, vol. 52, no. 4, pp. 282–288, 2015.

[57] R. Daneshjou, Z. Zappala, K. Kukurba et al., "PATH-SCAN: a reporting tool for identifying clinically actionable variants," *Pacific Symposium on Biocomputing*, pp. 229–240, 2014.

[58] W. Zhou, H. Zhao, Z. Chong et al., "ClinSeK: a targeted variant characterization framework for clinical sequencing," *Genome Medicine*, vol. 7, no. 1, article 34, 2015.

[59] P. N. Robinson, S. Köhler, A. Oellrich et al., "Improved exome prioritization of disease genes through cross-species phenotype comparison," *Genome Research*, vol. 24, no. 2, pp. 340–348, 2014.

[60] A. Antanaviciute, C. M. Watson, S. M. Harrison et al., "OVA: integrating molecular and physical phenotype data from multiple biomedical domain ontologies with variant filtering for enhanced variant prioritization," *Bioinformatics*, vol. 31, no. 23, pp. 3822–3829, 2015.

[61] E. M. Ramos, C. Din-Lovinescu, J. S. Berg et al., "Characterizing genetic variants for clinical action," *American Journal of Medical Genetics, Part C: Seminars in Medical Genetics*, vol. 166, no. 1, pp. 93–104, 2014.

[62] J. A. Tennessen, A. W. Bigham, T. D. O'Connor et al., "Evolution and functional impact of rare coding variation from deep sequencing of human exomes," *Science*, vol. 336, no. 6090, pp. 64–69, 2012.

[63] P. Danecek, A. Auton, G. Abecasis et al., "The variant call format and VCFtools," *Bioinformatics*, vol. 27, no. 15, Article ID btr330, pp. 2156–2158, 2011.

[64] M. J. Bamshad, S. B. Ng, A. W. Bigham et al., "Exome sequencing as a tool for Mendelian disease gene discovery," *Nature Reviews Genetics*, vol. 12, no. 11, pp. 745–755, 2011.

[65] Y. Guo, F. Ye, Q. Sheng, T. Clark, and D. C. Samuels, "Three-stage quality control strategies for DNA re-sequencing data," *Briefings in Bioinformatics*, vol. 15, no. 6, pp. 879–889, 2014.

[66] N. Gharani, M. A. Keller, C. B. Stack et al., "The Coriell personalized medicine collaborative pharmacogenomics appraisal, evidence scoring and interpretation system," *Genome Medicine*, vol. 5, no. 10, article 93, 2013.

[67] M. V. Relling and T. E. Klein, "CPIC: clinical pharmacogenetics implementation consortium of the pharmacogenomics research network," *Clinical Pharmacology and Therapeutics*, vol. 89, no. 3, pp. 464–467, 2011.

[68] J. J. Swen, M. Nijenhuis, A. de Boer et al., "Pharmacogenetics: from bench to byte—an update of guidelines," *Clinical Pharmacology and Therapeutics*, vol. 89, no. 5, pp. 662–673, 2011.

[69] S. M. Teutsch, L. A. Bradley, G. E. Palomaki et al., "The evaluation of genomic applications in practice and prevention (EGAPP) initiative: methods of the EGAPP working group," *Genetics in Medicine*, vol. 11, no. 1, pp. 3–14, 2009.

[70] I. A. Adzhubei, S. Schmidt, L. Peshkin et al., "A method and server for predicting damaging missense mutations," *Nature Methods*, vol. 7, no. 4, pp. 248–249, 2010.

[71] W. McLaren, B. Pritchard, D. Rios, Y. Chen, P. Flicek, and F. Cunningham, "Deriving the consequences of genomic variants with the Ensembl API and SNP Effect Predictor," *Bioinformatics*, vol. 26, no. 16, Article ID btq330, pp. 2069–2070, 2010.

[72] B. Reva, Y. Antipin, and C. Sander, "Predicting the functional impact of protein mutations: application to cancer genomics," *Nucleic Acids Research*, vol. 39, no. 17, article e118, 2011.

[73] N.-L. Sim, P. Kumar, J. Hu, S. Henikoff, G. Schneider, and P. C. Ng, "SIFT web server: predicting effects of amino acid substitutions on proteins," *Nucleic Acids Research*, vol. 40, no. 1, pp. W452–W457, 2012.

[74] F. Gnad, A. Baucom, K. Mukhyala, G. Manning, and Z. Zhang, "Assessment of computational methods for predicting the effects of missense mutations in human cancers," *BMC Genomics*, vol. 14, supplement 3, article S7, 2013.

[75] S. E. Flanagan, A.-M. Patch, and S. Ellard, "Using SIFT and PolyPhen to predict loss-of-function and gain-of-function mutations," *Genetic Testing and Molecular Biomarkers*, vol. 14, no. 4, pp. 533–537, 2010.

[76] S. Castellana and T. Mazza, "Congruency in the prediction of pathogenic missense mutations: state-of-the-art web-based tools," *Briefings in Bioinformatics*, vol. 14, no. 4, pp. 448–459, 2013.

[77] D. K. Crockett, E. Lyon, M. S. Williams, S. P. Narus, J. C. Facelli, and J. A. Mitchell, "Utility of gene-specific algorithms for predicting pathogenicity of uncertain gene variants," *The Journal of the American Medical Informatics Association*, vol. 19, no. 2, pp. 207–211, 2012.

[78] G. P. Jarvik, L. A. Amendola, H. McLaughlin et al., "Performance of ACMG variant classification guidelines within and across 9 CLIA labs in the Clinical Sequeuncing Exploratory Research (CSER) Consortium; (Abstract/Program #1986)," in *Proceedings of the 65th Annual Meeting of the American Society of Human Genetics*, Baltimore, Md, USA, October 2015.

[79] H. L. Rehm, S. J. Bale, P. Bayrak-Toydemir et al., "ACMG clinical laboratory standards for next-generation sequencing," *Genetics in Medicine*, vol. 15, no. 9, pp. 733–747, 2013.

[80] N. Aziz, Q. Zhao, L. Bry et al., "College of American Pathologists' laboratory standards for next-generation sequencing clinical tests," *Archives of Pathology & Laboratory Medicine*, vol. 139, no. 4, pp. 481–493, 2015.

[81] M. M. Weiss, B. Van der Zwaag, J. D. H. Jongbloed et al., "Best practice guidelines for the use of next-generation sequencing applications in genome diagnostics: a national collaborative study of dutch genome diagnostic laboratories," *Human Mutation*, vol. 34, no. 10, pp. 1313–1321, 2013.

[82] A. S. Gargis, L. Kalman, D. P. Bick et al., "Good laboratory practice for clinical next-generation sequencing informatics pipelines," *Nature Biotechnology*, vol. 33, no. 7, pp. 689–693, 2015.

[83] B. M. Welch, S. R. Loya, K. Eilbeck, and K. Kawamoto, "A proposed clinical decision support architecture capable of supporting whole genome sequence information," *Journal of Personalized Medicine*, vol. 4, no. 2, pp. 176–199, 2014.

[84] A. N. Kho, L. V. Rasmussen, J. J. Connolly et al., "Practical challenges in integrating genomic data into the electronic health record," *Genetics in Medicine*, vol. 15, no. 10, pp. 772–778, 2013.

[85] A. O'Driscoll, J. Daugelaite, and R. D. Sleator, "'Big data,' Hadoop and cloud computing in genomics," *Journal of Biomedical Informatics*, vol. 46, no. 5, pp. 774–781, 2013.

[86] B. Langmead, M. C. Schatz, J. Lin, M. Pop, and S. L. Salzberg, "Searching for SNPs with cloud computing," *Genome Biology*, vol. 10, no. 11, article R134, 2009.

[87] A. McKenna, M. Hanna, E. Banks et al., "The genome analysis toolkit: a MapReduce framework for analyzing next-generation DNA sequencing data," *Genome Research*, vol. 20, no. 9, pp. 1297–1303, 2010.

[88] M. Niemenmaa, A. Kallio, A. Schumacher, P. Klemelä, E. Korpelainen, and K. Heljanko, "Hadoop-BAM: directly manipulating next generation sequencing data in the cloud," *Bioinformatics*, vol. 28, no. 6, pp. 876–877, 2012.

[89] M. Lawler, L. L. Siu, H. L. Rehm et al., "All the world's a stage: facilitating discovery science and improved cancer care through the global alliance for genomics and health," *Cancer Discovery*, vol. 5, no. 11, pp. 1133–1136, 2015.

[90] B. Paten, M. Diekhans, B. J. Druker et al., "The NIH BD2K center for big data in translational genomics," *Journal of the American Medical Informatics Association*, vol. 22, no. 6, pp. 1143–1147, 2015.

[91] R. Hazin, K. B. Brothers, B. A. Malin et al., "Ethical, legal, and social implications of incorporating genomic information into electronic health records," *Genetics in Medicine*, vol. 15, no. 10, pp. 810–816, 2013.

[92] J. J. P. C. Rodrigues, I. de La Torre, G. Fernández, and M. López-Coronado, "Analysis of the security and privacy requirements of cloud-based electronic health records systems," *Journal of Medical Internet Research*, vol. 15, no. 8, article e186, 2013.

[93] P. L. Peissig, A. Nikolai, and M. Brilliant, "Personalized medicine," in *Drug Discovery and Evaluation: Pharmacological Assays*, F. J. Hock, Ed., pp. 1–16, Springer, 2015.

[94] J. F. Peterson, E. Bowton, J. R. Field et al., "Electronic health record design and implementation for pharmacogenomics: a local perspective," *Genetics in Medicine*, vol. 15, no. 10, pp. 833–841, 2013.

[95] B. H. Shirts, J. S. Salama, S. J. Aronson et al., "CSER and eMERGE: current and potential state of the display of genetic information in the electronic health record," *Journal of the American Medical Informatics Association*, vol. 22, no. 6, pp. 1231–1242, 2015.

# 15

# Two Different Maintenance Strategies in the Hospital Environment: Preventive Maintenance for Older Technology Devices and Predictive Maintenance for Newer High-Tech Devices

**Mana Sezdi**

*Department of Biomedical Device Technology, Istanbul University, 34320 Istanbul, Turkey*

Correspondence should be addressed to Mana Sezdi; mana@istanbul.edu.tr

Academic Editor: Manuel Doblaré

A maintenance program generated through the consideration of characteristics and failures of medical equipment is an important component of technology management. However, older technology devices and newer high-tech devices cannot be efficiently managed using the same strategies because of their different characteristics. This study aimed to generate a maintenance program comprising two different strategies to increase the efficiency of device management: preventive maintenance for older technology devices and predictive maintenance for newer high-tech devices. For preventive maintenance development, 589 older technology devices were subjected to performance verification and safety testing (PVST). For predictive maintenance development, the manufacturers' recommendations were used for 134 high-tech devices. These strategies were evaluated in terms of device reliability. This study recommends the use of two different maintenance strategies for old and new devices at hospitals in developing countries. Thus, older technology devices that applied only corrective maintenance will be included in maintenance like high-tech devices.

## 1. Introduction

Medical technology includes all medical equipment used by health organizations for diagnosis, therapy, monitoring, rehabilitation, and care. Therefore, medical technology management plays a key role in health care. Effective medical device management is required to ensure high-quality patient care [1, 2]. Efficient and accurate equipment provides a high degree of patient safety. Accomplished medical device management will greatly assist in the reduction of adverse incidents and medical device-related accidents. For medical technology management, hospitals must have activities for maintaining, inspecting, and testing all medical equipment in the inventory. These activities must be performed within the scope of a program called "maintenance program." The Medicine and Healthcare Products Regulatory Agency declares that maintenance activities and their intervals should be planned in accordance with the manufacturers' recommendations or strategies listed in an alternative equipment maintenance program [3]. These alternative program strategies must be based on valid standards of practice.

A maintenance program, generated by considering the characteristics and failures of medical equipment, is important with regard to usability and efficiency. However, it is inefficient to use the same strategies for the management of older technology devices and newer high-tech devices because of their different characteristics. The new high-tech devices functional control activities planned in accordance with the manufacturers' recommendations and daily programmed self-tests should be done. These devices are tested against their specifications presented by their manufacturers. According to the 2007/47/EC Directive, these tests must be planned by the manufacturers. The directive states that "The instructions for use must contain details of the nature and frequency of the maintenance and calibration needed to ensure that the devices operate properly and safely at all times" [4]. For this reason, daily checks, including visual controls and specific device tests, are described in the user guide and carried out by users.

Unlike new high-tech devices, the manufacturers' recommendations for older technology devices are not applicable because of the long usage time and device age. Generally, in developing countries, such as Turkey, older technology equipment mainly receives corrective maintenance. For example, a device is repaired when damaged or nondurable parts are replaced. In other words, maintenance is not specific to each device. Yearly maintenance contracts with manufacturers are only set for high-tech devices. This study investigated whether older technology devices could be included in maintenance strategies similar to those used for high-tech devices.

The quality of older technology medical devices can be ensured through periodical performance verification and safety testing (PVST) in accordance with international standards. PVST uses a standard measurement system with known accuracy to measure the accuracy of medical equipment [5–7]. PVST which includes qualitative and quantitative tests is performed by qualified biomedical personnel. During PVST, if a device is identified as not compatible with international standards, the hidden failures are determined and recorded by the biomedical staff. These failures are repaired by the hospital's biomedical staff or service technicians employed by manufacturers. This process discloses the possible failures of medical equipment.

All test results indicate causation, a tremendously important factor in the prevention of adverse incidents and generation of an effective maintenance program. Valuable lessons can be learned from an analysis of failures and these can be applied to maintenance programs [6]. Therefore, failure analysis is the main activity of a maintenance program.

Recently, the demand for medical device management is increasing as the number of medical devices increases. Therefore, the development of more effective maintenance programs has achieved prominence.

The initial purpose of this study was to generate a maintenance program comprising two different maintenance strategies, one each for older technology devices and newer high-tech devices, utilizing the manufacturers' recommendations and PVST results, respectively, and to determine the success rate of this program using the indicators. Accordingly, old technology devices will be included in the maintenance systems through separate testing.

The Food and Drug Administration maintains a database of medical equipment failures and has conducted some preventive studies for all medical sectors [8]. Several reports have analyzed medical failures and preventive maintenance [9–20]. However, very little information about hidden failures was available in the literature when the collection of hidden failure data was initiated for this study. Wallace and Kuhn presented an analysis of software-related medical device failures that led to manufacturer recalls, but they caused no deaths or injuries [9]. In addition, Bliznakov et al. reported medical device recalls due to software failures. The authors collected data related to software failures and performed an analysis via failure classification [10]. Many other studies

have presented alternative maintenance strategies for each piece of equipment. Ridgway et al. classified failures in an attempt to reduce equipment downtime [11]. Santos and Almeida prepared maintenance schedules using mean intervals between failures [12]. Taghipour et al. studied a multicriteria decision-making model to prioritize medical devices according to criticality [13]. Taghipour et al. also described a periodic inspection optimization model for complex repairable systems [14, 15]. Hamdi et al. presented a new approach to work-order prioritization for medical equipment maintenance requests [16]. Taghipour and Banjevic modeled an optimal periodic inspection interval in a preventive maintenance [17]. Khalaf et al. presented evidence-based maintenance using a mixed integer model [18]. Miniati et al. analyzed the technical data from medical devices with support from technology managers [19]. Lastly, Saleh et al. used quality function deployment to solve problems related to preventive maintenance prioritization [20]. The present study differs from previous studies because it presents a maintenance program created using two different strategies. The first strategy incorporates daily checks for new high-tech devices, whereas the second implements PVST as the sole performance measurement for older technology devices. To the best of our knowledge, no previous study has focused on hidden medical device failures determined during the PVST of medical devices.

## 2. Methods

This study included a total of 723 high-risk medical devices maintained by the Medical Faculty of Istanbul University [21]. Low-risk devices were excluded from the study. The high-risk devices were classified as older technology devices and newer high-tech devices. This classification was performed because of the lack of service or user manuals, and corresponding lack of manufacturer recommendations for many older technology devices. This lack makes it impossible to apply the same procedures to old technology and new high-tech devices. Thus, different procedures were applied to old technology and new high-tech devices in order to develop maintenance. As seen in Figure 1, old technology devices (589 devices) comprised of electrocardiography (ECG) devices, pulse oximetry devices, sphygmomanometers, infant incubators, phototherapy units, defibrillators, surgical aspirators, and electrosurgical units. These devices were tested by applying PVST. The second group (134 devices), which mostly contained imaging devices, comprised computerized tomography (CT), angiography, mammography, C-arm radiography, magnetic resonance (MR), and positron emission tomography and gamma cameras. The second group also included ventilators and anesthesia devices used in intensive care departments. Accordingly, these devices had a 24-hour workload. The devices in the first group, excluding those used in intensive care and emergency departments, had 8-hour workloads. The groups were investigated separately and two different maintenance strategies were developed: predictive maintenance for newer high-tech devices and preventive maintenance for older technology devices.

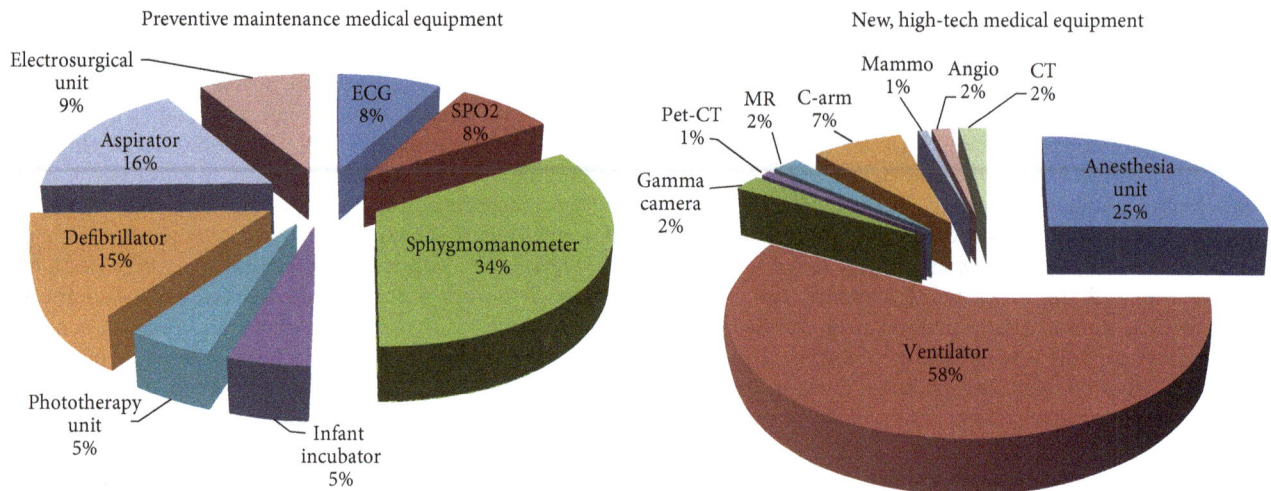

FIGURE 1: Medical devices in the old technology and new high-tech device groups.

The development of preventive maintenance for older technology devices required a long procedural duration, whereas predictive maintenance for newer high-tech devices was developed in accordance with the manufacturers' recommendations.

*2.1. Predictive Maintenance for Newer High-Tech Devices.* A predictive maintenance program for newer high-tech devices was developed by applying maintenance time schedules created according to the manufacturers' recommendations. Under this program, predictive maintenance was conducted for each device through a contract with the manufacturer's technical service and cooperation of the biomedical department of the hospital. The hospital's biomedical personnel also attended the maintenance activities. After each service session, maintenance reports were delivered to the biomedical staff by the manufacturer's technical service department.

Users performed daily checks of the devices. They were trained in the performance of daily checks through user training provided by the manufacturer. Users reported failures identified during daily checks. The most important point in this section was the collection of regular feedback from all device users. Training aimed to ensure that the smallest failure would be reported. Although the exact training success and feedback rates were not determined, an increase in feedback was observed. In addition, failures occurring during work hours were reported to the manufacturer's technical service by the hospital's biomedical personnel. Staffs also attended to failure detection and provided failure reports. As a result, data were obtained and used to evaluate predictive maintenance.

*2.2. Preventive Maintenance for Older Technology Devices.* A preventive maintenance program for older technology devices was developed via analysis of the PVST results of the equipment. The following PVST steps were performed in sequence by the hospital's biomedical personnel [5]:

(i) determination of the PVST intervals,

(ii) application of the PVST,

(iii) interpretation of the PVST results according to the acceptance criteria stated in international standards.

*2.2.1. PVST Intervals.* PVST intervals were determined by calculating the Equipment Management Number (EMN), which is described in the Clinical Equipment Management standards of the Technology and Safety Management series developed by the Joint Commission. Given the lack of the manufacturers' recommendation for the old technology devices investigated in this study, the EMN was used with a general approach to determine the initial PVST interval. PVST intervals accepted by industry could have been used if the manufacturers' recommendations were present [22]. The EMN technique, introduced by Fennigkoh and Smith, classifies equipment using three parameters: function, risk, and maintenance requirements [23]. A numerical value is assigned to each device type by classifying the above-mentioned parameters. The scores used to calculate EMN can be seen in Table 1. Specifically, the EMN is the sum of the Equipment Function Score, Equipment Risk Score, and Maintenance Requirement Score. PVST intervals range from 6 to 12 months, depending on the EMN. According to the standards, EMN can have a maximum value of 20. If the calculated number is 12 or higher, the equipment is incorporated into the annual PVST plan. In addition, if the EMN is greater than 17, the device must be controlled every 6 months.

The calculated EMN and PVST intervals determined for the medical equipment investigated in this study are shown in Table 2.

*2.2.2. PVST Procedures.* PVST was performed according to the procedures of Inspection and Preventive Maintenance (IPM), prepared by the Emergency Care Research Institute [24]. In this study, testing parameters for medical devices

TABLE 1: Scores used to calculate the Equipment Management Number.

| Score | Function | Risk | Maintenance requirement |
|---|---|---|---|
| 10 | Life recovery | — | — |
| 9 | Surgical and intensive care | — | — |
| 8 | Physical therapy | — | — |
| 7 | Surgical and intensive care | — | — |
| 6 | Other physiological monitors | — | — |
| 5 | Analytical laboratory | Patient death | Very important |
| 4 | Laboratory equipment | Patient-staff injury | Moderately important |
| 3 | Computers | Wrong diagnosis | Less important |
| 2 | Belong to the patients | Treatment delays | The least important |
| 1 | Other equipment pieces | Risk not important | Minimally important |

TABLE 2: PVST parameters and PVST intervals of medical devices (FP: function point, RP: risk point, MR: maintenance requirement, and EMN: equipment management number).

| Medical device | PVST parameters | Simulator analyzer measurement device | FP | RP | MR | EMN | Test interval |
|---|---|---|---|---|---|---|---|
| Electrocardiography | Linearity sensitivity 1 mV pulse intensity Paper speed | Patient Simulator (Fluke MPS450) | 7 | 3 | 4 | 14 | 12 months |
| Pulse oximeter | ECG BPM test Oxygen saturation | SPO2 Analyzer (Fluke Index 2 XLF) | 7 | 3 | 4 | 14 | 12 months |
| Sphygmomanometer | Pressure leakage Pressure accuracy | NIBP Simulator (Fluke BP Pump 2L) | 6 | 3 | 4 | 13 | 12 months |
| Infant incubator | Temperature test Humidity test Noise test Baby probe test | Patient Simulator (Fluke MPS450) | 10 | 5 | 5 | 20 | 6 months |
| Phototherapy unit | Intensity | Phototherapy Analyzer (Dale 40) | 8 | 4 | 5 | 17 | 6 months |
| Defibrillator | ECG BPM test ECG amplitude test ECG arrhythmia test Energy test Charge time test Sync. discharge test | Defibrillator Analyzer (Fluke QED 6H) | 10 | 5 | 5 | 20 | 6 months |
| Aspirator | Max. free flow Rate of vacuum rise Max. vacuum Vac. gauge accuracy | Flow Analyzer (Fluke VT Plus) | 9 | 3 | 4 | 16 | 12 months |
| Electrosurgical unit | Cutting-power test Coag. power test Bipolar-power test HF leakage test REM alarm test | Electrosurgical Unit Analyzer (Rigel UNITHERM) | 9 | 5 | 5 | 19 | 6 months |

TABLE 3: Data list screen (8 records; total: 589 records).

| Location | Device name | Brand code | Serial number | Status | Error |
|---|---|---|---|---|---|
| ECG room | ECG | Nihon Kohden | 4971 | Passed | No problem |
| Service | SPO2 | Massimo | N43378 | Passed | No problem |
| Emergency | Sphygmomanometer | Riester | 091250123 | Failed | High pressure leakage |
| Infant intensive care unit | Infant incubator | Fanem | CI1649 | Failed | High temperature |
| Infant intensive care unit | Phototherapy unit | Medix | 560-09 | Passed | No problem |
| Emergency | Defibrillator | Nihon Kohden | 07728 | Failed | Low battery |
| Operation room | Aspirator | Bıçakcılar | 1598 | Failed | Low vacuum |
| Operation room | Electrosurgical unit | Martin | BO 88 74 | Failed | Power circuit error |

In total, the data of 589 medical devices were listed.

measured during PVST were determined from IPM procedures. The procedures comprised both quantitative and qualitative tests. The qualitative test evaluated the device's physical parameters (e.g., connectors, battery, and electrodes). The quantitative test includes functional controls. The main principle was the evaluation of all functional parameters of the medical device. Although the qualitative test was general, the quantitative test was specific for each device. The quantitative test parameters measured for each device in this study are listed in Table 2.

Tests were performed with a low level of uncertainty, which was calculated using the procedures declared in the Guide to the Expression of Uncertainty in Measurement (GUM).

*2.2.3. Interpretation of the PVST Results.* To interpret the PVST results, the acceptance criteria in the IPM procedures were considered. Medical devices for which measurement results fell within the acceptable range were considered appropriate with respect to international standards and were labeled with green stickers. This designation indicated that the medical equipment passed the inspection and could be used. Test results were accordingly recorded as "Passed" (P) in documentation and the database. Medical devices for which measurement results fell outside of the acceptable range were considered inappropriate with respect to international standards and were labeled with red stickers. The red sticker indicated the presence of failures and stated that the device should not be used. The corresponding PVST result was recorded as "Failed" (F) in documentation and the database.

Clinical staffs were trained with regard to their responses to each label color. According to the procedure applied for red label devices, staffs were prohibited from using the device, which was sent to the clinical engineering department to

identify and remove any hidden failures that did not completely disable the primary device functions. After correction and a second PVST, the device could be returned for use in the department.

All data regarding information about the equipment, such as the equipment name, location, serial number, interpretation results (Passed or Failed), and failure definition, were entered in the operation page. A sample page is shown in Table 3.

PVST, when performed at a determined interval, provides a large statistical failure dataset that could be used to establish a maintenance interval. The preventive maintenance time schedule was planned using data obtained from PVST results. Hidden failures detected during PVST that could affect device performance were considered during preventive maintenance planning. For example, a 3-month interval was planned for maintenance of the most common hidden failures detected in incubators during PVST. A 6-month interval was planned for maintenance of less frequently encountered failures. Maintenance checklists were prepared and required nondurable parts for continuous medical equipment service were determined. The maintenance process with regard to the qualitative and quantitative device parameters was defined using maintenance checklists. The defined processes included control, cleaning, calibration, replacement, and measurement. The checklist stated which part was to be subjected to which process. Notably, the same part may include more than one process. For example, batteries are initially checked and subsequently changed. Similarly, pedals are controlled, cleaned, and changed if necessary.

*2.3. Evaluation of the Maintenance Program.* The performance of maintenance strategies for older technology devices and newer high-tech devices was assessed in terms of progress in achieving the expectation defined by the program. Maintenance activities were evaluated using a failure rate indicator. A 6-month validation phase was planned to monitor whether the failure rates of old technology devices and new high-tech devices would decrease with the application of the maintenance plan. This phase was selected because defibrillators and electrosurgical units selected pilot devices for the evaluation of the preventive maintenance and have a 6-month PVST interval.

No preventive maintenance was conducted in the hospital before this study. However, medical devices were subjected to PVST before the study. The hidden failures of all medical devices were recorded. To evaluate preventive maintenance, the results of PVST during preventive maintenance were compared with the results of PVST before maintenance. In addition, the predictive maintenance results were evaluated by comparing the failures that occurred within 6 months of prepredictive maintenance and those that occurred during predictive maintenance. Data of failures that occurred before predictive maintenance were extracted from each device's failure history which was available in the hospital documentation.

A reporting system was planned in which an archive of all devices' failure histories would be created. This reporting system enabled the monitoring of all medical device information. To this end, biomedical personnel collected user checklists and technical service forms from the manufacturers' technical services. Data in these documents were entered on device information cards to generate a failure history for each device. Hence, this method provided a reporting system comprising the collection of data from checklists. Parameters related to failures, such as the failure definition, repair time, and replaced parts, were followed easily. In particular, unwanted data, such as the maximum repair time and more frequent failure rate, were identified. These data were reported to the decision-maker to explain the overall situation. For this, a one-page report was designed to supporting decision-makers in the allocation of an increased budget for technology procurement, new maintenance contracts, or more biomedical personnel. A sample report form for decision-makers is shown as follows:

*Executive Summary*

*Medical Devices Predictive and Preventative Maintenance Report*

Number of Total Medical Device:

Number of Total Medical Device subject to Preventative Maintenance:

Number of Total Medical Device subject to Predictive Maintenance:

(1) Failed devices often

Location

—

—

Device

—

—

Manufacturer

—

—

Model

—

—

Serial Number

—

—

(2) The failed devices in the warranty period

Location

—

—

Device

—

—

Manufacturer

—

—

Model

—

—

Serial Number

—

—

(3) Failed end-of-support devices

Location

—

—

Device

—

—

Manufacturer

—

—

Model

—

—

Serial Number

—

—

(4) Parts which were need to be replaced but not included in the annual maintenance contract

Location

—

—

Device

—

—

Manufacturer

—

—

Model

—

—

Serial Number

—

—

(5) Devices which could not be found their non-durable parts and could not be repaired

Location

—

—

Device

—

—

Manufacturer

—

—

Model

—

—

Serial Number

—

—

(6) Non-durable parts which have been changed again in the warranty period although they had been changed before

Location

—

—

Device

—

—

Manufacturer

—

—

Model

—

—

Serial Number

—

—

(7) The devices which can not get technical service from their contracted firm

Location

—

—

Device

—

—

Manufacturer

—

—

Model

—

—

TABLE 4: Predictive maintenance time schedule including newer high-tech devices.

| Device | Brand | Model | Daily | Every 1 m | Every 3 m | Every 4 m | Every 6 m | Every 12 m |
|---|---|---|---|---|---|---|---|---|
| | | | | Predictive maintenance time schedule | | | | |
| CT | Philips | Brilliance CT 16-Slice | × | | | × | | |
| | Siemens | Somatom Sensation 4 | × | | | × | | |
| | Toshiba | Aquilion 64 | × | | × | | | |
| Angio | Philips | MultiDiagnost Eleva | × | | | × | | |
| | Siemens | Axiom Artis dtA | × | | | × | | |
| Mammo | IMS | Giotto SDL | × | | | × | | |
| C-arm | Siemens | Arcadis Varic | × | | | | × | |
| | Siemens | Arcadis Varic Gen 2 | × | | | | × | |
| | Siemens | Siremobil Compact | × | | | | × | |
| | Siemens | Siremobil Compact L | × | | | | × | |
| | Philips | BV Endura | × | | | | × | |
| MR | Siemens | Magnetom Symphony | × | | | × | | |
| | Philips | Achieva 1,5 T | × | | | × | | |
| | Philips | Achieva 3,0 T | × | | | × | | |
| Pet-CT | Siemens | Biograph 6 TruePoint | × | | × | | | |
| Gamma | Siemens | E-Cam Extended Gantry | × | | × | | | × |
| Camera | Mediso | Nucline DHV-2 Sprit | × | × | × | | × | × |
| | Mediso | Nucline TH-22 | × | × | × | | × | × |
| Ventilator | Maquet | Servo-s | × | | | | × | |
| | Maquet | Servo-i | × | | | | × | |
| | Draeger | Babylog 8000 plus | × | | | | × | |
| | Draeger | Evita 4 Neoflow | × | | | | × | |
| | GE | Engström | × | | | | × | |
| Anesthesia unit | Draeger | Fabius | × | | | | × | |
| | Draeger | Fabius GC | × | | | | × | |
| | Draeger | Julian | × | | | | × | |
| | Draeger | Primus | × | | | | × | |
| | GE Datex | Avannce S5 | × | | | | × | |
| | GE Datex | Aestiva 5 | × | | | | × | |

Istanbul University Hospitals.
Predictive Maintenance Program 2014.

Serial Number

—

—

This report will help decision-makers to define short- and long-term priority plans for technology investments based on safety aspects.

## 3. Results

This study planned predictive maintenance for 134 newer high-tech devices and preventive maintenance for 589 older technology devices.

*3.1. Predictive Maintenance.* Planned predictive maintenance involved the usage of daily checklists created by the manufacturers. These daily checklists which included simple, mandatory pre- and post-use tasks, were presented to the device users. Maintenance time schedules were planned according to the manufacturers' recommendations provided in the user guides. Table 4 shows a sample maintenance time schedule, including each device brand and model. The devices were also subjected to monthly maintenance, in addition to the recommended maintenance period. Since annual maintenance fee payments are divided into 12 months in accordance with the Turkish currency system, the contracted company must visually maintain the device every month. This visual maintenance comprises short-term maintenance, especially device cleaning.

*3.2. Preventive Maintenance.* For older technology devices, preventive maintenance was planned by analyzing PVST results. Accordingly, failures were detected in 126 (22%) of the 589 medical devices from different departments in the Medical Faculty at Istanbul University; they were marked as

TABLE 5: Medical device failures.

| Medical device | Total # | Number | Errors | Error code |
|---|---|---|---|---|
| Electrocardiogram | 50 | 2 | Not working | ECG01 |
| | | 1 | Power circuit error | ECG02 |
| | | 1 | Paper speed error | ECG03 |
| | | 3 | Electrode error | ECG04 |
| | | 1 | Sensitivity error | ECG05 |
| Pulse oximeter | 46 | 3 | Not working | SPO01 |
| | | 1 | Low BPM | SPO02 |
| | | 1 | High BPM | SPO03 |
| | | 2 | Low oxygen saturation | SPO04 |
| | | 2 | High oxygen saturation | SPO05 |
| | | 5 | Probe error | SPO06 |
| Sphygmomanometer | 200 | 12 | Not working | SPG01 |
| | | 15 | High pressure leakage | SPG02 |
| | | 8 | Cuff error | SPG03 |
| | | 4 | Broken manometer | SPG04 |
| | | 5 | Missing piece | SPG05 |
| Infant incubator | 28 | 3 | Not working | INC01 |
| | | 2 | Over temperature | INC02 |
| | | 1 | Display error | INC03 |
| | | 1 | Baby probe error | INC04 |
| | | 2 | Broken cover | INC05 |
| Phototherapy unit | 30 | 3 | Not working | PHT01 |
| | | 2 | Low intensity | PHT02 |
| Defibrillator | 86 | 3 | Not working | DEF01 |
| | | 1 | Low/high energy | DEF02 |
| | | 3 | Low battery | DEF03 |
| | | 2 | Electrode error | DEF04 |
| | | 1 | Paddle error | DEF05 |
| | | 2 | BPM error | DEF06 |
| | | 2 | Synchronization error | DEF07 |
| Aspirator | 97 | 6 | Not working | ASP01 |
| | | 4 | High vacuum | ASP02 |
| | | 3 | Low vacuum | ASP03 |
| | | 3 | Maximum vacuum | ASP04 |
| | | 2 | Vacuum rise error | ASP05 |
| Electrosurgical unit | 52 | 1 | Not working | ESU01 |
| | | 3 | Power circuit error | ESU02 |
| | | 3 | High/low cut power | ESU03 |
| | | 2 | High/low coag. power | ESU04 |
| | | 1 | High/low bipolar power | ESU05 |
| | | 2 | Foot switching error | ESU06 |
| | | 2 | Patient electrode error | ESU07 |

"Failed," and the remaining 463 were marked as "Passed." When the "Failed" devices were analyzed according to their errors, several technical hidden failures were observed. The failures are summarized in Table 5 according to error code. In addition, Figure 2 presents the distribution of hidden failures.

PVST results were used to plan a preventive maintenance time schedule for old technology devices. This preventive maintenance time schedule indicates the maintenance interval for the device. The adequate interval for effective maintenance was determined for each device and nondurable part. Equipment with recorded failures was assigned a more frequent maintenance schedule. The time schedules for old technology devices are shown in Table 6.

Preventive maintenance checklists were prepared for the devices. These checklists defined the maintenance process of the qualitative and quantitative device parameters.

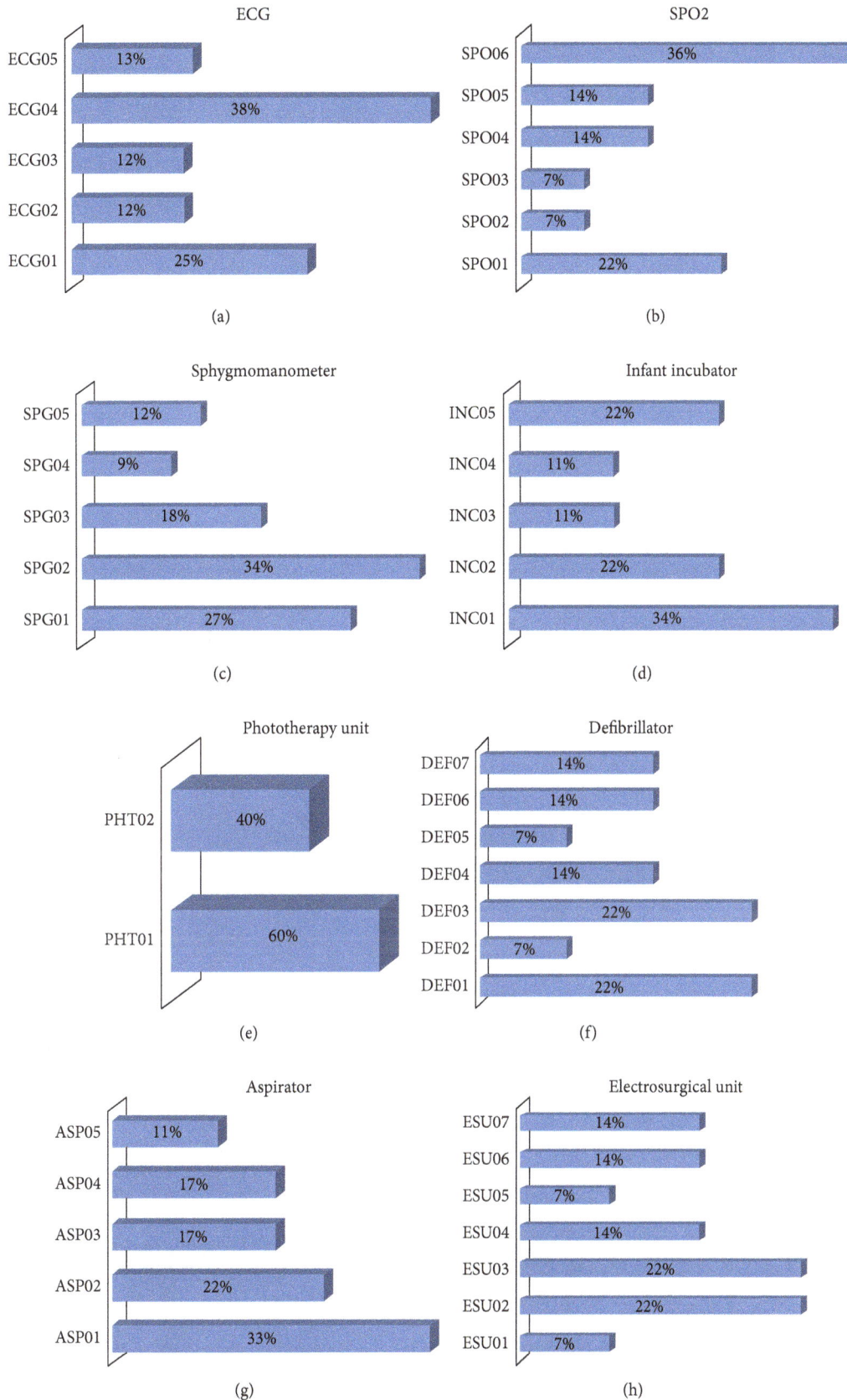

FIGURE 2: Failures specific for each type of older technology medical device.

TABLE 6: Preventive maintenance time schedule including older technology devices.

| Device | | Preventive maintenance time schedule | | | | | |
| --- | --- | --- | --- | --- | --- | --- | --- |
| | | Daily | Weekly | Every 3 m | Every 6 m | Every 12 m | As needed |
| Infant incubator | Baby temperature probe | | | × | | | |
| | Air filter | | | × | | | |
| | Electrical fuse | | | × | | | |
| | Switch | | | × | | | |
| | Breaker relay | | | × | | | |
| | Fan motor | | | | × | | |
| | Vacuum compressor motor | | | | × | | |
| | Pressure sensor | | | | × | | |
| | Noise sensor | | | | × | | |
| | Air circulation sensor | | | | × | | |
| | Humidity sensor | | | | × | | |
| | Temperature sensor | | | | × | | |
| | Accumulator | × | | | | | |
| | Gasket | | | | | | × |
| Aspirator | Air input filter | | | × | | | |
| | Pump motor | | | × | | | |
| | Fan motor | | | × | | | |
| | Air hose | | × | | | | |
| | Fluid suction hose | × | | | | | |
| Defibrillator | Battery | | × | | | | |
| | Spoon connection cable | | × | | | | |
| | Fibrillation detection sensor | | | | × | | |
| | Charging transformer | | | | | | × |
| | Heart beat sensor | | | | × | | |
| | ECG sensor | | | | × | | |
| | Leakage relay | | | × | | | |
| | Electrical fuse | | | × | | | |
| | Defibrillation time sensor | | | | × | | |
| Pulse oximeter | Probes | | | × | | | |
| | Optic sensor | | | | × | | |
| | Battery | | × | | | | |
| | Connector | | | | | | × |

Istanbul University Hospitals
Preventive Maintenance Program 2014.

The checklist also stated which part was to be subjected to which process. The required visual, functional, and electrical controls were explained in the checklist. In addition, nondurable parts requiring replacement were identified in the checklist.

The PVST analysis revealed that nondurable parts (e.g., ECG patient electrodes, oximeter probes, cuffs, defibrillator batteries, and ultraviolet lamps) must be stocked for each piece of medical equipment. Both the number and features of the nondurable parts required for each type of medical device were determined. However, spare parts were not stocked for devices maintained by manufacturers' technical services.

*3.3. Performance of the Maintenance Program.* The primary focus of preventive and predictive maintenance is the reliability of medical devices [25]. Therefore, reliability was analyzed to evaluate the performance of preventive and predictive maintenance. Indicators such as failure rates per old technology devices and per new technology devices were determined to evaluate the equipment reliability.

The success of preventive maintenance was evaluated by analyzing the results of PVST performed after preventive maintenance. The results of PVST performed before and after preventive maintenance were then compared. Since preventive maintenance includes old technology devices, the failure rate of sample devices provides information about the failure rate of old technology devices. The defibrillator and electrosurgical units were selected as pilot medical devices. Before preventive maintenance, 86 defibrillators and 52 electrosurgical units were inspected, and their results

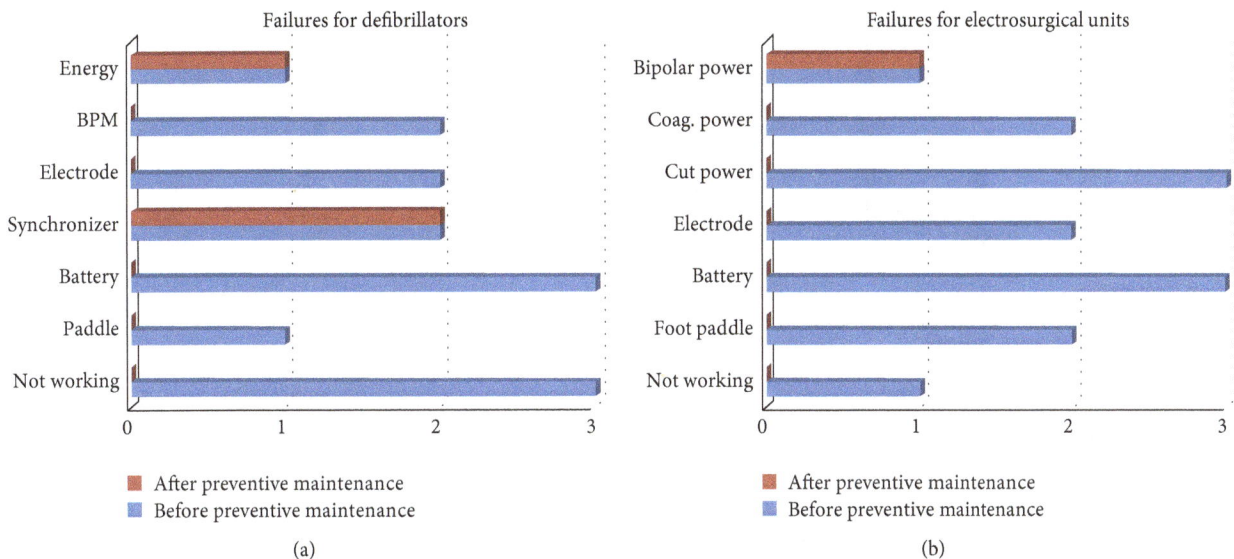

FIGURE 3: (a) Failures of the defibrillators and (b) of the electrosurgical units before and after preventive maintenance.

were analyzed to develop preventive maintenance. After maintenance, the devices were inspected again after a period of 6 months. Figures 3(a) and 3(b) show the results of the qualitative and quantitative tests performed before and after preventive maintenance, respectively. In addition, PVST results obtained after preventive maintenance indicated that the minor and major defects detected during PVST were largely rectified. Traditional preventive maintenance (TPM) of some components was also performed. For example, batteries were replaced before complete depletion, and paddles were lubricated to increase conductivity. Therefore, in contrast to the results of PVST performed before preventive maintenance, fewer failed components were identified after preventive maintenance.

The defibrillator is a high-risk device with regard to patient safety. The patient's life is at risk if the device fails completely or does not provide sufficient energy to the patient when in use. The parameters measured during PVST reflect the risks of the defibrillator. In particular, the quantitative parameters such as "output energy," "charge time," and "energy after 60 sec" are important parameters that may pose a serious threat to the patient. During the evaluation of preventive maintenance, the incidence of these failures was found to have decreased. The qualitative parameters of defibrillators are related to physical specifications. Although they are considered to have a lesser impact on patient safety, quantitative parameters are also important because they are directly related to defibrillator function. This is one reason why the defibrillator was used as a pilot device during preventive maintenance evaluation. All parameters affect defibrillator operation directly and patient safety indirectly. The above-described situation is also valid for the second pilot device, the electrosurgical unit. The other devices investigated in this study, such as ECG, pulse oximeter, and aspirator, might cause some inconvenience to the patient, but they do not pose a serious risk. In these devices, the determined failures were

hidden and indicated deviations from the devices' functional performance specifications. Hidden failure repair is required to prevent serious failures and to ensure standard service from the device but is not essential for the patient safety.

For both pilot devices, problems related to quantitative parameters that were determined by PVST before preventive maintenance were resolved during preventive maintenance (Figure 3). The three nonworking defibrillators were restored to a working condition. Batteries, pedals, and electrodes with issues were changed. Only problems related to the synchronizers of two defibrillators could not be resolved by the hospital's biomedical staff and required manufacturer's technical service. In addition, an issue with the output energy of one defibrillator was also not resolved during preventive maintenance (Figure 3(a)) and the device was sent to the manufacturer's technical service. Similar to the defibrillators, all hidden failures in the electrosurgical units were resolved during preventive maintenance, except for a bipolar power-related problem (Figure 3(b)).

The success of predictive maintenance was evaluated by analyzing medical equipment failure reports after predictive maintenance. The gamma camera and ventilator were selected as pilot medical devices. Their failure rates could be assumed to represent the failure rate of new high-tech devices. Failures occurring within 6 months of pre- and postpredictive maintenance were extracted from the devices' failure histories, which were available in the hospital documentation. Figures 4 and 5 present the failures of gamma cameras and ventilators occurring pre- and postpredictive maintenance, respectively. The failures were classified into two categories: those reported during daily checks and those occurring during work. The latter group caused the devices to stop working. In contrast, the former group was generally noticed during daily checks and generally related to the device's physical condition or software. Accordingly, such failures had no or little influence on the device's functioning.

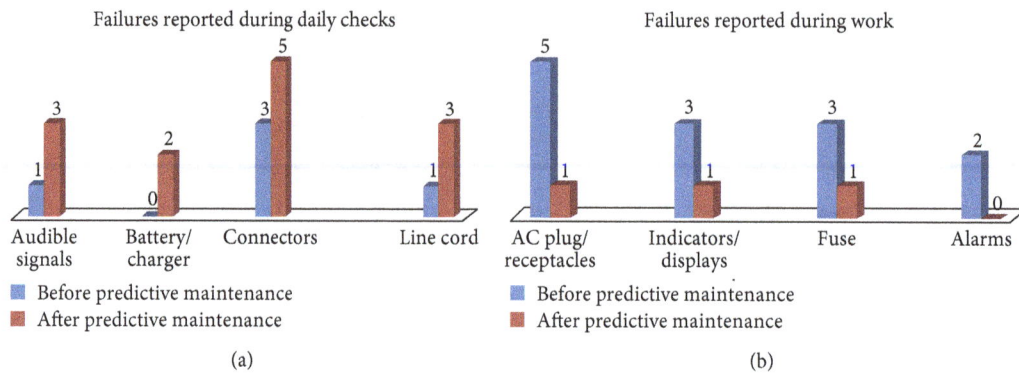

FIGURE 4: Failures of the gamma camera before and after predictive maintenance. (a) Failures reported during daily checks. (b) Failures reported during work.

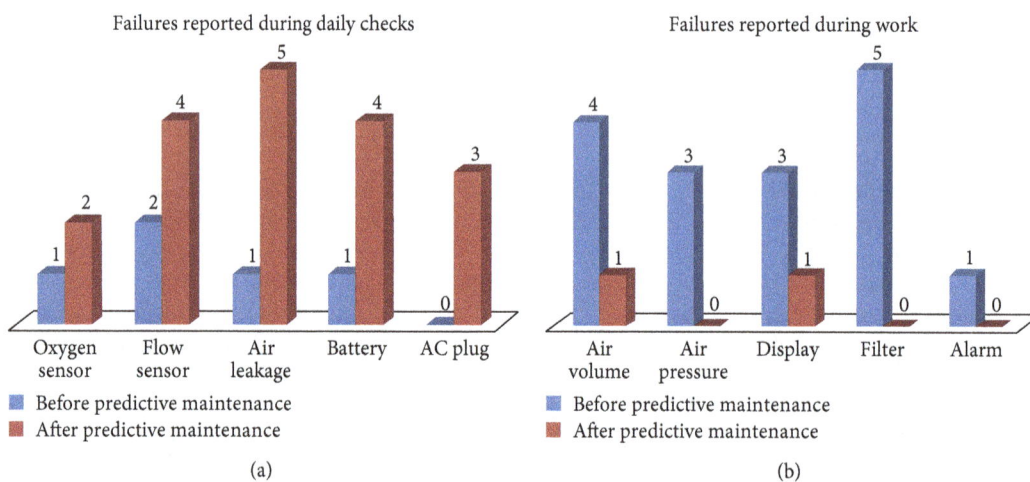

FIGURE 5: Failures of the ventilator before and after predictive maintenance. (a) Failures reported during daily checks. (b) Failures reported during work.

As shown in Figures 4 and 5, a greater number of failures were reported during daily checks after predictive maintenance. This might be attributed to failures being ignored by users during daily checks prior to predictive maintenance. The increased reporting of failures during daily checks indicates the user support of predictive maintenance. In contrast, a greater number of failures occurring during work were reported before predictive maintenance. This indicates that some failures during work were prevented by applying predictive maintenance.

## 4. Discussion

This report describes the formation of a maintenance program using the PVST results for older technology medical devices and the manufacturers' recommendations for newer high-tech devices. The resulting maintenance program forms a basis for quality assurance practices.

This study differs from other studies reported in the literature on two points. The first point is that older technology devices and newer high-tech devices were investigated separately. This led to the use of two different methodologies: PVST for older technology devices and the manufacturers' recommendations for newer high-tech devices. It is important to overcome such failures before they occur and thus avoid harming the patient. Unresolved failures may lead to several types of important medical equipment accidents. Accordingly, use of the PVST results was preferred for the development of a maintenance program for older technology devices.

The second point is that this study examined hidden medical equipment failures arising from noncompliance with international standards. Although other studies investigated hardware or software failures of medical devices, the present study addressed hidden failures that affect the quality of the medical device and patient safety. Wallace and Kuhn [9] and Bliznakov et al. [10] also presented an analysis of failures. But, these failures were related to software and resulted in device recalls by the manufacturers. In the present study, hidden failures were analyzed to develop a preventive maintenance protocol, and failures detected during daily checks and usages were analyzed to develop a predictive maintenance protocol.

Ridgway et al. classified failures in terms of repair calls. According to the authors, calls related to failures were classified as follows [11]:

(i) user-related calls,

(ii) accessory- or connectivity-related calls,

(iii) physical-stress-related calls,

(iv) environmental-stress-related calls,

(v) human-interference-related calls.

After classification, the authors recommended user training, a well-managed battery-care program, availability of the proper accessories, and maintenance of the environmental conditions specified by the equipment manufacturer. In this study, failures were classified and analyzed in terms of technology levels (older technology devices and newer high-tech devices). Since failures were detected through daily checks, the failures used to develop predictive maintenance were related to user competence, accessories, connectivity, or environmental stress. In addition, since hidden failures were detected during PVST, failures used to develop preventive maintenance were related to accessories, connectivity, and environmental stress. Therefore, it can be stated that both preventive and predictive maintenance require a plan for maintaining the availability of proper accessories, as recommended by Ridgway et al. However, in the present study, the battery-care program was included in accessories planning rather than as a separate plan. In addition, biomedical staff competence with regard to PVST is more important than user competence in our model.

Taghipour and Banjevic used the mean time between failures to prepare maintenance schedules. The authors determined the maintenance activity intervals of devices in terms of intensity of use. They reported that devices with a high intensity of use require maintenance more frequently than devices with a low intensity of use [17]. In the present study, the maintenance schedule was prepared in accordance to the rate of device failure. Devices with high failure rates were scheduled to receive more frequent maintenance.

The present study and a small component of a study conducted by Taghipour [25] are only similar in terms of the PVST results analysis. Taghipour analyzed the PVST results of infusion pumps before and after preventive maintenance and noted that medical devices included in a maintenance program have smaller errors than other devices. Similarly, as shown in Figures 3(a) and 3(b) in the present study, fewer hidden failures were identified after preventive maintenance. This was in contrast to the results of PVST performed before preventive maintenance.

As mentioned above, the present study included two different maintenance strategies: predictive and preventive maintenance. Programmed maintenance based on the manufacturers' recommendations for new high-tech medical devices represented the predictive maintenance strategy. Predictive maintenance is known as time-based maintenance and is defined as a maintenance strategy wherein maintenance activities are performed at scheduled time intervals recommended by manufacturers [25]. In contrast,

programmed maintenance based on an analysis of the performance inspection results of old technology medical devices represented the preventive maintenance strategy. Preventive maintenance is also known as condition-based maintenance and is defined as a maintenance strategy that involves periodic and continuous equipment condition monitoring to detect equipment degradation [25]. The information obtained from PVST results was used to determine the maintenance requirements and maintenance time schedule. For example, decision regarding filter replacement before the manufacturer's recommended replacement interval was based on equipment PVST results.

Whereas the predictive maintenance strategy was applied to individual components of new high-tech devices in consideration of the equipment brand and model, the preventive maintenance strategy was applied to groups of equipment such as defibrillators and oximeters.

Maintenance programs require resources such as budgets and test equipment. Predictive maintenance requires a budget to facilitate contracts with the manufacturer technical services, whereas preventive maintenance requires sensors and special equipment to conduct PVST.

In the predictive maintenance program, the user is responsible for reporting problems. If the user reports a problem, it will be added to the database. However, biomedical staffs conduct the PVST of equipment included in a preventive maintenance program. The analyzed failures are directly related to the device. This does not cover faults caused by the users.

Predictive maintenance may not always be optimal. Since a time-based schedule is implemented a device may receive more or less maintenance than required. However, using the preventive maintenance program, it is possible to track medical devices' hidden failures and to determine the most appropriate maintenance in terms of required nondurable parts and elapsed time. The replacement of components with failures was included in this model, as devices with nondurable parts fail if those parts are not replaced or restored. Preventive maintenance activities were performed by the hospital's biomedical personnel. These personnel also replaced nondurable parts. Nondurable parts requiring replacement at regular intervals should be stocked to ensure uninterrupted maintenance. These parts are supplied with a storage period of 1 year. For nondurable parts that are replaced twice yearly, a stock of two should be kept and a stock of three should be kept for parts replaced thrice yearly. Otherwise, maintaining a supply of expired nondurable parts extends the maintenance process and disrupts preventive maintenance.

As mentioned above, the current program helps to prevent problems prior to medical equipment failure and to maintain a stock of required nondurable parts. This feature increases the performance and efficiency of biomedical staffs. Medical equipment can be better tracked by repeating PVST throughout the year, as the database of equipment failures will contain PVST histories of older technology devices.

Preventive maintenance involves relatively old technology. Since the number of older technology devices in a hospital is greater than the number of new high-tech devices, the scope of preventive maintenance is more extensive than that of predictive maintenance. The distribution of failures might change because some old devices will be removed from use. By adding new devices to the inventory, the scope of preventive maintenance will become narrower, and the scope of predictive maintenance will become broader. However, new high-tech devices are also more expensive than older technology devices. Accordingly, predictive maintenance will be more costly than preventive maintenance.

This study has some limitations, because it was limited to high-risk devices in terms of patient safety and cost. Devices that pose risks to patients and users, old devices, and complex devices such as radiology devices are frequently considered for maintenance. Accordingly, the study did not include low-risk devices such as nebulizers and flow meters. The scope of the study could be extended to include other high-risk devices. For example, anesthesia units and vaporizers might be included in the preventive maintenance category. Although all endoscopy systems, including colonoscopy, gastroscopy, bronchoscopy, and laryngoscopy devices, could be incorporated into a preventive maintenance strategy, they do not undergo PVST. Rather, these devices are controlled via fluid leakage tests after each use. If there is any leakage, corrective maintenance is implemented. Operating tables and electrical patient beds requiring only electrical safety measurements may be incorporated into preventive maintenance.

In addition, all newly acquired equipment will be included in a maintenance program after considering its technology level.

The other limitation of the proposed model is that the criteria suggested by Fennigkoh and Smith [23] were used to determine the PVST interval. The EMN was used because this parameter has been accepted as a supervision criterion by the Ministry of Health in Turkey.

This study predicted that the reliability and failure patterns of a device would be affected by external factors such as the expertise level of users and biomedical staffs. Accordingly, the users were trained in the performance of daily checks through user training provided by the manufacturer. In addition, the clinical staffs were also trained about their responses to the different colored label on the devices after PVST. Both types of training were important for successful maintenance.

## 5. Conclusion

This paper proposes two different maintenance strategies: preventive maintenance for old technology devices and predictive maintenance for new high-tech devices. The first strategy takes into account the results of performance verification and safety testing. The second strategy considers the manufacturer recommendations.

Although preventive and predictive maintenance strategies differ in many ways, a maintenance program comprising both strategies yielded positive results. The maintenance strategy evaluation demonstrated that strategies based on PVST results and the manufacturers' recommendations led to a significant reduction in equipment failures and a significant increase in corrective maintenance.

The usage of different maintenance strategies for older devices and newer high-tech technology devices to develop maintenance strategies is important in terms of its consequences.

Firstly, the older technology devices that applied only corrective maintenance in developing countries will be included in the maintenance strategies like newer high-tech devices.

Secondly, the inclusion of both old and new technology devices to the maintenance system provides a wider range of maintenance that covers all medical devices in hospitals with many old technology devices.

Thirdly, the performance verification and safety testing earn importance to develop maintenance strategies for devices without manufacturer recommendations.

Lastly, considering carefully all outcomes of the medical equipment failures and existence of a detailed history for every device help decision-makers to manage medical equipment.

The next plan is to continue the study of failures of other medical devices excluded from this initial study.

## Competing Interests

The authors declare that they have no competing interests.

## Acknowledgments

A part of the measurements was performed by using test devices bought in the scope of the projects supported by The Research Fund of the University of Istanbul. The project numbers are BYP-39624 and YADOP-38953. Additionally, the authors are grateful to the biomedical personnel of the medical calibration group at the Biomedical and Clinical Engineering Department at Istanbul University for their help during the performance verification and safety testing of the medical equipment.

## References

[1] P. Derrico, M. Ritrovato, F. Nocchi, C. Capussotto, T. Franchin, and L. De Vivo, "Clinical engineering," in *Applied Biomedical Engineering*, G. Gargiulo, Ed., pp. 169–196, InTech, Rijeka, Croatia, 2011.

[2] R. Miniati, F. Dori, and M. F. Medici, "Health technology management," in *Advanced Technologies*, K. Jayanthakumaran, Ed., pp. 187–209, InTech, 2009.

[3] Medicines and Healthcare Products Regulatory Agency, *Managing Medical Devices*, MHRA, London, UK, 2014.

[4] European Union, *European Medical Devices Directive 2007/47/EC*, Strasburg, France, 2007.

[5] M. Sezdi, "Medical technology management and patient safety," in *Roadmap of Biomedical Engineers and Milestones*, S. Kara, Ed., pp. 183–208, InTech, Rijeka, Croatia, 2012.

[6] M. Sezdi, "Performance analysis for medical devices," *Biomedical Engineering Research*, vol. 2, no. 3, pp. 139–146, 2013.

[7] M. Sezdi and E. Ozdemir, "BMED: a web based application to analyze the performance of medical devices," *Biomedical Engineering: Applications, Basis and Communications*, vol. 26, no. 3, pp. 10–18, 2014.

[8] N. Lowe and W. L. Scott, *Medical Device Reporting for User Facilities*, Food and Drug Administration, Silver Spring, Md, USA, 1996.

[9] D. R. Wallace and D. R. Kuhn, "Lessons from 342 medical device failures," in *Proceedings of the 4th IEEE International Symposium on High-Assurance Systems Engineering (HASE '99)*, pp. 123–131, Washington, DC, USA, November 1999.

[10] Z. Bliznakov, G. Mitalasand, and N. Pallikarakis, "Analysis and classification of medical device recalls," *IFMBE Proceedings*, vol. 14, no. 25, pp. 3782–3785, 2007.

[11] M. Ridgway, L. R. Atles, and A. Subhan, "Reducing equipment downtime: a new line of attack," *Journal of Clinical Engineering*, vol. 34, no. 4, pp. 200–204, 2009.

[12] R. P. Santos and R. M. Almeida, "Hospital medical equipment maintenance schedules using the mean time between failures," *Cadernos Saude Coletiva*, vol. 18, no. 2, pp. 309–314, 2010.

[13] S. Taghipour, D. Banjevic, and A. K. S. Jardine, "Prioritization of medical equipment for maintenance decisions," *Journal of the Operational Research Society*, vol. 62, no. 9, pp. 1666–1687, 2011.

[14] S. Taghipour, D. Banjevic, and A. K. S. Jardine, "Periodic inspection optimization model for a complex repairable system," *Reliability Engineering and System Safety*, vol. 95, no. 9, pp. 944–952, 2010.

[15] S. Taghipour and D. Banjevic, "Periodic inspection optimization models for a repairable system subject to hidden failures," *IEEE Transactions on Reliability*, vol. 60, no. 1, pp. 275–285, 2011.

[16] N. Hamdi, R. Oweis, H. A. Zraiq, and D. A. Sammour, "An intelligent healthcare management system: a new approach in work-order prioritization for medical equipment maintenance requests," *Journal of Medical Systems*, vol. 36, no. 2, pp. 557–567, 2012.

[17] S. Taghipour and D. Banjevic, "Optimum inspection interval for a system under periodic and opportunistic inspections," *IIE Transactions*, vol. 44, no. 11, pp. 932–948, 2012.

[18] A. Khalaf, K. Djouani, Y. Hamam, and Y. Alaylı, "Evidence-based mathematical maintenance model for medical equipment," in *Proceedings of the International Conference on Electronic Devices, Systems and Applications (ICEDSA '10)*, pp. 222–226, Kuala Lumpur, Malaysia, April 2010.

[19] R. Miniati, F. Dori, E. Iadanza, M. M. Fregonara, and G. B. Gentili, "Health technology management: a database analysis as support of technology managers in hospitals," *Technology and Health Care*, vol. 19, no. 6, pp. 445–454, 2011.

[20] N. Saleh, A. A. Sharawi, M. A. Elwahed, A. Petti, D. Puppato, and G. Balestra, "Preventive maintenance prioritization index of medical equipment using quality function deployment," *IEEE Journal of Biomedical and Health Informatics*, vol. 19, no. 3, pp. 1029–1035, 2015.

[21] M. Sezdi, "The quality control system of medical devices in Cerrahpasa Health Faculty at Istanbul University," in *Proceedings of the 4th International Conference on Quality in Healthcare Accreditation and Patient Safety*, pp. 21–22, Antalya, Turkey, 2010.

[22] Healthcare Technology Management Community, "Choosing appropriate PM intervals," HTM ComDoc 6, November 2015, http://www.htmcommunitydb.org.

[23] L. Fennigkoh and B. Smith, "Clinical Equipment Management," in *JCAHO Plant*, vol. 2 of *Technology & Safely Management Series*, pp. 5–14, 1989.

[24] Emergency Care Research Institute, "Inspection and Preventive Maintenance System Procedures (Biomedical Benchmark)," August 2014, http://www.ecri.org.

[25] S. Taghipour, *Reliability and maintenance of medical devices [Ph.D. thesis]*, University of Toronto, Toronto, Canada, 2011.

# 16

# Using the Integration of Discrete Event and Agent-Based Simulation to Enhance Outpatient Service Quality in an Orthopedic Department

**Cholada Kittipittayakorn[1] and Kuo-Ching Ying[2]**

[1]*Graduate Institute of Industrial and Business Management, National Taipei University of Technology, No. 1, Section 3, Zhongxiao E. Road, Taipei 10608, Taiwan*
[2]*Department of Industrial Engineering and Management, National Taipei University of Technology, No. 1, Section 3, Zhongxiao E. Road, Taipei 10608, Taiwan*

Correspondence should be addressed to Kuo-Ching Ying; kcying@ntut.edu.tw

Academic Editor: John S. Katsanis

Many hospitals are currently paying more attention to patient satisfaction since it is an important service quality index. Many Asian countries' healthcare systems have a mixed-type registration, accepting both walk-in patients and scheduled patients. This complex registration system causes a long patient waiting time in outpatient clinics. Different approaches have been proposed to reduce the waiting time. This study uses the integration of discrete event simulation (DES) and agent-based simulation (ABS) to improve patient waiting time and is the first attempt to apply this approach to solve this key problem faced by orthopedic departments. From the data collected, patient behaviors are modeled and incorporated into a massive agent-based simulation. The proposed approach is an aid for analyzing and modifying orthopedic department processes, allows us to consider far more details, and provides more reliable results. After applying the proposed approach, the total waiting time of the orthopedic department fell from 1246.39 minutes to 847.21 minutes. Thus, using the correct simulation model significantly reduces patient waiting time in an orthopedic department.

## 1. Introduction

The concept of improving the quality of healthcare service has been repeatedly discussed in recent years. Healthcare providers try to provide patients with better service and excellent treatment. Patients who are satisfied with their service experience are more likely to come back to the hospital in the future [1]. Many studies have regarded patient waiting time as a significant component of patient satisfaction/dissatisfaction [2–7]. Bernhart et al. [8] presented the relative importance of various patient satisfaction factors, finding the service waiting time to be one of the key factors. Patient satisfaction is an important indicator of healthcare outcomes and plays a key role in improving healthcare service quality to attract patients [9].

Patient satisfaction and patient waiting time are important factors in the field of healthcare service. A long waiting time reflects negatively on the quality of the hospital and cripples its competitive advantages [10]. Outpatient waiting time means the time spent by an outpatient in a queue waiting to be served. Throughput time is the amount of time required for a patient to pass through a hospital process. The throughput time includes process time, service time, move time, and waiting time. Utilization rate means the percentage of time a doctor spends doing diagnosis. A direct way to improve patient satisfaction and service quality is to reduce the waiting time. Groome and Mayeaux Jr. [7] explained some factors that affect waiting time, including arrival time, failure to show up for appointments, consultation time, and registration time. Bailey [11] and Welch [12] proposed a single-block/individual system in which the best scheduling policy for patient waiting time is to place two patients at the beginning of the period and then schedule patients evenly over the intervals based on average service time.

Wijewickrama and Takakuwa [13] analyzed the long-waiting-time problem in outpatient clinics with a mixed-type registration, using the simulation approach to test four scheduling rules in comparison with the original case. They found that implementing the rule that "first priority is given to shorter processing of patients for consultation with a physician" can achieve the best waiting-time performance. Su and Shih [14] applied the simulation approach to test four assumed models, such as changing patient sequencing and assigning an interval time for scheduled patients. Reynolds et al. [15] tested eight cases to determine how different numbers of doctors and nurses affect waiting time. Baril et al. [16] applied a simulation model to improve performance at an outpatient orthopedic clinic, focusing on the relationships and interactions among patient flows, resource capacity (number of consulting rooms and number of nurses), and appointment scheduling rules. In short, there are different ways to improve patient waiting time amongst which healthcare providers should select the approach that best fits their situation.

Operation-management tools, which are well known in industrial engineering, are being effectively used in the healthcare industry for enhancing both the use of limited resources and system efficiency [17–19]. Recently, the use of computing simulation for achieving a more effective decision-making has exhibited a rising trending [20]. Computer simulation uses computer software to simulate an abstract model of a specific system representing real-world situations. Computer simulation was applied to hospital systems in 1979 to improve the scheduling of staff members [21]. Rohleder et al. [2] used a simulation model to identify certain elements, such as staffing level, patient scheduling, and promptness of service that could reduce patient waiting time at an orthopedic outpatient clinic. Reilly et al. [22] proposed a delay-scheduling model for patients in a walk-in clinic and applied computer simulation to evaluate the clinical performance with different physician staffing patterns and different rules for delay scheduling.

DES is a computer-based methodology that provides an intuitive and flexible approach for representing complex systems. It allows users to estimate the impact of operational changes before expending resources to implement those changes [23]. A DES model can represent the patient visit process, identify process bottlenecks, and adjust resource allocation, without disturbing the actual system [24]. Gul and Guneri applied a DES model to determine the optimal staff level to reduce the patient average length of stay (LOS) in an emergency department, as well as to improve patient throughput and utilization of resources [25]. Lu et al. [26] employed DES to improve outpatient service quality in an orthopedic surgery department. Kim et al. [27] improved a mental health clinic design by using DES.

Entities built into a DES model are typically simple, reactive, and limited in decision-making [28]. Moreover, human capabilities such as multitasking need to be used to set up a validated model [29]. Thus, using only DES is insufficient to model human behavior since the possible path of the entity is predetermined in a DES model [30]. ABS has been proposed to model the human discretion factor in a simulation model [31]. It is a new approach for modeling systems of autonomous, interacting agents [32]. An agent can be described as an autonomous entity that makes decisions based on a set of rules [33]. In the system, agents communicate with one another; they adapt and change their behavior based on the outcome of the interaction [34]. Crooks and Hailegiorgis [35] developed ABS further to explore the spread of cholera. They modeled the spread of cholera by explicitly representing the interaction between humans and their environment.

In outpatient clinic modeling, behaviors related to patients and healthcare providers can be modeled to investigate patient flow, in order to improve waiting time. Aburukba et al. [36] used a distributed multiagent approach to model an intelligent dynamic scheduling solution in advertisement. They believed that the agent-based model is appropriate due to its ability to support both dynamic behavior and distributed structure. Hutzschenreuter et al. [37] demonstrated an agent-based simulation and evaluation tool for patient admission scheduling, with the aim of achieving the efficient use of hospital resources through the combination of different profiles of resource use.

The main aim of this work is to improve clinical services by reducing patient waiting time in an orthopedic department. The integration of DES and ABS is used to determine the optimal scheduling for each consultation session. To the best of our knowledge, this paper is the first study applying the integration of DES and ABS models to solve the operational problem in a hospital. The integration of DES and ABS can take advantage of both approaches [38]. DES provides an environment for agents as well as work rules. The orthopedic outpatient clinic environment can be constructed by using DES for orthopedic outpatient flow and by applying ABS for human decision-making.

The rest of the paper is organized as follows. Section 2 describes the patient flow at the outpatient clinic of an orthopedic department and explains a simulation model. Section 3 shows the results after applying the proposed approach. Section 4 discusses the results before and after applying the proposed approach. Finally, Section 5 presents our conclusions.

## 2. Methods

The community hospital in this research is a 689-patient-bed medical center with more than 20 clinical departments and has approximately seven hundred employees, including one hundred physicians, three hundred nurses, and three hundred staff members. The patient volume in the orthopedic department at this community hospital is over 5500 per year and faces the challenge of increasing patient visits. The department, which has nine doctors, is divided into three different teams: hand and foot, trauma, and sports. Current data show that the outpatients on average spend only about 14 minutes to get serviced but almost two hours (104 minutes) waiting in line; waiting time accounts for over 88% of the total process time.

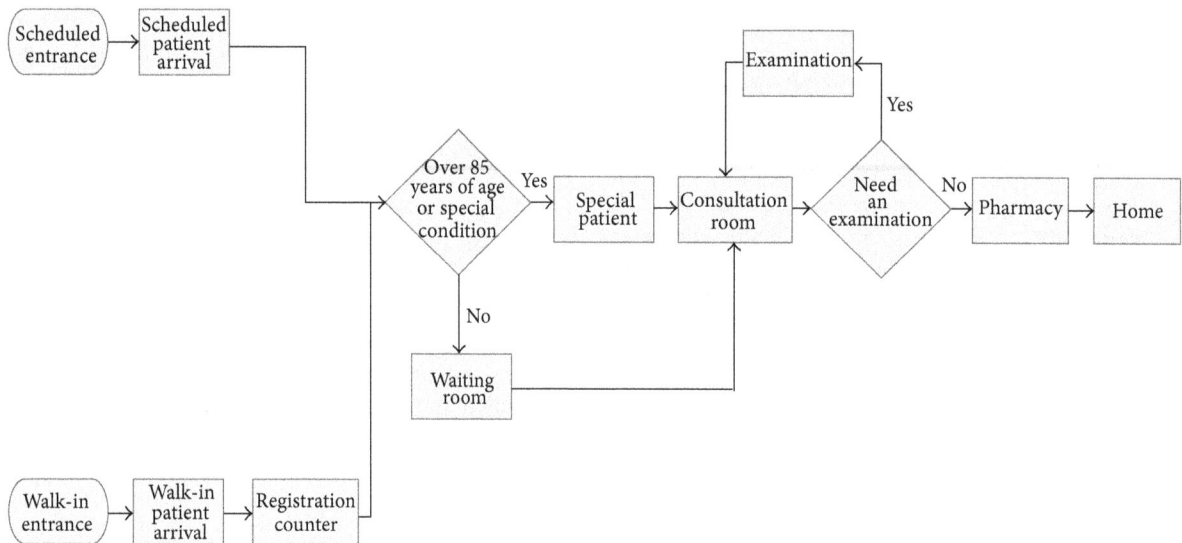

FIGURE 1: Patient flow at the outpatient clinic of the orthopedic department.

*2.1. Description of the Outpatient Orthopedic Department.* The orthopedic department operates from 8:30 a.m. to 10:00 p.m. on weekdays and has 12 consultation sessions per week. The five consultation sessions are treated by doctors from the sports team, the four consultation sessions are treated by doctors from the trauma team, and the three consultation sessions are treated by doctors from the hand and foot team. The types of patients for each consultation session depend on the doctor team. For instance, if the session is seen by a doctor from the trauma team, then most patients in this session would be injured patients. Based on the observations of this department, we formulate a patient flowchart, as shown in Figure 1. The following processes are typical for an orthopedic outpatient visit:

(i) A walk-in patient stands in line for registration; during registration, basic information such as name, birth date, and identity number is collected.

(ii) After registration, the walk-in patient goes to the orthopedic clinic and waits for consultation.

(iii) A scheduled patient can go directly to the clinic and wait for consultation.

(iv) Both types of patients can be seen according to their registered numbers.

(v) For current scheduling policy, odd numbers are assigned to walk-in patients and even numbers are assigned to scheduled patients (a doctor will see one walk-in patient and then one scheduled patient).

(vi) The orthopedic department has a special policy: patients who are over 85 years of age or have a special condition have first priority to see a doctor. In this study, we define these patients as "special patients."

(vii) Appointments for patients who arrive late will be postponed until the following three patients have been seen.

(viii) After a patient consults a doctor, it is decided whether the patient needs to have a medical examination. If so, the patient goes for the examination and will return to see the doctor again. The doctor will prescribe medicine if required. The patient then receives the medicine and leaves the hospital or receives a prescription, picks up the drug, and leaves the hospital.

*2.2. System Analysis.* The department's operations and details of each consultation section were investigated through interviews with staff members, close observations of the department's daily operations, and collecting the hospital database. Focus groups were formed, including orthopedic surgeons, nurses, healthcare assistants, and radiologists.

The orthopedic department contains different zones, including registration area, waiting area, treatment area, examination room, and pharmacy. The department shares the examination room and pharmacy with other departments. Figure 2 shows the layout of the department.

All data were collected from Monday to Friday from the orthopedic department over a two-month period (June to July) by hospital staff. Different orthopedic department areas were observed with the purpose of analyzing and taking notes about how the different processes take place, and data were collected on registration time, patient queues, clinic start time, consultation period, clinic end time, arrival time, consultation time, late rate, no-show rate, examination time, and examination rate. The collected data were formed into two groups. The June data were denoted as model-building data and were used to build a simulation model. The July data were used to validate the simulation model. All data were analyzed statistically and used to construct a simulation model.

*2.3. Orthopedic Department Modeling.* Developing a simulation model consists of the following steps: describing a problem, formulating a problem, collecting and processing

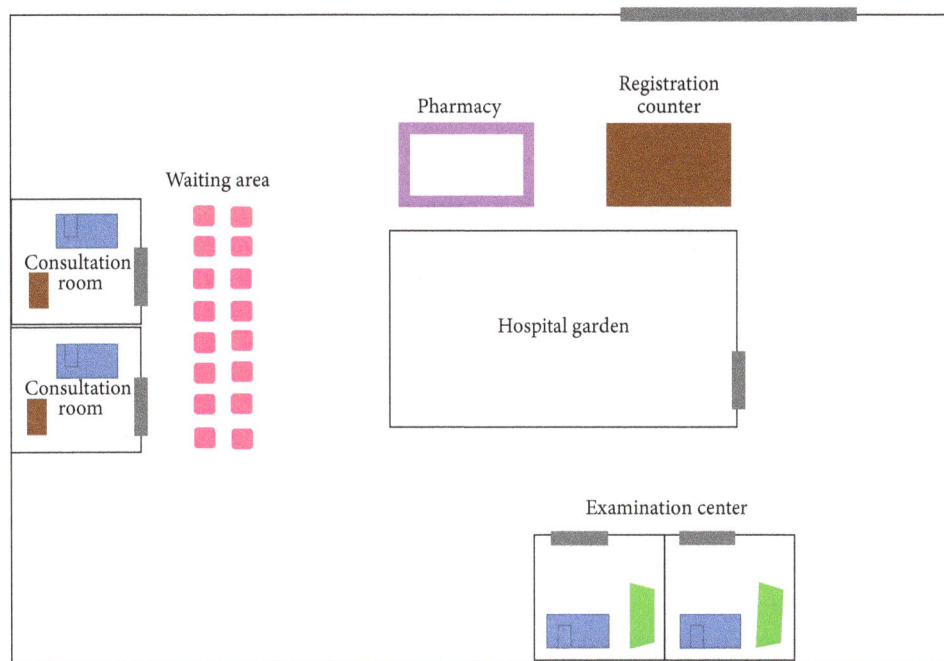

FIGURE 2: Orthopedic department layout.

real system data, formulating and developing a model, verifying and validating a model, documenting a model for future use, selecting appropriate experimental design, establishing experimental conditions for runs, performing simulation runs, and interpreting results [39]. The orthopedic department model defined by this study is an integration of ABS and DES, incorporating a population of simulated real-world outpatient-use data with a discrete event simulation of an orthopedic department. We observe that the orthopedic department processes consist of continuous changes, so that when we analyze these processes, it is better to divide a continuous process into discrete parts to simplify the analysis. In this case, DES is the best choice when the system under analysis can naturally be described as a sequence of operations.

Since the orthopedic department is a dynamic environment with full human interactions, human behaviors affect the outcome of those interactions. The entities of an orthopedic department, such as doctors, nurses, and administration staff, are humans with emotions and reasoning abilities. These agents adapt and change their behavior during the simulation. ABS allows us to explore the system, which has a natural representation consisting of interacting agents. In this situation, it is best to apply agent-based modeling to capture emergent phenomena. For modeling purposes, patients are considered as static objects. This study develops a simulation model using AnyLogic 7 to represent the patient flow in the orthopedic department. We choose AnyLogic 7, because it supports DES and ABS and allows us to efficiently combine it with other modeling approaches. The simulation of the current system without any changes is run as the case-based

model. The results of the simulation provide a baseline for comparing operational changes.

*2.4. Simulation and Implementation.* The simulation model is implemented in AnyLogic 7. This is the only simulation tool that supports all of the most common simulation methodologies, such as system dynamics and discrete event and agent-based modeling, and enables the user to capture the complexity and heterogeneity of business, economic, and social systems to any desired level of detail.

The current version of the simulator includes the registration counter, waiting room, consultation room, examination center, and pharmacy. Through the information obtained during interviews carried out with the orthopedic staff, this study identifies two kinds of agents: active agents and passive agents [40]. The active agents in this simulation are orthopedic outpatients, doctors, nurses, healthcare assistants, radiologists, biomedical scientists, and administration staffs. The passive agents represent solely reactive aspects of the system, such as the patient information system, examination center, and loudspeaker system.

In the simulation model, orthopedic outpatients arrive at the orthopedic clinic by their own means and go to the registration counter. In the simulation the input information is read from a text file within the data given by the hospital. Once the registration process has been carried out, the patients go to the waiting area. Patients who are over 85 years of age or have a condition can be seen by a doctor first. The patients' scheduling changes depending on the numbers of walk-in patients and scheduled patients inside the waiting area. Once the patient is seen by a doctor, the doctor decides whether the patient needs an examination. After seeing a doctor, the patient goes to the pharmacy and then leaves the hospital.

## 3. Results

*3.1. Model Validation.* The model validation ensures that the model correctly represents the real world. The simulation model is validated by comparing data generated by the model and data collected from the orthopedic department. Table 1 shows confidence intervals of the simulation outputs at the 95% ($\alpha$ = 0.05) confidence level and the actual values obtained from the collected data. The comparison verifies that, for waiting time, throughout time, and utilization, there are no significant differences between the results obtained using the simulation and those that occurred in the real system. We conclude that the model is truly representative of the existing environment. Therefore, the validated model can be used for subsequent analysis.

*3.2. Main Results.* This research applies the integration of DES and ABS to an orthopedic clinic. The different consultation sessions yield different results, which are shown in Table 2. To further verify the effectiveness of the proposed approach, the study performs the paired *t*-test on the average real-world waiting time to compare the waiting times before and after applying the approach. At the confidence level $\alpha$ = 0.05, the results in Table 3 clearly confirm the superiority of the proposed approach.

## 4. Discussion

The main objective of this study is to reduce the outpatient waiting time in the orthopedic department. After applying the proposed approach, the results show that the waiting time dropped significantly: for consultation session 1, the waiting time fell to 39.28 minutes (32.47%); for consultation session 2, the waiting time fell to 43.72 minutes (35.16%); for consultation session 3, the waiting time fell to 21.97 minutes (27.89%); for consultation session 4, the waiting time fell to 16.75 minutes (26.35%); for consultation session 5, the waiting time fell to 22.27 minutes (27.64%); for consultation session 6, the waiting time fell to 35.67 minutes (30.51%); for consultation session 7, the waiting time fell to 23.85 minutes (28.60%); for consultation session 8, the waiting time fell to 55.97 minutes (38.23%); for consultation session 9, the waiting time fell to 22.8 minutes (29.34%); for consultation session 10, the waiting time fell to 37.79 minutes (31.78%); for consultation session 11, the waiting time fell to 56.62 minutes (37.65%); for consultation session 12, the waiting time fell to 22.5 minutes (26.64%). The average waiting time after applying the proposed approach of 12 consultation sessions fell to 33.27 minutes (32.03%).

It is obvious from Tables 2 and 3 that the proposed approach is very effective for improving clinical services by reducing patient waiting time in the orthopedic department. These results underscore the benefits of modeling operational changes before implementation, particularly under a resource limitation situation. This study shows that simulation models can be useful decision-support tools for healthcare provider management, not only for waiting time reduction in an orthopedic department, but also for the hospital as a whole.

## 5. Conclusions

Service quality, which always influences hospital patient satisfaction, has recently become an important index in the healthcare field. Our previous study has shown that waiting time is a key performance index of patient satisfaction. Computer simulation is an efficient approach to study such a complex system. The increasing interest in the integration of simulation approaches may be explained by the increasingly complex nature of the problems being faced. Several problems involve interacting elements of a different nature. Thus, modelers face the choice of identifying the best single paradigm or adopting multiple paradigms, such as an integration of the simulation approach and applying it to the whole system.

In this paper we have integrated DES and ABS simulation models to evaluate proposed strategies applied toward an orthopedic department so as to reduce patient waiting time. The integration of DES and ABS allows us to utilize the advantages of both simulations. DES helps us to understand the orthopedic department processes and to replicate the orthopedic department system, whereas ABS allows us to consider the variation in individual behavior in order to model a situation with interdependencies between work entities. The simulation model herein correctly emulates the patient flow in the orthopedic department and can be used to analyze the effects of potential improvement policies. The research results indicate that the proposed approach achieves a considerable reduction in waiting time. Moreover, the reduction in waiting time does not need any additional resources.

Although our results suggest that the integration of DES and ABS can improve the waiting time in an orthopedic clinic, there are several important limitations to discuss. First, since this research provides only one example, more case studies implementing the model are needed for external validity. Second, the proposed simulation model only generates a method of evaluating a solution but does not generate solutions themselves. Finally, the proposed simulation model does not yield an answer. It merely provides a set of the system's responses to different operating conditions, and so the results need to be well interpreted and understood before any changes are implemented.

The approach of this research not only is applicable to the orthopedic department at this hospital but also can be applied to reduce patient waiting time at other orthopedic departments nationwide. Furthermore, the results can be helpful for other hospital departments in addition to orthopedics.

TABLE 1: Validation of simulation model by a comparison between simulated and collected data.

| | Simulation model | Confidence interval | Collected data | Difference (%) |
|---|---|---|---|---|
| Consultation session variable 1 | | | | |
| Average waiting time (minute) | 124.36 | [105.08, 143.64] | 121.77 | 2.083 |
| Average throughput time (minute) | 132.54 | [120.27, 144.81] | 134.12 | 1.192 |
| Average utilization (%) | 92.16 | [76.26, 106.06] | 93.51 | 1.46 |
| Consultation session variable 2 | | | | |
| Average waiting time (minute) | 122.57 | [100.66, 144.48] | 125.98 | 2.78 |
| Average throughput time (minute) | 129.92 | [118.53, 141.31] | 131.45 | 1.18 |
| Average utilization (%) | 88.56 | [74.54, 102.58] | 84.97 | 1.79 |
| Consultation session variable 3 | | | | |
| Average waiting time (minute) | 77.75 | [48.84, 106.68] | 75.41 | 3.00 |
| Average throughput time (minute) | 85.47 | [71.45, 99.49] | 86.68 | 1.42 |
| Average utilization (%) | 85.63 | [54.95, 116.31] | 82.78 | 3.33 |
| Consultation session variable 4 | | | | |
| Average waiting time (minute) | 65.15 | [49.37, 80.93] | 66.13 | 1.50 |
| Average throughput time (minute) | 72.31 | [50.4, 94.22] | 74.14 | 2.53 |
| Average utilization (%) | 91.53 | [76.19, 106.87] | 90.23 | 1.42 |
| Consultation session variable 5 | | | | |
| Average waiting time (minute) | 81.36 | [61.64, 101.08] | 79.65 | 2.10 |
| Average throughput time (minute) | 89.37 | [71.23, 107.51] | 90.98 | 1.80 |
| Average utilization (%) | 87.67 | [72.24, 103.1] | 86.36 | 1.49 |
| Consultation session variable 6 | | | | |
| Average waiting time (minute) | 116.3 | [107.01, 125.59] | 117.24 | 0.81 |
| Average throughput time (minute) | 137.0 | [126.92, 147.08] | 138.38 | 1.01 |
| Average utilization (%) | 91.7 | [70.66, 112.74] | 89.68 | 2.20 |
| Consultation session variable 7 | | | | |
| Average waiting time (minute) | 85.1 | [66.79, 103.41] | 86.76 | 1.95 |
| Average throughput time (minute) | 102.0 | [86.97, 117.03] | 103.51 | 1.48 |
| Average utilization (%) | 92.6 | [88.66, 96.54] | 92.57 | 0.03 |
| Consultation session variable 8 | | | | |
| Average waiting time (minute) | 145.3 | [137.41, 153.19] | 144.12 | 0.81 |
| Average throughput time (minute) | 156.0 | [137.33, 174.67] | 158.98 | 1.91 |
| Average utilization (%) | 95.5 | [78.85, 112.15] | 93.97 | 1.60 |
| Consultation session variable 9 | | | | |
| Average waiting time (minute) | 75.3 | [59.43, 91.17] | 74.12 | 1.57 |
| Average throughput time (minute) | 90.0 | [72.66, 107.34] | 88.32 | 1.87 |
| Average utilization (%) | 91.8 | [66.47, 117.13] | 94.21 | 2.63 |
| Consultation session variable 10 | | | | |
| Average waiting time (minute) | 122.1 | [115.08, 129.12] | 122.97 | 0.71 |
| Average throughput time (minute) | 130.63 | [117.6, 143.66] | 132.45 | 1.39 |
| Average utilization (%) | 89.84 | [75.2, 104.48] | 88.41 | 1.59 |
| Consultation session variable 11 | | | | |
| Average waiting time (minute) | 151.51 | [136.08, 166.94] | 154.01 | 1.65 |
| Average throughput time (minute) | 159.83 | [145.63, 174.03] | 157.63 | 1.38 |
| Average utilization (%) | 96.09 | [74.09, 118.09] | 98.34 | −2.34 |
| Consultation session variable 12 | | | | |
| Average waiting time (minute) | 82.82 | [72.5, 93.14] | 83.68 | 1.04 |
| Average throughput time (minute) | 95.52 | [74.39, 116.65] | 97.66 | 2.24 |
| Average utilization (%) | 94.21 | [71.71, 116.71] | 91.96 | 2.39 |

TABLE 2: Waiting time improvement for the orthopedic department.

| Consultation session | Average real-world waiting time | Average waiting time after applying the proposed approach | Waiting time improvement (%) |
|---|---|---|---|
| 1 | 2:00:59* | 1:21:42 | 32.47 |
| 2 | 2:04:21 | 1:20:38 | 35.16 |
| 3 | 1:18:46 | 0:56:48 | 27.89 |
| 4 | 1:03:34 | 0:46:49 | 26.35 |
| 5 | 1:20:34 | 0:58:18 | 27.64 |
| 6 | 1:56:54 | 1:21:14 | 30.51 |
| 7 | 1:23:24 | 0:59:33 | 28.60 |
| 8 | 2:26:24 | 1:30:26 | 38.23 |
| 9 | 1:17:42 | 0:54:54 | 29.34 |
| 10 | 1:58:55 | 1:21:08 | 31.83 |
| 11 | 2:30:23 | 1:33:46 | 37.65 |
| 12 | 1:24:27 | 1:01:57 | 26.64 |

*hh:mm:ss.

TABLE 3: Paired $t$-tests performed on average real-world waiting time (after applying the approach versus before applying the approach).

| After applying the approach | Before applying the approach |
|---|---|
| Difference | 1995.5 |
| Dof | 11 |
| $t$-value | −8.347 |
| One-tail significance | <0.0001 |

## Competing Interests

The authors declare that there is no competing interests.

## Acknowledgments

The authors would like to thank the Ministry of Science and Technology of the Republic of China, Taiwan, for financially supporting this research under Contract no. MOST104-2221-E-027-045.

## References

[1] K. Freeman and S. A. Denham, "Improving patient satisfaction by addressing same day surgery wait times," *Journal of Perianesthesia Nursing*, vol. 23, no. 6, pp. 387–393, 2008.

[2] T. R. Rohleder, P. Lewkonia, D. P. Bischak, P. Duffy, and R. Hendijani, "Using simulation modeling to improve patient flow at an outpatient orthopedic clinic," *Health Care Management Science*, vol. 14, no. 2, pp. 135–145, 2011.

[3] C. A. Feddock, A. R. Hoellein, C. H. Griffith III et al., "Can physicians improve patient satisfaction with long waiting times?" *Evaluation & the Health Professions*, vol. 28, no. 1, pp. 40–52, 2005.

[4] G. M. Eilers, "Improving patient satisfaction with waiting time," *Journal of American College Health*, vol. 53, no. 1, pp. 41–43, 2004.

[5] O. A. Soremekun, J. K. Takayesu, and S. J. Bohan, "Framework for analyzing wait times and other factors that impact patient satisfaction in the emergency department," *The Journal of Emergency Medicine*, vol. 41, no. 6, pp. 686–692, 2011.

[6] E. D. Boudreaux and E. L. O'Hea, "Patient satisfaction in the emergency department: a review of the literature and implications for practice," *The Journal of Emergency Medicine*, vol. 26, no. 1, pp. 13–26, 2004.

[7] L. J. Groome and E. J. Mayeaux Jr., "Decreasing extremes in patient waiting time," *Quality Management in Health Care*, vol. 19, no. 2, pp. 117–128, 2010.

[8] M. H. Bernhart, I. G. P. Wiadnyana, H. Wihardjo, and I. Pohan, "Patient satisfaction in developing countries," *Social Science & Medicine*, vol. 48, no. 8, pp. 989–996, 1999.

[9] A. B. Tehrani, S. R. Feldman, F. T. Camacho, and R. Balkrishnan, "Patient satisfaction with outpatient medical care in the United States," *Health Outcomes Research in Medicine*, vol. 2, no. 4, pp. e197–e202, 2011.

[10] B.-L. Chen, E.-D. Li, K. Yamawuchi, K. Kato, S. Naganawa, and W.-J. Miao, "Impact of adjustment measures on reducing outpatient waiting time in a community hospital: application of a computer simulation," *Chinese Medical Journal*, vol. 123, no. 5, pp. 574–580, 2010.

[11] N. T. J. Bailey, "A study of queues and appointment systems in hospital outpatient departments, with special reference to waiting-times," *Journal of the Royal Statistical Society*, vol. 14, no. 2, pp. 185–199, 1952.

[12] J. D. Welch, "Appointment system in hospital outpatient department," *Operational Research Quarterly*, vol. 15, no. 3, pp. 224–232, 1964.

[13] A. K. A. Wijewickrama and S. Takakuwa, "Simulation analysis of an outpatient department of internal medicine in a university hospital," in *Proceedings of the Winter Simulation Conference (WSC '06)*, pp. 425–432, IEEE, Monterey, Calif, USA, December 2006.

[14] S. Su and C.-L. Shih, "Managing a mixed-registration-type appointment system in outpatient clinics," *International Journal of Medical Informatics*, vol. 70, no. 1, pp. 31–40, 2003.

[15] J. Reynolds, Z. Zeng, J. Li, and S.-Y. Chiang, "Design and analysis of a health care clinic for homeless people using simulations,"

*International Journal of Health Care Quality Assurance*, vol. 23, no. 6, pp. 607–620, 2010.

[16] C. Baril, V. Gascon, and S. Cartier, "Design and analysis of an outpatient orthopaedic clinic performance with discrete event simulation and design of experiments," *Computers & Industrial Engineering*, vol. 78, pp. 285–298, 2014.

[17] J. L. Wiler, R. T. Griffey, and T. Olsen, "Review of modeling approaches for emergency department patient flow and crowding research," *Academic Emergency Medicine*, vol. 18, no. 12, pp. 1371–1379, 2011.

[18] P. M. Carter, J. S. Desmond, C. Akanbobnaab et al., "Optimizing clinical operations as part of a global emergency medicine initiative in Kumasi, Ghana: application of lean manufacturing principals to low-resource health systems," *Academic Emergency Medicine*, vol. 19, no. 3, pp. 338–347, 2012.

[19] P. P. Reid, W. D. Compton, J. H. Grossman, and G. Fanjiang, *Building a Better Delivery System: A New Engineering/Health Care Partnership*, National Academies Press, Washington, DC, USA, 2005.

[20] S. H. Jacobson, S. N. Hall, and J. R. Swisher, "Discrete-event simulation of health care systems," in *Patient Flow: Reducing Delay in Healthcare Delivery*, R. W. Hall, Ed., vol. 91 of *International Series in Operations Research & Management Science*, pp. 211–252, Springer, New York, NY, USA, 2006.

[21] W. M. Hancock and P. F. Walter, "The use of computer simulation to develop hospital systems," *ACM SIGSIM Simulation Digest*, vol. 10, no. 4, pp. 28–32, 1979.

[22] T. A. Reilly, V. P. Marathe, and B. E. Fries, "A delay-scheduling model for patients using a walk-in clinic," *Journal of Medical Systems*, vol. 2, no. 4, pp. 303–313, 1978.

[23] W. Abo-Hamad and A. Arisha, "Simulation-based framework to improve patient experience in an emergency department," *European Journal of Operational Research*, vol. 224, no. 1, pp. 154–166, 2013.

[24] T. Wang, A. Guinet, A. Belaidi, and B. Besombes, "Modelling and simulation of emergency services with ARIS and Arena. Case study: the emergency department of Saint Joseph and Saint Luc hospital," *Production Planning & Control*, vol. 20, no. 6, pp. 484–495, 2009.

[25] M. Gul and A. F. Guneri, "A computer simulation model to reduce patient length of stay and to improve resource utilization rate in an emergency department service system," *Journal of Industrial Engineering International*, vol. 19, no. 5, pp. 221–231, 2012.

[26] T.-P. Lu, J.-T. Shih, C. Kittipittayakorn, and G.-F. Lian, "Improving outpatient service quality in department of orthopedic surgery by using collaborative approaches," in *Proceedings of the IEEE 17th International Conference on Computer Supported Cooperative Work in Design (CSCWD '13)*, pp. 515–520, IEEE, British Columbia, Canada, June 2013.

[27] B. Kim, Y. Elstein, B. Shiner, R. Konrad, A. S. Pomerantz, and B. V. Watts, "Use of discrete event simulation to improve a mental health clinic," *General Hospital Psychiatry*, vol. 35, no. 6, pp. 668–670, 2013.

[28] C. A. Chung, *Simulation Modeling Handbook: A Practical Approach*, CRC Press, New York, NY, USA, 2003.

[29] T. J. Schriber, D. T. Brunner, and J. S. Smith, "How discrete-event simulation software works and why it matters," in *Proceedings of the Winter Simulation Conference (WSC '12)*, pp. 15–22, IEEE, Berlin, Germany, December 2012.

[30] M. M. Gunal and M. Pidd, "Understanding accident and emergency department performance using simulation," in *Proceedings of the Winter Simulation Conference (WSC '06)*, pp. 446–452, Monterey, Calif, USA, December 2006.

[31] B. Dubiel and O. Tsimhoni, "Integrating agent based modeling into a discrete event simulation," in *Proceedings of the Winter Simulation Conference*, pp. 9–15, IEEE, December 2005.

[32] M. J. North and C. M. Macal, "Agent-based modeling and systems dynamics model reproduction," *International Journal of Simulation and Process Modeling*, vol. 5, no. 3, pp. 256–271, 2009.

[33] P. Escudero-Marin and M. Pidd, "Using ABMS to simulate emergency departments," in *Proceedings of Winter Simulation Conference (WSC '11)*, vol. 1, pp. 1239–1250, Phoenix, Ariz, USA, December 2011.

[34] E. Cabrera, E. Luque, M. Taboada, F. Epelde, and M. L. Iglesias, "ABMS optimization for emergency departments," in *Proceedings of the Winter Simulation Conference (WSC '12)*, pp. 1–12, IEEE, Berlin, Germany, December 2012.

[35] A. T. Crooks and A. B. Hailegiorgis, "An agent-based modeling approach applied to the spread of cholera," *Environmental Modelling & Software*, vol. 62, pp. 164–177, 2014.

[36] R. Aburukba, H. Ghenniwa, and W. Shen, "Agent-based approach for dynamic scheduling in content-based networks," in *Proceedings of the IEEE International Conference on e-Business Engineering (ICEBE '06)*, pp. 425–432, Shanghai, China, October 2006.

[37] A. K. Hutzschenreuter, P. A. N. Bosman, I. Blonk-Altena, J. van Aarle, and H. La Poutré, "Agent-based patient admission scheduling in hospitals," in *Proceedings of the 7th International Joint Conference on Autonomous Agents and Multiagent Systems: Industrial Track (AAMAS '08)*, pp. 45–52, International Foundation for Autonomous Agents and Multiagent Systems, Estoril, Portugal, May 2008.

[38] B. Dubiel and O. Tsimhoni, "Integrating agent based modeling into a discrete event simulation," in *Proceedings of Winter Simulation Conference*, pp. 9–15, Orlando, Fla, USA, December 2005.

[39] M. Anu, "Introduction to modeling and simulation," in *Proceedings of the 29th Conference on Winter Simulation (WSC '97)*, pp. 7–13, Atlanta, Ga, USA, December 1997.

[40] M. Taboada, E. Cabrera, M. L. Iglesias, F. Epelde, and E. Luque, "An agent-based decision support system for hospitals emergency departments," *Procedia Computer Science*, vol. 4, pp. 1880–1889, 2011.

# 17

# A Computer-Aided Detection System for Digital Chest Radiographs

**Juan Manuel Carrillo-de-Gea,**[1] **Ginés García-Mateos,**[1]
**José Luis Fernández-Alemán,**[1] **and José Luis Hernández-Hernández**[2]

[1]*Computer Science and Systems Department, Faculty of Computer Science, University of Murcia, 30100 Murcia, Spain*
[2]*Academic Unit of Engineering, Autonomous University of Guerrero, 39087 Chilpancingo, GRO, Mexico*

Correspondence should be addressed to Ginés García-Mateos; ginesgm@um.es

Academic Editor: Yinkwee Ng

Computer-aided detection systems aim at the automatic detection of diseases using different medical imaging modalities. In this paper, a novel approach to detecting normality/pathology in digital chest radiographs is proposed. The problem tackled is complicated since it is not focused on particular diseases but anything that differs from what is considered as normality. First, the areas of interest of the chest are found using template matching on the images. Then, a texture descriptor called local binary patterns (LBP) is computed for those areas. After that, LBP histograms are applied in a classifier algorithm, which produces the final normality/pathology decision. Our experimental results show the feasibility of the proposal, with success rates above 87% in the best cases. Moreover, our technique is able to locate the possible areas of pathology in nonnormal radiographs. Strengths and limitations of the proposed approach are described in the Conclusions.

## 1. Introduction

Medical imaging is a key field in healthcare engineering, which aims to help medical professionals to identify lesions and diseases. Early attempts at computerized analysis of medical images were made in the 1960s, such as diagnosis of primary bone tumor [1] and detection of abnormalities in mammograms [2]. In the 1980s a new concept emerged, *computer-aided diagnosis* (CAD) which assumed that the computer output could be utilized to assist physicians, but not to replace them. Currently, CAD systems are employed in the early detection of pathologies, that is, to obtain a "second opinion" and help them make the final decision [3–6]. A CAD system can also be very useful to provide some basic information when the human expert monitoring is not possible.

Each biomedical image technique is appropriate for certain diagnostics. For example, MRI enables the spatial localisation required for cross-sectional imaging whereas ultrasound images allow physicians the visualisation of soft tissues and have revolutionised obstetric care [7]. However, digital radiology is still the backbone of diagnostic bioimaging, mainly due to three reasons: (1) its capability to detect unsuspected pathologies; (2) being not invasive; and (3) having a low radiation dose and low cost [8].

The majority of the studies related to CAD research have been concerned with some organs such as chest, breast, colon, and liver [5, 9–11]. The objective of this paper is to perform an automatic normality/pathology classification of posteroanterior (PA) digital chest radiographs. The proposed method is not specialized in a given set of types of lesions or diseases but is able to detect anything that differs from normality. A sample view of the radiographs under study is shown in Figure 1.

Although there is much computer vision research in CAD techniques, the problem studied here has received little attention so far. For example, we can cite some interesting research on CAD systems that work with mammography for breast nodule detection [12, 13]. Also, there are examples of systems focused on lung nodule detection using computer tomography [14, 15] or radiography [16–18]. These research

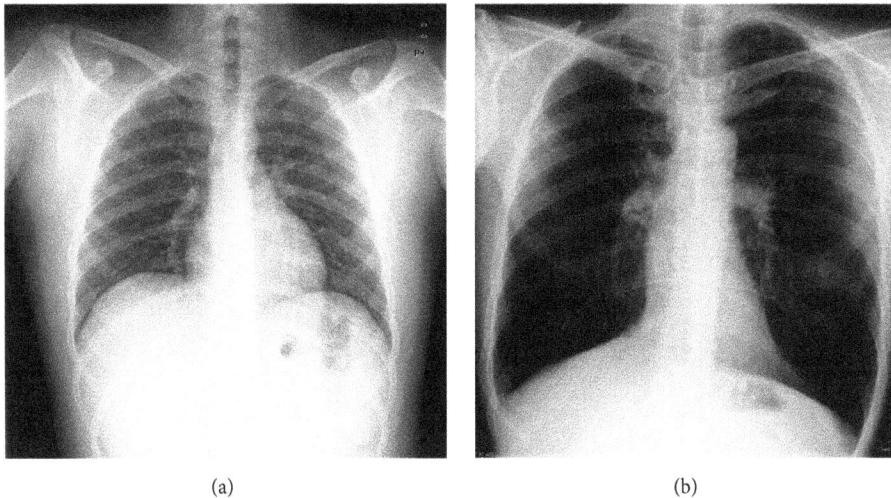

(a)                                    (b)

FIGURE 1: Sample chest radiographs in posteroanterior view. (a) Normal. (b) Pathological.

efforts have resulted in commercial systems available in clinical practice [19].

Besides, some authors have proposed CAD systems capable of recognizing diseases such as polyps in the colon [20], acute intracranial haemorrhage [21], and severe respiratory syndrome [22]. Due to its importance in CAD systems, much research work has been devoted to the segmentation of anatomical regions of the body. Related to thoracic medical imaging, attention is directed particularly to the lungs [8, 23, 24], the lung fields, the heart and the clavicles [25], certain lung structures as hilar region [26], and the liver and neighboring abdominal organs [10, 11]; the latter two methods do not use simple radiographs, but other 3D image modalities such as CT and MRI. Some authors are also investigating how to segment the bony structures of the chest [27, 28], often to eliminate the shadows projected on the lung parenchyma.

On the other hand, much less research has been dedicated to the generic problem of discriminating normality from pathology. In this field, we can find the approach described in [29], which tackles the classification normal/nonnormal of radiographies of the chest. A $k$-nearest neighbors ($k$-NN) classifier is proposed using as input features the responses to a set of Gabor wavelet filters. Another interesting work is [30] that used computed tomographies (CT) for the problem of lung texture recognition. They used a LBP operator extended to 3D, performing a comparison of LBP histograms. These authors also presented a texture classification-based system for emphysema quantification in CT images comprising three classes: normal tissue, centrilobular emphysema, and paraseptal emphysema [31]. The present paper is an extension of the preliminary work described in [32], with a substantial improvement in the proposed method and the experimental validation.

## 2. Materials and Methods

A sample of 48 high resolution DICOM images of chest radiographs (25 males and 23 females) were provided by the Hospital General Universitario Reina Sofía de Murcia

(HGURSM), Spain, to perform tests. The local Ethics Committees of the HGURSM approved the study, and written informed consent was obtained from the radiologist in charge of the diagnostic procedure at HGURSM. The images have a resolution of 3000 × 3000 pixels and a depth of 12 bits per pixel. In the available images, there are 25 normal (12 males and 13 females) and 23 pathologic (13 males and 10 females) samples. The ages of the subjects range from 15 to 93 years, with an average of 55.

The proposed image classification method is described in the following subsections. A global view of the developed system is shown in Figure 2.

*2.1. Preprocessing and Segmentation.* The first stage of the system is preprocessing and segmentation. In this step, the input DICOM files are reduced in pixel depth, from 12 to 8 bits per pixel. After that, decimation is applied to the images using supersampling interpolation, reducing the size to 1000 × 1000 pixels, that is, the standard resolution for the following steps.

In general, segmentation procedures are used to identify regions containing certain kinds of lesions [34]. In our system, the image is segmented to locate the position of both lungs in the radiographs, in order to determine the areas of interest. The proposed segmentation method is based on the template matching algorithm [35], which is a well-known technique in computer vision. This process consists in searching for a given template in all possible locations of an image, applying a predefined similarity measure for each location.

Samples of right and left lungs, extracted from the training set, are used as templates in the matching process. Different patterns of lungs are used to cope with the variety of aspects they can adopt due to sex, age, or individuals. The value applied in the matching algorithm is a correlation coefficient [36], which produces normalized values near 1 for the optimal location of the matching. Therefore, the location with maximum correlation is selected as the expected position of each lung. Afterwards, left and right lungs are segmented in square grids of 3 × 4 regions, as depicted

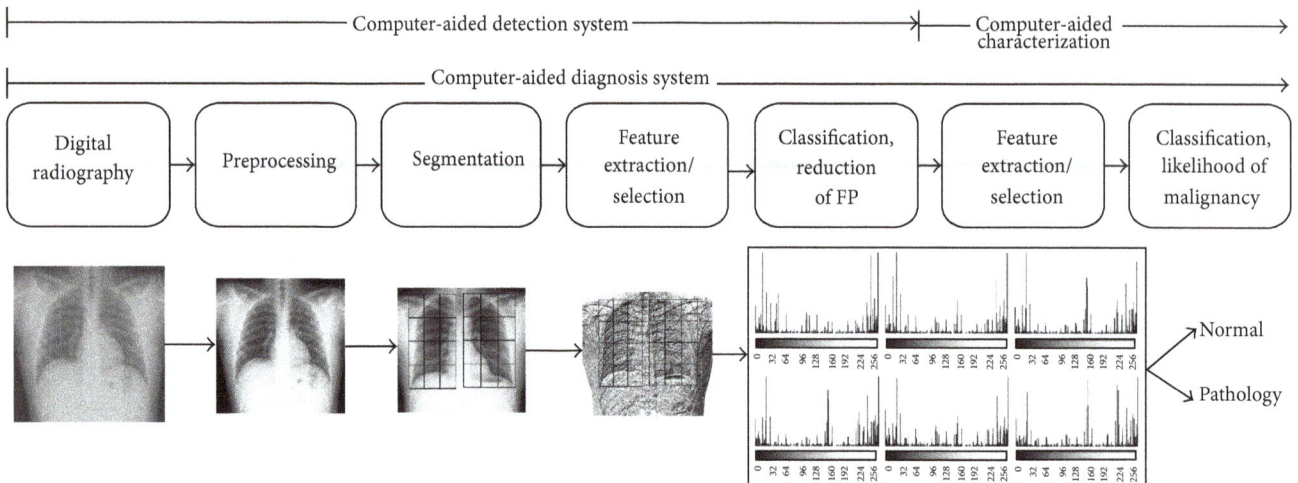

FIGURE 2: Typical scheme of a CAD system as proposed by [33]. Below each generic step, a sample image of the proposed method is shown.

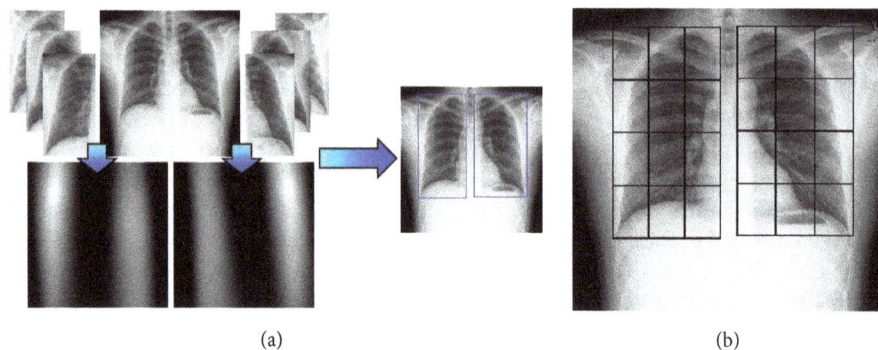

(a)                                                                                          (b)

FIGURE 3: Lung location and segmentation in a radiograph. (a) Application of template matching to a radiography (left and right patterns), matching maps, and the obtained optimal location. (b) The detected lungs are divided into two grids of regions.

in Figure 3. Observe that the proposed method does not produce a precise segmentation of the lungs contour, but a bounding box for each lung, which is sufficient for the subsequent processes.

*2.2. Feature Extraction with LBP.* The aim of this step is to produce meaningful texture descriptors for the regions of interest. Different kinds of features have been used for biomedical images such as Fourier transform, wavelet filters, and SIFT features. The technique proposed in this paper is based on LBP features, which were introduced in [37]. LBP are an invariant texture descriptor that produces a value for each pixel in the images. Let us consider a single channel image, $I$, with an arbitrary photometric resolution. The LBP computation for a pixel $I(x, y)$ takes into account the 8 pixels surrounding point $(x, y)$, using the following equation:

$$\text{LBP}(x, y) = \sum_{n=0}^{7} 2^n t\left(I(x, y) - I(\text{neigh}(n, x, y))\right),$$

$$\text{with } t(v) = \begin{cases} 0, & v \geq 0 \\ 1, & v < 0, \end{cases} \tag{1}$$

where neigh iterates the neighbors of pixel $(x, y)$, that is, $\{(x-1, y-1), (x, y-1), (x+1, y-1), (x-1, y), (x+1, y), (x-1, y+1), (x, y+1), (x+1, y+1)\}$, and $t(v)$ is a function that thresholds its parameter $v$. Figure 4 shows a graphical representation of the computation of the LBP for a single pixel.

Each $\text{LBP}(x, y)$ can take 256 values, from 0 to 255, encoding gray-level information with respect to the central pixel $(x, y)$. These values are not taken individually; instead, they are aggregated in histograms for each region of interest. Given a region $R$, which consists of a set of pixels, the corresponding histogram $H_R$ is given by

$$H_R(i) = \frac{1}{|R|} \sum_{p \in R} eq(i, \text{LBP}(p)),$$

$$\text{with } eq(a, b) = \begin{cases} 1, & a = b \\ 0, & a \neq b, \end{cases} \tag{2}$$

where $i$ goes from 0 to 255. Observe that the histograms are normalized dividing the result by $|R|$, that is, the size of the region in pixels. A sample application of LBP histograms is shown in Figure 5, as compared to the histogram of gray levels of the original radiography. Note that all bits of the LBP image contain relevant information, but this may not be clearly seen

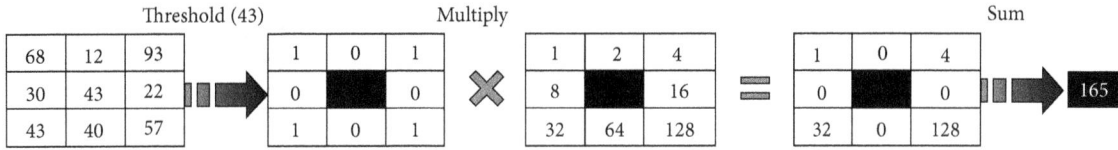

FIGURE 4: Example of a LBP calculation.

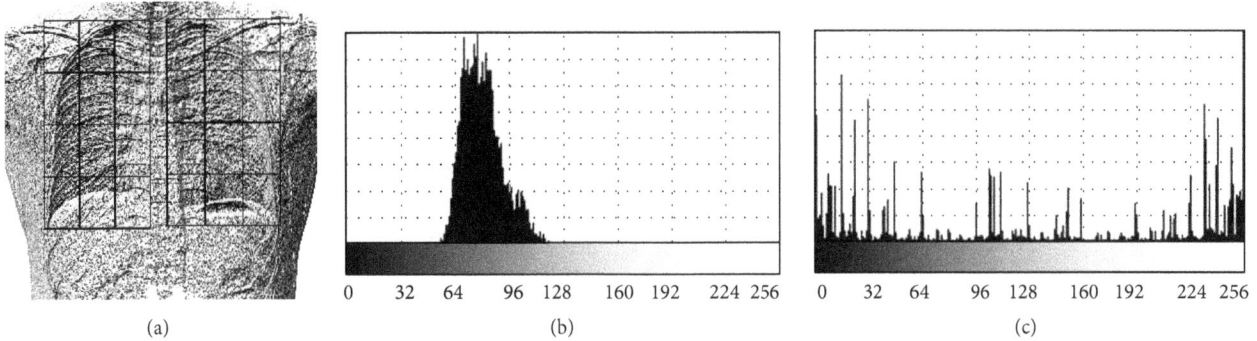

FIGURE 5: Sample application of LBP to a radiography. (a) LBP image of the radiography in Figure 3. (b) Histogram of gray levels of the original image. (c) LBP histogram for the same region.

in the image (only the most significant bits are appreciated in a visual inspection by humans).

As mentioned before, the input radiography is divided into a grid of 3 × 4 regions for both lungs, which are determined according to the segmentation step. The LBP histogram of each region is obtained, producing a feature vector of 24 histograms of 256 bins. Figure 6 presents an example of this stage.

*2.3. Classification of the Features.* Classifiers typically used in most of the procedures for analyzing medical images can be divided into the following categories: conventional classifiers, artificial neural networks [3, 6, 38, 39], fuzzy systems [40], and support vector machines [41, 42]. A key aspect to consider is the problem known as the *curse of dimensionality*: a classifier with a high dimensionality requires a large number of training samples to avoid overfitting. However, in our case, the number of available samples is very reduced, so simple classifiers based on distances between histograms are applied.

In particular, the Bhattacharyya distance [42] is used to provide a measure of the similarity of two histograms. Considering two histograms $H_1$ and $H_2$, this distance is defined by

$$d\left(H_1, H_2\right) = \sqrt{1 - \sum_{i=0}^{255} \sqrt{H_1\left(i\right) \cdot H_2\left(i\right)}}. \quad (3)$$

Let us assume a training set of $n$ radiographs, $T = \{T_1, T_2, \ldots, T_n\}$, and a new radiograph $I$ to classify. The 24 LBP histograms of all the images are computed (both training set and $I$). Then, each histogram of $I$ is compared with $n$ corresponding histograms in $T$ using (3). After that, the difference between the minimum distance to the normal radiographs of $T$ and the minimum distance to the pathological radiographs

of $T$ is computed. That is, the system calculates for each region $R$ in image $I$:

$$v\left(R\right) = \min_{o \in \text{normal}} d\left(H_R\left(I\right), H_R\left(T_o\right)\right)$$
$$- \min_{p \in \text{pathologic}} d\left(H_R\left(I\right), H_R\left(T_p\right)\right), \quad (4)$$

where normal is the set of normal radiographies in $T$ and pathologic is the set of pathologic ones. The values $v(R)$ can be interpreted as *votes* to either normality or pathology; a high negative value should be obtained for regions similar to the normal samples and a high positive value for the nonnormal samples. Therefore, the set of 24 values, $\{v(1), v(2), \ldots, v(24)\}$, provides information that has to be combined in a final classification. Three different approaches are proposed for this purpose:

(1) *GDAV: Greater Difference in Absolute Value.* This technique consists of obtaining the maximum value of $|v(R)|$ for all $R$ in $\{1, 2, \ldots, 24\}$. If the corresponding $v(R)$ is a negative number, then image $I$ is classified as normal; otherwise, it is classified as pathologic. This method considers that the region which has a greater difference is the one that contains most information for the problem.

(2) *DV: Discrete Voting.* In this case, all regions contribute to the final classification. The sign of each $v(R)$ is considered as a vote to normality (negative sign) or to pathology (positive sign). The class with the most votes provides the final classification for $I$.

(3) *CV: Continuous Voting.* A potential drawback of DV method is that relevant information can be lost when discretizing the values of $v(R)$. To avoid this problem, CV takes the sum $v(1) + v(2) + \cdots + v(24)$. If the

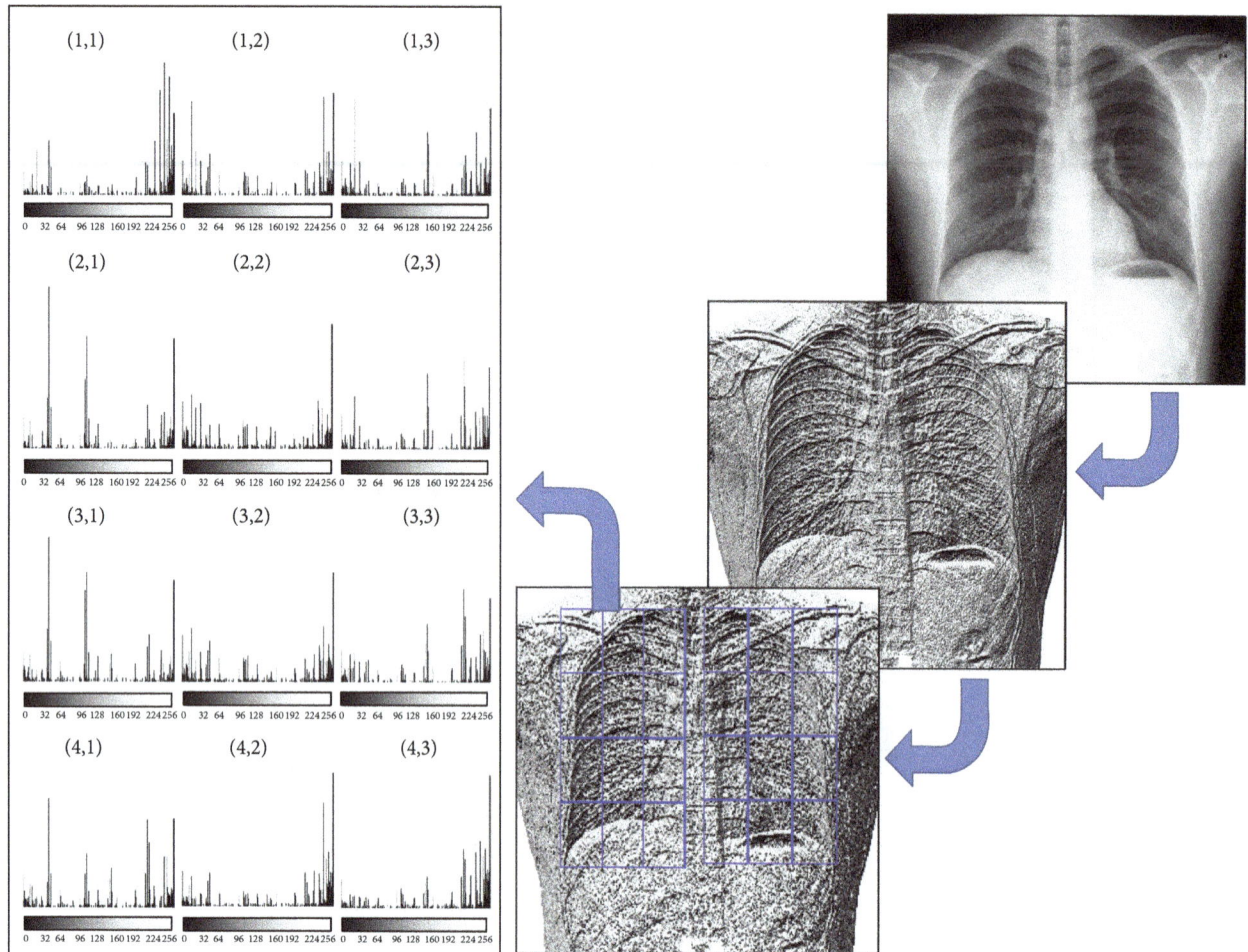

FIGURE 6: Calculation of LBP histograms in a sample chest radiograph. From right to left: input radiograph; computed LBP image; segmented regions; and LBP histograms obtained for each region of the left lung.

sum is positive, image $I$ is considered as pathologic and otherwise normal. In fact, the optimum decision threshold is not necessarily 0, but it can be slightly biased. This threshold determines the compromise between false positive and false negative errors.

These three classification techniques assume that all the regions of the images have the same information for the problem. However, this could not be the case if some areas are more discriminant than others. Therefore, we have studied the use of matrix that weighs the relative importance of each region of interest. It is called *discrimination matrix* and can be defined as a function $w(R)$ of real values from 0 to 1, for each $R$ in $\{1, 2, \ldots, 24\}$. These weights are obtained from the same set of training data. When using the discrimination matrix in classification, all the $v(R)$ are substituted by the product $v(R)w(R)$. The three classifiers described above are evaluated both using the weighted values and not using them.

## 3. Results and Discussion

The set of 48 digital chest radiographs (25 normal and 23 pathologic) described in Section 2 has been used in the experimental validation of the proposed method. The testing

procedure performs a leave-one-out process, which consists in removing one image from the data set, $I$, and takes the rest of images as the training set, $T$. Image $I$ is classified against $T$ using LBP histograms and the 6 classifiers described above (GDAV, DV, and CV; using discrimination matrix or not). If the predicted class is different from the real class of $I$, then there is a classification error. This process is repeated for all the available images. The *success rate* of a classifier is defined as the number of correctly classified images with respect to the total number of images.

*3.1. Experimental Results.* The success rates obtained for all the classifiers in the validation experiments of the technique are presented in Table 1. These results are indicated for males, females, and using all individuals.

We were also interested in studying the effect of the threshold in the voting methods. Figure 7 shows a graphical comparison of the three classifiers, with and without weighting matrix, using different thresholds for DV and CV methods.

*3.2. Discussion of the Results.* In a problem of binary classification, as the present one, the expected error rate of

TABLE 1: Success rates (as a percentage from 0 to 1) of classification using GDAV, DV, and CV methods, with and without discrimination matrix. The best result for each classifier is marked in bold. In the male/female tests, only those classes are included in the training and testing process.

| | Without discr. matrix | | | With discr. matrix | | |
| --- | --- | --- | --- | --- | --- | --- |
| | Male | Female | All | Male | Female | All |
| GDAV | 0.48 | 0.65 | 0.69 | 0.68 | **0.74** | 0.65 |
| DV | 0.56 | 0.69 | 0.56 | 0.72 | 0.74 | **0.79** |
| CV | 0.56 | 0.61 | 0.56 | 0.64 | **0.87** | 0.71 |

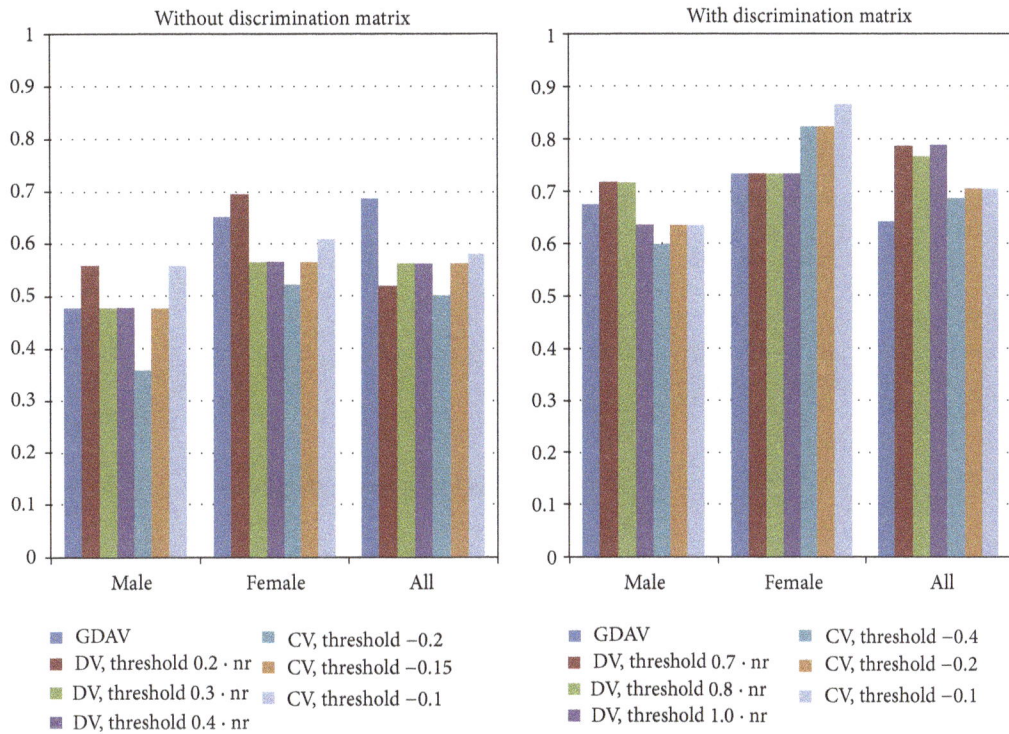

FIGURE 7: Success rates of the classifiers with and without discrimination matrix and using different thresholds. nr represents the number of existing radiographs in the training set.

a completely random classifier would be 50%. The fact that some experiments, for example, GDAV method in the male subset, produce a higher error is an evidence of the complexity of the tackled problem. Besides the implicit difficulty of the problem, the small number of images available poses an additional challenge. To get a sample of all possible variations of sex, age, pathologies, and so forth, some thousands of radiographs would be necessary. For example, some classifiers in Table 1 produce better results with the complete set than with only the male/female set.

There is not a method clearly yielding the best accuracy for all the tests, although voting schemes, DV and CV, usually obtain less error rates. Figure 7 shows that the correct selection of the threshold, specially in CV method, can affect greatly its effectiveness. In CV, the optimum threshold appears to be near 0, as it would be expected.

Regarding the comparison between using or not the discrimination matrix, there is very strong evidence that using it has a big benefit in the obtained results. Almost all methods achieve a significant improvement applying the

matrix of weights, with an average of 21% higher accuracy. The best result is obtained with CV method, giving 87% of correct classifications. Considering the set of all images, the optimum classifier is DV with discrimination matrix, producing 79% of accuracy.

A relevant limitation of our data set is that the areas of abnormality are not marked in the available pathological images; indeed, these radiographs may contain many normal regions. This fact hinders the distinction of normality. The improvement achieved by using the discrimination matrix shows that this problem has a great effect in the results. A greater benefit could be obtained if pathological areas were precisely marked in the training samples.

*3.3. Hypothesis Testing.* In this subsection, information is provided on the procedure followed to conduct an experiment to investigate if the proportion of cases which were correctly classified is the same for all the classifiers (GDAV, DV, and CV). The following hypotheses are proposed in this study:

TABLE 2: Results of the hypothesis testing on the GDAV, DV, and CV classifiers, without and with discrimination matrix, and using male, female, and all radiographs. $N$ is the sample size, and df means degrees of freedom.

| | Without discr. matrix | | | With discr. matrix | | |
| --- | --- | --- | --- | --- | --- | --- |
| | Male | Female | All | Male | Female | All |
| $N$ | 25 | 23 | 48 | 25 | 23 | 48 |
| Cochran's Q | 1.14 | 0.75 | 2.05 | 0.46 | 2.57 | 5.28 |
| df | 2 | 2 | 2 | 2 | 2 | 2 |
| Asymptotic significance | 0.56 | 0.68 | 0.35 | 0.79 | 0.27 | 0.07 |

(H0)  *Null Hypothesis.* The classifiers GDAV, DV, and CV are equally effective.

(H1)  *Alternative Hypothesis.* There is a difference in effectiveness among the classifiers GDAV, DV, and CV.

The metric selected to measure classifiers effectiveness was correct detection (normality/pathology). Thus, classifier effectiveness is the dependent variable, and the kind of classifier is the independent variable. Since the dependent variable is dichotomous, Cochran's Q nonparametric statistical test is employed to verify if the three classifiers have identical effects.

Table 2 shows the results obtained using SPSS 19.0 statistical software package. Based on the observed significance levels, we can reject the null hypothesis; that is, there are statistically significant differences with regard to the correct detections among the classifiers, for the set *All* $\chi^2(2) = 5.28$ ($p = 0.07$) with discrimination matrix. However, Cochran's Q test did not indicate any differences among the three classifiers (value higher than 0.1) in all the other cases.

## 4. Conclusions

A new approach for detecting normality/pathology in chest radiographies has been presented. Our method is based on LBP as a simple but powerful texture descriptor. LBP histograms of different lung regions are classified and then combined to produce the final classification. Different combination schemes have been compared, and a statistical analysis has found that in some cases there is a significant difference among them.

In general, the use of a discrimination matrix yields an average improvement around 20% in the success rates. This fact indicates that not all regions have the same importance in the pathology detection. Moreover, when a pathology is detected, the obtained distances could be used to identify the regions with most probability of abnormality. This can be helpful to the medical professionals, which can center their attention in the suspicious areas.

The obtained success rate is near 90% for the best classifiers. There is clearly an important margin for improvement, since the developed system is a prototype for research purposes. In order to be introduced in the context of a hospital, a better accuracy would be required. One disadvantage of the proposed approach is that it requires a large number of images, in order to have enough samples of all appearances for different sex, age, kinds of pathologies, and so forth. Therefore, a large set of chest radiographs would be needed to improve the results. Moreover, as discussed above, these images should be marked more precisely with the areas of pathology. Another limitation of the method is that it relies only on texture information. Some types of diseases, for example, affecting only the intensity of the images, would not be detected. To overcome this issue, the combination of other image descriptors could be applied, such as scale-invariant features or deep learning methods. In any case, we have to recall that these kinds of systems are designed to help radiologists, not to replace them.

## Competing Interests

The authors indicated no potential competing interests.

## Acknowledgments

This work was supported by the Spanish MINECO, as well as European Commission FEDER funds, under Grants TIN2015-66972-C5-3-R and TIN2015-70259-C2-2-R.

## References

[1]  G. S. Lodwick, C. L. Haun, W. E. Smith, R. F. Keller, and E. D. Robertson, "Computer diagnosis of primary bone tumors," *Radiology*, vol. 80, no. 2, pp. 273–275, 1963.

[2]  F. Winsberg, M. Elkin, J. Macy, V. Bordaz, and W. Weymouth, "Detection of radiographic abnormalities in mammograms by means of optical scanning and computer analysis," *Radiology*, vol. 89, no. 2, pp. 211–215, 1967.

[3]  M. Peker, B. Şen, and D. Delen, "Computer-aided diagnosis of Parkinson's disease using complex-valued neural networks and mRMR feature selection algorithm," *Journal of Healthcare Engineering*, vol. 6, no. 3, pp. 281–302, 2015.

[4]  J. Zhang, H. Li, L. Lv, X. Shi, F. Guo, and Y. Zhang, "A computer-aided method for improving the reliability of Lenke classification for scoliosis," *Journal of Healthcare Engineering*, vol. 6, no. 2, pp. 145–158, 2015.

[5]  S. P. Singh and S. Urooj, "An improved CAD system for breast cancer diagnosis based on generalized Pseudo-Zernike moment and Ada-DEWNN classifier," *Journal of Medical Systems*, vol. 40, no. 4, article 105, pp. 1–13, 2016.

[6]  T. J. Hirschauer, H. Adeli, and J. A. Buford, "Computer-aided diagnosis of parkinson's disease using enhanced probabilistic neural network," *Journal of Medical Systems*, vol. 39, no. 11, article 179, 2015.

[7]  P. Morris and A. Perkins, "Diagnostic imaging," *The Lancet*, vol. 379, no. 9825, pp. 1525–1533, 2012.

[8]  P. Campadelli and E. Casiraghi, "Lung field segmentation in digital postero-anterior chest radiographs," in *Pattern Recognition*

and Image Analysis, S. Singh, M. Singh, C. Apte, and P. Perner, Eds., vol. 3687 of Lecture Notes in Computer Science, pp. 736–745, Springer, Heidelberg, Germany, 2005.

[9] K. Doi, "Computer-aided diagnosis in medical imaging: historical review, current status and future potential," Computerized Medical Imaging and Graphics, vol. 31, no. 4-5, pp. 198–211, 2007.

[10] P. Campadelli, E. Casiraghi, and A. Esposito, "Liver segmentation from computed tomography scans: a survey and a new algorithm," Artificial Intelligence in Medicine, vol. 45, no. 2-3, pp. 185–196, 2009.

[11] J. Wu, M. V. Kamath, M. D. Noseworthy, C. Boylan, and S. Poehlman, "Segmentation of images of abdominal organs," Critical Reviews in Biomedical Engineering, vol. 36, no. 5-6, pp. 305–334, 2008.

[12] R. A. Jadhav and R. A. Thorat, "Computer aided breast cancer analysis and detection using statistical features and neural networks," in Proceedings of the International Conference on Advances in Computing, Communication and Control (ICAC3 '09), pp. 283–288, ACM, Mumbai, India, January 2009.

[13] A. Oliver, X. Llado, J. Freixenet, and J. Marti, "False positive reduction in mammographic mass detection using local binary patterns," in Medical Image Computing and Computer-Assisted Intervention—MICCAI 2007, vol. 4791 of Lecture Notes in Computer Science, pp. 286–293, Springer, Heidelberg, Germany, 2007.

[14] J. Bi, S. Periaswamy, K. Okada et al., "Computer aided detection via asymmetric cascade of sparse hyperplane classifiers," in Proceedings of the 12th ACM SIGKDD International Conference on Knowledge Discovery and Data Mining (KDD '06), pp. 837–844, ACM, Philadelphia, Pa, USA, August 2006.

[15] Y. Nakamura, G. Fukano, H. Takizawa et al., "Eigen nodule: view-based recognition of lung nodule in chest X-ray CT images using subspace method," in Proceedings of the 17th International Conference on Pattern Recognition (ICPR '04), pp. 681–684, August 2004.

[16] P. Campadelli and E. Casiraghi, "Nodule detection in postero anterior chest radiographs," in Medical Image Computing and Computer-Assisted Intervention—MICCAI 2004, C. Barillot, D. R. Haynor, and P. Hellier, Eds., vol. 3217 of Lecture Notes in Computer Science, pp. 1048–1049, Springer, Heidelberg, Germany, 2004.

[17] P. Campadelli and E. Casiraghi, "Pruning the nodule candidate set in postero anterior chest radiographs," in Biological and Artificial Intelligence Environments, pp. 37–43, Springer, Amsterdam, The Netherlands, 2005.

[18] R. C. Hardie, S. K. Rogers, T. Wilson, and A. Rogers, "Performance analysis of a new computer aided detection system for identifying lung nodules on chest radiographs," Medical Image Analysis, vol. 12, no. 3, pp. 240–258, 2008.

[19] M. Kallergi, "Evaluation strategies for medical-image analysis and processing metodologies," in Medical Image Analysis Methods, pp. 433–471, CRC Press, Boca Raton, Fla, USA, 2005.

[20] L. Bogoni, P. Cathier, M. Dundar et al., "Computer-aided detection (CAD) for CT colonography: a tool to address a growing need," British Journal of Radiology, vol. 78, pp. S57–S62, 2005.

[21] B. Hao, C. K.-S. Leung, S. Camorlinga et al., "A computer-aided change detection system for paediatric acute intracranial haemorrhage," in Proceedings of the C3S2E Conference (C3S2E '08), pp. 109–111, ACM, Montreal, Canada, May 2008.

[22] M. Freedman, B. Lo, F. Lure, H. Zhao, J. Lin, and M. Yeh, "Computer-aided detection of severe acute respiratory syndrome (SARS) on chest radiography," International Congress Series, vol. 1268, pp. 908–910, 2004.

[23] M. Antonelli, B. Lazzerini, and F. Marcelloni, "Segmentation and reconstruction of the lung volume in CT images," in Proceedings of the 20th Annual ACM Symposium on Applied Computing (SAC '05), pp. 255–259, ACM, Santa Fe, New Mexico, March 2005.

[24] S. Chen, L. Cao, J. Liu, and X. Tang, "Automatic segmentation of lung fields from radiographic images of SARS patients using a new graph cuts algorithm," Proceedings of the 18th International Conference on Pattern Recognition (ICPR '06), vol. 1, pp. 271–274, 2006.

[25] B. van Ginneken, M. B. Stegmann, and M. Loog, "Segmentation of anatomical structures in chest radiographs using supervised methods: a comparative study on a public database," Medical Image Analysis, vol. 10, no. 1, pp. 19–40, 2006.

[26] M. Park, J. S. Jin, and L. S. Wilson, "Detection and measurement of hilar region in chest radiograph," in Proceedings of the Pan-Sydney Workshop on Visualisation (VIP '02), pp. 83–87, Australian Computer Society, 2002.

[27] J. Ramachandran, M. Pattichis, and P. Soliz, "Pre-classification of chest radiographs for improved active shape model segmentation of ribs," in Proceedings of the 5th IEEE Southwest Symposium on Image Analysis and Interpretation (SSIAI '02), pp. 188–192, IEEE, 2002.

[28] G. Simkó, G. Orbán, P. Máday, and G. Horváth, "Elimination of clavicle shadows to help automatic lung nodule detection on chest radiographs," in Proceedings of the 4th European Conference of the International Federation for Medical and Biological Engineering (ECIFMBE '08), J. V. Sloten, P. Verdonck, M. Nyssen, and J. Haueisen, Eds., vol. 22 of IFMBE Proceedings, pp. 488–491, Antwerp, Belgium, November 2008.

[29] M. Park, J. S. Jin, and L. S. Wilson, "Detection of abnormal texture in chest X-rays with reduction of ribs," in Proceedings of the Pan-Sydney Area Workshop on Visual Information Processing (VIP '04), pp. 71–74, Australian Computer Society, 2004.

[30] L. Sørensen, S. B. Shaker, and M. de Bruijne, "Texture classification in lung CT using local binary patterns," in Medical Image Computing and Computer-Assisted Intervention—MICCAI 2008, D. Metaxas, L. Axel, G. Fichtinger, and G. Székely, Eds., vol. 5241 of Lecture Notes in Computer Science, pp. 934–941, Springer, Heidelberg, Germany, 2008.

[31] L. Sørensen, S. B. Shaker, and M. de Bruijne, "Quantitative analysis of pulmonary emphysema using local binary patterns," IEEE Transactions on Medical Imaging, vol. 29, no. 2, pp. 559–569, 2010.

[32] J. M. Carrillo-De-Gea and G. García-Mateos, "Detection of normality/pathology on chest radiographs using LBP," in Proceedings of the 1st International Conference on Bioinformatics (BIOINFORMATICS '10), pp. 167–172, January 2010.

[33] A. N. Papadopoulos, M. E. Plissiti, and D. I. Fotiadis, "Medical-image processing and analysis for CAD systems," in Medical Image Analysis Methods, The Electrical Engineering and Applied Signal Processing Series, chapter 2, pp. 51–86, CRC Press, Boca Raton, Fla, USA, 2005.

[34] C.-W. Bong and M. Rajeswari, "Multi-objective nature-inspired clustering and classification techniques for image segmentation," Applied Soft Computing, vol. 11, no. 4, pp. 3271–3282, 2011.

[35] S. Theodoridis and K. Koutroumbas, "Template matching," in *Pattern Recognition*, chapter 8, pp. 481–519, Academic Press, Boston, Mass, USA, 4th edition, 2009.

[36] K. Briechle and U. Hanebeck, "Template matching using fast normalized cross correlation," in *Optical Pattern Recognition XII*, vol. 4387 of *Proceedings of SPIE*, pp. 95–102, 2001.

[37] T. Ojala, M. Pietikäinen, and D. Harwood, "A comparative study of texture measures with classification based on feature distributions," *Pattern Recognition*, vol. 29, no. 1, pp. 51–59, 1996.

[38] P. Werbos, *The Roots of Backpropagation: From Ordered Derivatives to Neural Networks and Political Forecasting*, John Wiley & Sons, New York, NY, USA, 1994.

[39] F. Poggio, "Regularization theory, radial basis functions and networks," in *From Statistics to Neural Networks: Theory and Pattern Recognition Applications*, vol. 136 of *NATO ASI Series*, pp. 83–104, 1994.

[40] A. Bonarini, "Learning fuzzy classifier systems," in *Learning Classifier System: New Directions and Concepts*, pp. 83–106, Springer, Berlin, Germany, 2000.

[41] V. N. Vapnik, *Statistical Learning Theory*, John Wiley & Sons, New York, NY, USA, 1998.

[42] E. Choi and C. Lee, "Feature extraction based on the Bhattacharyya distance," *Pattern Recognition*, vol. 36, no. 8, pp. 1703–1709, 2003.

# 18

# Analysis of Cardiovascular Tissue Components for the Diagnosis of Coronary Vulnerable Plaque from Intravascular Ultrasound Images

**Ju Hwan Lee,[1] Yoo Na Hwang,[2] Ga Young Kim,[2] Eun Seok Shin,[3] and Sung Min Kim[1,2]**

[1]Department of Medical Devices Industry, Dongguk University-Seoul, 26 Pil-dong 3-ga, Jung-gu, Seoul 04620, Republic of Korea
[2]Department of Medical Biotechnology, Dongguk University-Bio Medi Campus, 32 Dongguk-ro, Ilsandong-gu, Goyang-si, Gyeonggi-do 10326, Republic of Korea
[3]Department of Cardiology, Ulsan University Hospital, University of Ulsan College of Medicine, 877 Bangeojinsunhwando-ro, Dong-gu, Ulsan 44033, Republic of Korea

Correspondence should be addressed to Sung Min Kim; smkim@dongguk.edu

Academic Editor: Feng-Huei Lin

The purpose of this study was to characterize cardiovascular tissue components and analyze the different tissue properties for predicting coronary vulnerable plaque from intravascular ultrasound (IVUS) images. For this purpose, sequential IVUS image frames were obtained from human coronary arteries using 20 MHz catheters. The plaque regions between the intima and media-adventitial borders were manually segmented in all IVUS images. Tissue components of the plaque regions were classified into having fibrous tissue (FT), fibrofatty tissue (FFT), necrotic core (NC), or dense calcium (DC). The media area and lumen diameter were also estimated simultaneously. In addition, the external elastic membrane (EEM) was computed to predict the vulnerable plaque after the tissue characterization. The reliability of manual segmentation was validated in terms of inter- and intraobserver agreements. The quantitative results found that the FT and the media as well as the NC would be good indicators for predicting vulnerable plaques in IVUS images. In addition, the lumen was not suitable for early diagnosis of vulnerable plaque because of the low significance compared to the other vessel parameters. To predict vulnerable plaque rupture, future study should have additional experiments using various tissue components, such as the EEM, FT, NC, and media.

## 1. Introduction

Vulnerable plaques are defined as nonobstructive atherosclerotic lesions that are prone to rupture, causing acute coronary syndromes [1, 2]. Thin-cap fibroatheroma (TCFA), the hallmark of a vulnerable plaque, is characterized as a large lipid pool with an overlying thin fibrous cap (<65 $\mu$m) and is heavily infiltrated by inflammatory cells and macrophages which deteriorate plaque stability [3–6].

Intravascular ultrasound (IVUS) is the gold standard for evaluating coronary plaque, lumen, and vessel characteristics [7, 8], and IVUS is an invasive imaging modality which allows the visualization of plaque morphology and collection of morphological information about the arterial wall [9]. However, although visual interpretation of grayscale IVUS can extract information on calcified tissue within plaques, and because of IVUS's inability to accurately differentiate specific plaque components, it is not easy to identify a vulnerable plaque [8, 10]. The addition of spectral analysis—virtual histology (VH)—has demonstrated a potential to provide more detailed quantitative information on plaque composition and morphology of fibrous tissue (FT), fibrofatty tissue (FFT), necrotic core (NC), and dense calcium (DC) [11]. In particular, VH-IVUS has allowed for detection of TCFA as a lesion corresponding to two criteria in at least three sequential

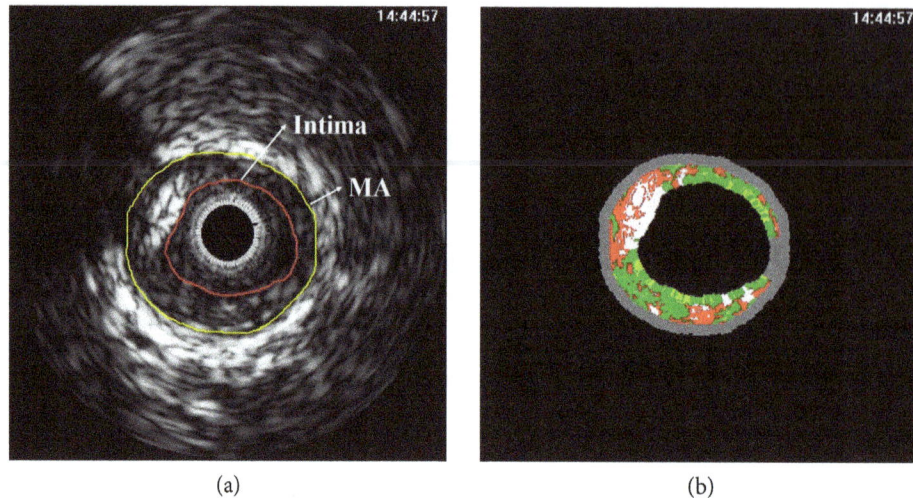

FIGURE 1: One example of the recorded IVUS images: (a) grayscale and (b) corresponding VH-IVUS images (MA: media to adventitia).

frames: (1) focal NC lesions > 10% without evident overlying FT and (2) plaque volume ≥ 40% [12].

VH-IVUS, however, has several limitations in identifying a vulnerable plaque. First, VH-IVUS cannot visualize the TCFA due to its limited spatial resolution (>100 $\mu$m). Therefore, the diagnostic accuracy for a vulnerable plaque is relatively low (≈76%) [13, 14], since it depends on the plaque characterization results, and these may not be adequate. A second limitation of VH-IVUS is from its electrocardiogram- (ECG-) gated acquisition. To minimize both radio frequency (RF) attenuation and shifting due to the presence of blood and a large amount of data, VH-IVUS depends on an ECG-gated procedure [15]. As a consequence, the RF spectrum from only one IVUS frame in each cardiac cycle is recorded which is synchronized with the R-wave in the ECG. Assuming a pullback speed of 1 mm/s and a heart rate of 60 bpm, VH acquires only one frame/s in one cardiac cycle, located at the peak R-wave [16, 17]. Therefore, the longitudinal resolution of VH-IVUS is reduced to one image out of 30 frames/s compared to the rate of the grayscale IVUS [17].

Arterial remodeling (AR) can be a good solution to the above limitations. AR provides the compensatory vessel change corresponding to plaque growth caused by positive remodeling (PR) or negative remodeling (NR) [18]. PR is usually described for an outward plaque to the edge associated with the thinning of the arterial media, whereas the NR refers to "arterial wall shrinkage" at the plaque regions [19]. Patients with acute coronary syndrome more prevalently exhibit PR and a large plaque area, while patients with stable angina more often reveal NR and a smaller plaque area [20, 21]. Moreover, ex post facto studies for coronary artery disease have validated that plaques with PR had higher lipid content and characteristics of vulnerable plaques [22, 23]. Therefore, if the relationships between the AR and various cardiovascular parameters were analyzed quantitatively, it would be possible to improve diagnostic accuracy for vulnerable plaques.

The purpose of this study was to characterize cardiovascular tissue components and analyze the different tissue properties for predicting a coronary vulnerable plaque in IVUS images. The rest of this paper is organized as follows: Section 2 introduces the details of the image acquisition, evaluation parameters, and performance validation. Sections 3 and 4 present the experimental results and discussions, respectively. Finally, Section 5 concludes the paper and identifies future works.

## 2. Materials and Methods

*2.1. Image Acquisition.* 326 IVUS image frames were obtained from human coronary arteries of 14 acute coronary syndrome patients using an imaging system incorporating a 20 MHz Eagle Eye catheter (Volcano Therapeutics Inc., Rancho Cordova, CA, USA) (Figure 1). Sequential IVUS image frames were recorded along with the simultaneous ECG at 400 × 400 pixels with 8-bit grayscale. The motorized pullback speed was 0.5 mm/s, acquiring 30 frames/s. This study was approved by the Institutional Review Board (IRB) of Ulsan University Hospital, Republic of Korea.

*2.2. Evaluation Parameters.* A total of 12 evaluation parameters were estimated from the original IVUS images in order to analyze the similarities between different vessel properties (Table 1). Estimated parameters were divided into two groups including area and diameter. Lumen and vessel properties were estimated from the grayscale images, and the FT, FFT, NC, and DC parameters were obtained from the VH-IVUS images.

In addition, the external elastic membrane (EEM) was computed from all IVUS image frames to predict the vulnerable plaque after the tissue characterization. Theoretically, AR indicates dynamic changes of the EEM [24]. PR is significantly more frequent in patients with unstable coronary artery disease, whereas the NR mainly has an important role in restenosis [25]. In order to assess the extent and direction of remodeling, it is required to compare vessel size at the plaque site to an adjacent reference with minimal disease [26, 27]. PR and NR can be defined

TABLE 1: A total of 12 evaluation parameters obtained from the IVUS image sequences including area and diameter groups.

| Evaluation parameters | |
|---|---|
| Area | Lumen, fibrous, fibrolipidic, lipid core, calcified, media |
| Diameter | Maximum lumen diameter, minimum lumen diameter, average lumen diameter, maximum vessel diameter, minimum vessel diameter, average vessel diameter |

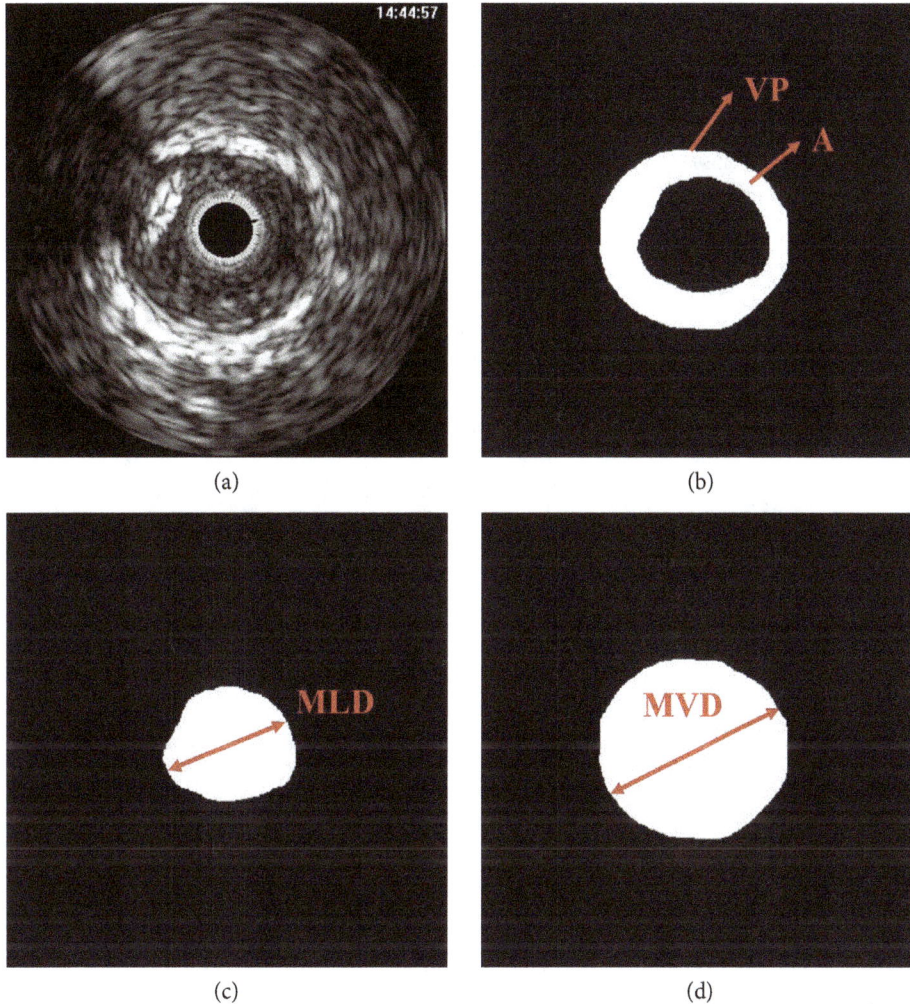

(a)　　　　(b)

(c)　　　　(d)

FIGURE 2: Validation indexes of the (a) original IVUS image, such as (b) area, vessel perimeter, (c) maximum lumen diameter, and (d) maximum vessel diameter.

as larger or smaller EEMs at the plaque site than at a reference site. Therefore, the EEMs were estimated for each IVUS image sequence and the correlations with various vessel properties were analyzed as a preliminary study to predict the vulnerable plaque.

*2.3. Performance Validation.* For all IVUS images, the intima and media to adventitial (MA) borders were manually traced by two independent experts twice within a month of one another. The reliability of the manual segmentation was validated in terms of the interobserver agreement (IEA) and intraobserver agreement (IRA) of the plaque regions. IEA

TABLE 2: IEA and IRA analyses of the manual tracing in terms of all validation indexes including A, VP, MLD, and MVD.

| | | A | VP | MLD | MVD |
|---|---|---|---|---|---|
| IEA | AD | $43.11 \pm 525.21$ | $2.284 \pm 5.68$ | $0.91 \pm 3.68$ | $2.44 \pm 3.64$ |
| | $r$ | 0.981 | 0.993 | 0.971 | 0.975 |
| IRA | AD | $38.77 \pm 584.86$ | $1.54 \pm 6.11$ | $1.02 \pm 3.90$ | $2.14 \pm 3.69$ |
| | $r$ | 0.977 | 0.991 | 0.967 | 0.974 |

Data: mean $\pm$ standard deviation, IEA: interobserver agreement, IRA: intraobserver agreement, AD: average difference, $r$: correlation coefficient, A: area, VP: vessel perimeter, MLD: maximum lumen diameter, and MVD: maximum vessel diameter. $p < 0.05$.

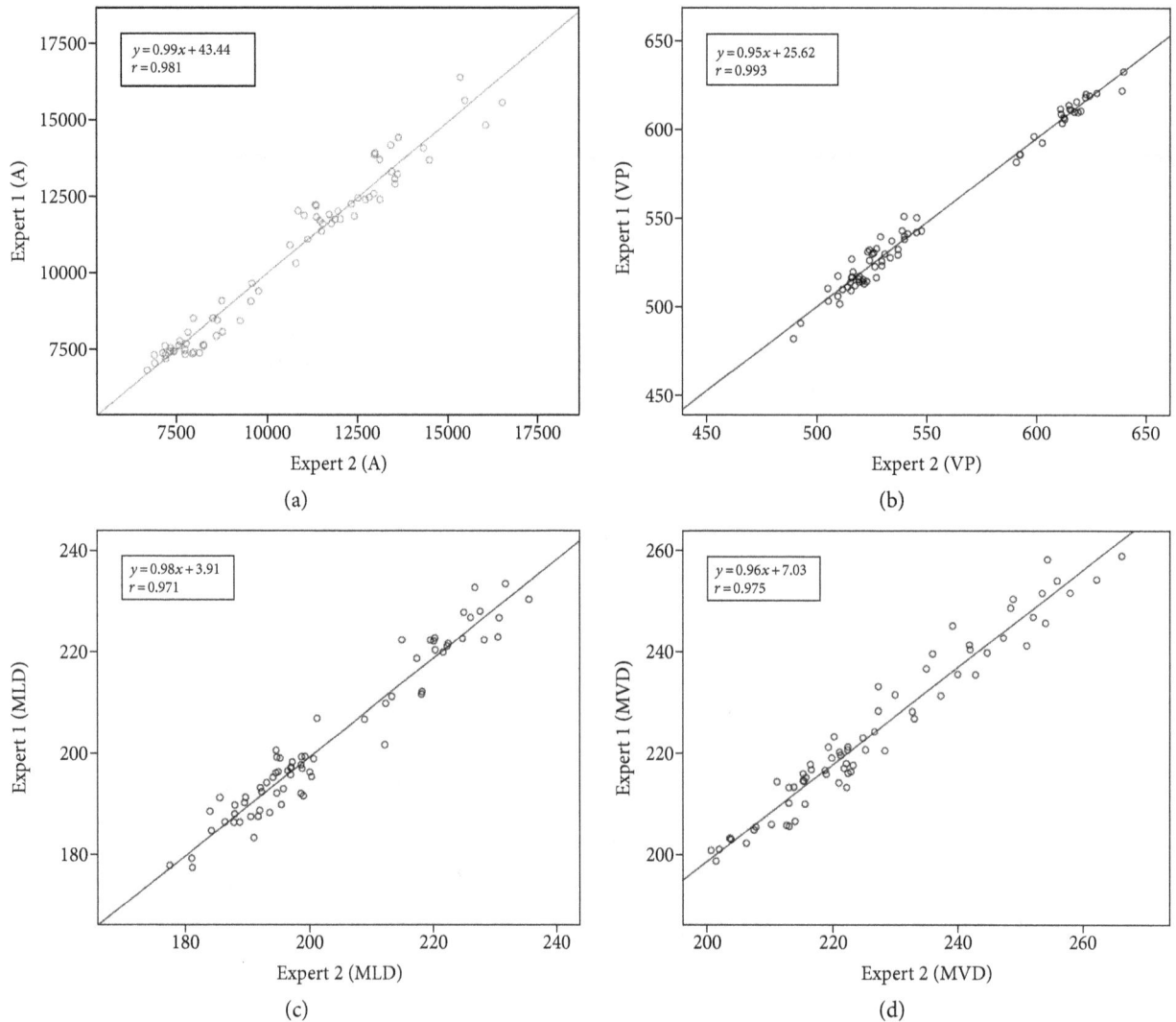

FIGURE 3: Linear regression plots for the manual segmentation between two experts (IEA) in terms of validation indexes including (a) A, (b) VP, (c) MLD, and (d) MVD.

was estimated by analyzing the between-experts results, and the within-experts results were investigated to determine the IRA. To quantify the reliability, the validation indexes including area (A), vessel perimeter (VP), maximum lumen diameter (MLD), and maximum vessel diameter (MVD) were computed from the segmented regions (Figure 2).

*2.4. Statistical Analyses.* For manual segmentation, the IEA and IRA were analyzed using the linear regression and Bland-Altman analysis. The data were analyzed by using a paired *t*-test with the SPSS Version 21 software (SPSS Inc., Chicago, IL, USA). A *p* value of less than 0.05 was considered to be significant.

## 3. Results

*3.1. IEA and IRA Variabilities for Manual Segmentation.* Table 2 shows the IEA and IRA results of the manual tracing for all validation indexes including A, VP, MLD, and MVD

for 20 MHz IVUS images. The overall average difference (AD) was greater in IEA group than that in IRA group; however, there were no significant differences. In addition, the A had the largest AD, while the MLD revealed the smallest value.

On the other hand, all ADs were distributed within the limits of agreement (±2 SD) and were close to zero. Bland-Altman analysis indicated that the manual segmentation performed with a low mean bias and less dispersion between and within the two experts. The linear analysis also revealed that the manual segmentation had a significantly high similarity (*r* > 0.967) for all IVUS images (Figures 3 and 4). These results supported the robustness of the manual tracing for comparing the similarities between tissue properties. Figures 3 and 4 depict the linear regression plots for the IEA and IRA in terms of validation indexes, respectively.

*3.2. Comparison of Similarities between the EEM and Evaluation Parameters.* Table 3 demonstrates statistical

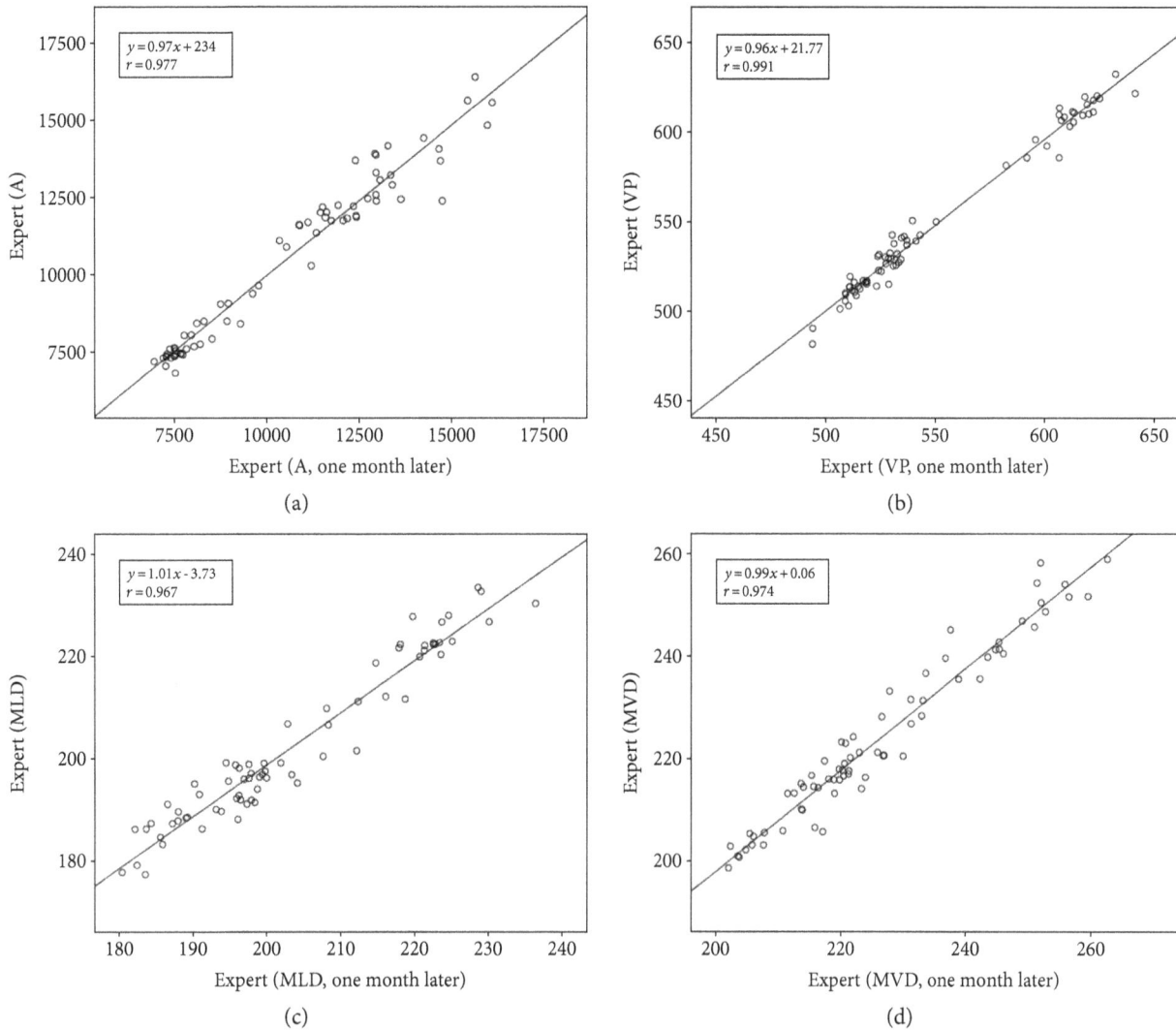

FIGURE 4: Linear regression plots for the manual segmentation within two experts (IRA) in terms of validation indexes including (a) A, (b) VP, (c) MLD, and (d) MVD.

significance levels between evaluation parameters and EEMs in terms of area and perimeter. The quantitative results revealed that the EEM was strongly correlated with the FT, NC, and media for all IVUS image sequences with a high degree of significance ($r > 0.748$), whereas the FFT and DC showed relatively low correlations ($r < 0.586$). Moreover, all lumen parameters including minimum, maximum, and average diameters had significantly low agreement compared to the EEM ($r < 0.515$). On the other hand, all vessel parameters showed significantly high correlations with the EEM area and EEM perimeter.

## 4. Discussion

Typically, VH-IVUS is regarded as the most effective method for diagnosing vulnerable plaques of acute coronary syndrome patients. Particularly, VH-IVUS can detect TCFA based on plaque compositions in at least three continuous images [12]. Although VH-IVUS is highly accurate for

identifying plaque components both in vitro and in vivo, its accuracy for detecting TCFA is approximately 76% [13, 16]. In this study, we attempted to improve the diagnostic accuracy of vulnerable plaques based on the fact that AR can reveal different dynamic changes according to cardiovascular lesion types. More specifically, correlations between EEMs and 12 evaluation parameters were investigated in this study to select optimum parameters for diagnosing vulnerable plaques.

Before tissue characterization, two independent experts manually traced each border (intima and MA) twice. The first and second estimations were within a month of one another to obtain accurate plaque regions. Manual segmentation based on Bland-Altman and linear regression analyses was used to evaluate parameters including A, VP, MLD, and MVD. Variabilities between segmentation results from the two experts were very small. Their correlation coefficients were significantly high for all evaluation parameters ($r > 0.96$). In addition, Bland-Altman plots revealed that the majority

TABLE 3: Comparison of the statistical significance levels between evaluation parameters and EEMs in terms of area and perimeter.

| Evaluation parameters | EEM area r | EEM area p | EEM perimeter r | EEM perimeter p |
|---|---|---|---|---|
| Lumen area | 0.502 | | 0.454 | |
| Fibrous area | 0.775 | | 0.791 | |
| Fibrolipidic area | 0.586 | | 0.580 | |
| Lipid core area | 0.748 | | 0.761 | |
| Calcified area | 0.520 | | 0.534 | |
| Media area | 0.855 | <0.001 | 0.859 | <0.001 |
| Minimum lumen diameter | 0.312 | | 0.271 | |
| Minimum vessel diameter | 0.974 | | 0.978 | |
| Maximum lumen diameter | 0.515 | | 0.480 | |
| Maximum vessel diameter | 0.979 | | 0.989 | |
| Average lumen diameter | 0.451 | | 0.411 | |
| Average vessel diameter | 0.993 | | 0.999 | |

$r$: correlation coefficient.

of average differences were within the limits of agreement. These findings support that manual reference data are useful for comparing tissue properties with the EEM.

Results of correlation analyses between EEMs and tissue properties revealed that FT, NC, and media had statistically significant correlations with the EEM whereas FFT and DC had relatively lower correlations with the EEM for all IVUS images. Pathologic features of vulnerable plaques include positively remodeled vessel (PR) defined as a large lipid and a thin fibrous cap (<65 $\mu$m) with macrophage infiltration [28, 29]. However, IVUS is unable to detect the thin fibrous cap and macrophage infiltration due to its limited spatial resolution. Therefore, it is important to find a key indicator that clearly reflects lipid characteristics for diagnosing vulnerable plaques. Regarding VH-IVUS, FFT and NC are typically regarded as lipid while FT is considered as densely packed collagen [11]. Therefore, clinicians can diagnose cardiovascular diseases based on the distribution of FFT and NC. However, our experimental results represented different aspects of plaque correlation. Although NC has been reported to be strongly correlated with PR in previous studies [30–32], FFT has relatively low correlations ($r < 0.586$) with PR. This might be due to the fact that FFT includes not only lipid components, but also collagen tissues which are not significantly correlated with PR. In other words, FFT has significant lipid interspread in collagen which may cause the abovementioned low correlation with PR. Based on these experimental results, it can be concluded that FFT is unsuitable for predicting vulnerable plaques from IVUS images.

Typically, a PR lesion has higher lipid content and macrophage count, both of which are markers of plaque vulnerability in necropsy study [22]. Results of the present study revealed that the EEM was strongly correlated with lipid content. FT and media were also found to be good indicators for diagnosing vulnerable plaques. This is a quite interesting result. As mentioned above, FT was not significantly correlated with vulnerable plaques. However, when the EEM was expanded, the volumes of plaques in lesion regions were

greatly increased with increasing collagen tissues (FT) which had the largest proportion of plaque components. For this reason, the correlation tendency of FT and PR was different from that of FFT and PR due to plaque composition, not tissue property. On the other hand, lumen parameters including minimum, maximum, and average diameters presented relatively low significances in their correlations with PR. The lumen site is usually not influenced by plaque growth until the lesion reaches 40% area stenosis [24]. Lee et al. [18] have also reported low correlations between the lumen area and PR/NR at minimal luminal area site ($p = 0.202$). Therefore, the lumen does not seem to relate with AR irrespective of the worst case.

## 5. Conclusions

The quantitative results of the present study revealed that the EEM was strongly correlated with the FT, NC, and media for all IVUS image sequences with a high degree of significance, whereas the FFT and DC showed relatively low correlations. Moreover, the lumen had significantly low agreement compared to the EEM. Based on these experimental results, it was found that the FT and the media as well as NC would be a good indicator for predicting vulnerable plaque in IVUS images. In addition, the lumen was not suitable for early diagnosis of vulnerable plaque because of the low significance compared to the other vessel parameters. To predict vessel rupture, future studies should have additional experiments using various tissue components, such as AR, FT, NC, and media.

## Competing Interests

There are no conflicts of interests.

## Acknowledgments

This work was supported by the International Collaborative R&D Program (N0000684) funded by the Ministry of Trade, Industry & Energy (MOTIE), Korea (N01150049, Developing high frequency bandwidth [40–60 MHz] high-resolution image system and probe technology for diagnosing cardiovascular lesion).

## References

[1] J. A. Schaar, J. E. Muller, E. Falk et al., "Terminology for high-risk and vulnerable coronary artery plaques," European Heart Journal, vol. 25, no. 12, pp. 1077–1082, 2004.

[2] L. G. Spagnoli, A. Mauriello, G. Sangiorgi et al., "Extracranial thrombotically active carotid plaque as a risk factor for ischemic stroke," JAMA, vol. 292, no. 15, pp. 1845–1852, 2004.

[3] C. Celeng, R. A. Takx, M. Ferencik, and P. Maurovich-Horvat, "Non-invasive and invasive imaging of vulnerable coronary plaque," Trends in Cardiovascular Medicine, vol. 26, no. 6, pp. 538–547, 2016.

[4] G. W. Stone, A. Maehara, A. J. Lansky et al., "A prospective natural-history study of coronary atherosclerosis," New England Journal of Medicine, vol. 364, no. 3, pp. 226–235, 2011.

[5] J. M. Cheng, H. M. Garcia-Garcia, S. P. de Boer et al., "In vivo detection of high-risk coronary plaques by radiofrequency intravascular ultrasound and cardiovascular outcome: results of the ATHEROREMO-IVUS study," *European Heart Journal*, vol. 35, no. 10, pp. 639–647, 2014.

[6] P. A. Calvert, D. R. Obaid, M. O'Sullivan et al., "Association between IVUS findings and adverse outcomes in patients with coronary artery disease: the VIVA (VH-IVUS in vulnerable atherosclerosis) study," *JACC: Cardiovascular Imaging*, vol. 4, no. 8, pp. 894–901, 2011.

[7] R. A. Nishimura, W. D. Edwards, C. A. Warnes et al., "Intravascular ultrasound imaging: in vitro validation and pathologic correlation," *Journal of the American College of Cardiology*, vol. 16, no. 1, pp. 145–154, 1990.

[8] R. J. Peters, W. E. Kok, M. G. Havenith, H. Rijsterborgh, A. C. van der Wal, and C. A. Visser, "Histopathologic validation of intracoronary ultrasound imaging," *Journal of the American Society of Echocardiography*, vol. 7, no. 3 Pt 1, pp. 230–241, 1994.

[9] A. Taki, Z. Najafi, A. Roodaki et al., "Automatic segmentation of calcified plaques and vessel borders in IVUS images," *International Journal of Computer Assisted Radiology and Surgery*, vol. 3, no. 3-4, pp. 347–354, 2008.

[10] E. N. Deliargyris, "Intravascular ultrasound virtual histology derived thin cap fibroatheroma," *Journal of the American College of Cardiology*, vol. 55, no. 15, pp. 1598–1599, 2010.

[11] A. Nair, B. D. Kuban, E. M. Tuzcu, P. Schoenhagen, S. E. Nissen, and D. G. Vince, "Coronary plaque classification with intravascular ultrasound radiofrequency data analysis," *Circulation*, vol. 106, no. 17, pp. 2200–2206, 2002.

[12] G. A. Rodriguez-Granillo, H. M. García-García, E. P. Mc Fadden et al., "In vivo intravascular ultrasound-derived thin-cap fibroatheroma detection using ultrasound radiofrequency data analysis," *Journal of the American College of Cardiology*, vol. 46, no. 11, pp. 2038–2042, 2005.

[13] A. Nair, M. P. Margolis, B. D. Kuban, and D. G. Vince, "Automated coronary plaque characterisation with intravascular ultrasound backscatter: ex vivo validation," *EuroIntervention*, vol. 3, no. 1, pp. 113–120, 2007.

[14] D. R. Obaid, P. A. Calvert, D. Gopalan et al., "Atherosclerotic plaque composition and classification identified by coronary computed tomography: assessment of computed tomography-generated plaque maps compared with virtual histology intravascular ultrasound and histology," *Circulation. Cardiovascular Imaging*, vol. 6, no. 5, pp. 655–664, 2013.

[15] A. Taki, H. Hetterich, A. Roodaki et al., "A new approach for improving coronary plaque component analysis based on intravascular ultrasound images," *Ultrasound in Medicine and Biology*, vol. 36, no. 8, pp. 1245–1258, 2010.

[16] K. Nasu, E. Tsuchikane, O. Katoh et al., "Accuracy of in vivo coronary plaque morphology assessment: a validation study of in vivo virtual histology compared with in vitro histopathology," *Journal of the American College of Cardiology*, vol. 47, no. 12, pp. 2405–2412, 2006.

[17] S. M. O'Malley, J. F. Granada, S. Carlier, M. Naghavi, and I. A. Kakadiaris, "Image-based gating of intravascular ultrasound pullback sequences," *IEEE Transactions on Information Technology in Biomedicine*, vol. 12, no. 3, pp. 299–306, 2008.

[18] C. S. Lee, Y. H. Seo, D. J. Yang et al., "Positive vascular remodeling in culprit coronary lesion is associated with plaque composition: an intravascular ultrasound-virtual histology study," *Korean Circulation Journal*, vol. 42, no. 11, pp. 747–752, 2012.

[19] J. C. Kaski, "Atheromatous plaque location and arterial remodelling," *European Heart Journal*, vol. 24, no. 4, pp. 291–293, 2003.

[20] M. Nakamura, H. Nishikawa, S. Mukai et al., "Impact of coronary artery remodeling on clinical presentation of coronary artery disease: an intravascular ultrasound study," *Journal of the American College of Cardiology*, vol. 37, no. 1, pp. 63–69, 2001.

[21] P. Schoenhagen, K. M. Ziada, S. R. Kapadia, T. D. Crowe, S. E. Nissen, and E. M. Tuzcu, "Extent and direction of arterial remodeling in stable versus unstable coronary syndromes: an intravascular ultrasound study," *Circulation*, vol. 101, no. 6, pp. 598–603, 2000.

[22] A. M. Varnava, P. G. Mills, and M. J. Davies, "Relationship between coronary artery remodeling and plaque vulnerability," *Circulation*, vol. 105, no. 8, pp. 939–943, 2002.

[23] A. P. Burke, F. D. Kolodgie, D. Weber, and R. Virmani, "Morphological predictors of arterial remodeling in coronary atherosclerosis," *Circulation*, vol. 105, no. 3, pp. 297–303, 2002.

[24] P. Schoenhagen, K. M. Ziada, D. G. Vince, S. E. Nissen, and E. M. Tuzcu, "Arterial remodeling and coronary artery disease: the concept of "dilated" versus "obstructive" coronary atherosclerosis," *Journal of the American College of Cardiology*, vol. 38, no. 2, pp. 297–306, 2001.

[25] D. Dash and R. Daggubati, "An update on clinical applications of intravascular ultrasound," *Journal of Cardiovascular Diseases and Diagnosis*, vol. 3, no. 5, 215 pages, 2015.

[26] D. D. McPherson, S. J. Sirna, L. F. Hiratzka et al., "Coronary arterial remodeling studied by high-frequency epicardial echocardiography: an early compensatory mechanism in patients with obstructive coronary atherosclerosis," *Journal of the American College of Cardiology*, vol. 17, no. 1, pp. 79–86, 1991.

[27] D. W. Losordo, K. Rosenfield, J. Kaufman, A. Pieczek, and J. M. Isner, "Focal compensatory enlargement of human arteries in response to progressive atherosclerosis. In vivo documentation using intravascular ultrasound," *Circulation*, vol. 89, no. 6, pp. 2570–2577, 1994.

[28] F. D. Kolodgie, R. Virmani, A. P. Burke et al., "Pathologic assessment of the vulnerable human coronary plaque," *Heart*, vol. 90, no. 12, pp. 1385–1391, 2004.

[29] R. Virmani, A. P. Burke, A. Farb, and F. D. Kolodgie, "Pathology of the vulnerable plaque," *Journal of the American College of Cardiology*, vol. 47, 8 Supplement, pp. C13–C18, 2006.

[30] D. Giroud, J. M. Li, P. Urban, B. Meier, and W. Rutishauer, "Relation of the site of acute myocardial infarction to the most severe coronary arterial stenosis at prior angiography," *American Journal of Cardiology*, vol. 69, no. 8, pp. 729–732, 1992.

[31] M. Nobuyoshi, M. Tanaka, H. Nosaka et al., "Progression of coronary atherosclerosis: is coronary spasm related to progression?" *Journal of the American College of Cardiology*, vol. 18, no. 4, pp. 904–910, 1991.

[32] R. Virmani, F. D. Kolodgie, A. P. Burke, A. Farb, and S. M. Schwartz, "Lessons from sudden coronary death: a comprehensive morphological classification scheme for atherosclerotic lesions," *Arteriosclerosis, Thrombosis, and Vascular Biology*, vol. 20, no. 5, pp. 1262–1275, 2000.

# 19

# Particle Size-Selective Assessment of Protection of European Standard FFP Respirators and Surgical Masks against Particles-Tested with Human Subjects

Shu-An Lee,[1] Dong-Chir Hwang,[1] He-Yi Li,[1] Chieh-Fu Tsai,[1]
Chun-Wan Chen,[2] and Jen-Kun Chen[3]

[1]Department of Environmental Engineering and Science, Feng Chia University, Taichung 40724, Taiwan
[2]Division of Occupational Hygiene, Institute of Labor, Occupational Safety and Health, Ministry of Labor,
 New Taipei City 22143, Taiwan
[3]Institute of Biomedical Engineering and Nanomedicine, National Health Research Institutes, Miaoli 35053, Taiwan

Correspondence should be addressed to Shu-An Lee; salee@fcu.edu.tw

Academic Editor: Saverio Affatato

This study was conducted to investigate the protection of disposable filtering half-facepiece respirators of different grades against particles between 0.093 and 1.61 μm. A personal sampling system was used to particle size-selectively assess the protection of respirators. The results show that about 10.9% of FFP2 respirators and 28.2% of FFP3 respirators demonstrate assigned protection factors (APFs) below 10 and 20, which are the levels assigned for these respirators by the British Standard. On average, the protection factors of FFP respirators were 11.5 to 15.9 times greater than those of surgical masks. The minimum protection factors (PFs) were observed for particles between 0.263 and 0.384 μm. No significant difference in PF results was found among FFP respirator categories and particle size. A strong association between fit factors and protection factors was found. The study indicates that FFP respirators may not achieve the expected protection level and the APFs may need to be revised for these classes of respirators.

## 1. Introduction

Respiratory protective devices (RPDs) are generally used to protect people from respiratory hazards, including chemical, biological, and radioactive materials. In the absence of engineering control and effective protection, RPDs can prevent workers in routine operations from life-threatening and health hazards. When RPDs cannot provide users with adequate protection, the risk of users' exposure to these respiratory hazards will increase and result in adverse health effects. Therefore, it is important to ensure that the RPDs provide adequate protection for users.

Disposable filtering half-facepiece respirators (DFHFRs), which are classified as air-purifying respirators, are widely used and accepted by workers in various industries and the general population. This is because DFHFRs are available in multiple sizes to fit a range of faces, are easy to maintain,

offer little hindrance to wearers [1], and have the highest rating and evaluation in weight and convenience [2]. Among DFHFRs, NIOSH-approved N95 filtering facepiece respirators or higher are recommended for healthcare workers against airborne infectious diseases such as Ebola [3]. The US National Institute for Occupational Safety and Health (NIOSH) classifies particulate filtering facepiece respirators (FFRs) into nine categories (N95, N99, N100, P95, P99, P100, R95, R99, and R100) [4]. N (not resistant to oil) means that the respirators cannot be used in an oil droplet environment; R (somewhat resistant to oil) and P (strongly resistant to oil) mean that this respirator can be used for protection against nonoily and oily aerosols. Numerical designations 95, 99, and 100 show the filter's minimum filtration efficiency with 95%, 99%, and 99.97%, respectively.

The European Standard (EN 149:2001) classifies FFRs into three classes: FFP1, FFP2, and FFP3 with corresponding minimum filtration efficiencies of 80%, 94%, and 99%. Therefore, FFP2 respirators are approximately equivalent to N95 FFRs, making them recommended for use in the prevention of airborne infectious diseases in the US and some other countries. However, because FFP3 respirators provide the highest level of protection, they are the only FFP class acceptable to the Health and Safety Executive (HSE) for protection against infectious aerosols in healthcare settings in the UK [5]. This poses a question. Do respirators with higher filtration efficiencies provide greater protection when human subjects don the respirators?

Surgical masks (SMs) are used to block large particles (such as droplets, splashes, sprays, or splatter) that may contain microorganisms (e.g., viruses and bacteria) from reaching the nose and mouth. And although they are primarily intended to protect patients from healthcare workers by minimizing exposure of saliva and respiratory secretions to the patients, they generally do not form a tight seal against the face skin and so are not recommended to protect people from airborne infectious diseases. Therefore, SMs have been relegated for protection against infection through fluid repellence only. The protection provided by SMs against particles (0.04–1.3 $\mu$m) is 8–12 times less than N95 FFRs [6], but they are both found to be equivalent for protection against influenza infection when the concentrations of infectious viruses are low [7]. SMs have been cleared by the Food and Drug Administration for sale in the US, while, in the UK, they must first comply with the Medical Devices Directive (MMD 93/42/EEC) [8] and be CE marked [9]. However, because N95/FFP2 respirators or above may be in short supply during a pandemic—or not available in many countries—it is important to know the protection efficiency of surgical masks.

The protection of respirators against microorganisms can be efficiently assessed by investigating respiratory protection against noninfectious particles of a corresponding particle size to infectious ones [10]. Therefore, the protection of the respirators is usually evaluated using sodium chloride (NaCl) and dioctyl phthalate (DOP) particles as challenge aerosols. NaCl particles are used to test filtration efficiencies against nonoily aerosols, while DOP particles are used for testing oily aerosols. N95 FFRs have been widely studied for filtration efficiency [11, 12], face seal leakage [12, 13], fit factors [14, 15], and protection factors [6, 10]. With respect to EN-specified FFP respirators, only the filtration efficiency was studied [16].

Because particles enter the respirator through face seal leaks and filter materials, respirator performance is assessed by fit testing, penetration testing, and total inward leakage (TIL) testing with human subjects. The TSI PortaCount® Plus with N95-Companion is commonly employed to quantify the respirator fit of N95 filtering facepiece respirators. However, the fit factor (FF) may not adequately reflect the true respiratory protection for a worker performing his/her actual work activities. As true workplace protection factors (WPFs) (during actual work activities) are often difficult to measure, NIOSH (2004) has proposed the use of the TIL test for assessing respirator performance as part of the certification process for a respirator [17]. The TIL test is meant to assess the protective level achieved by a respirator when contributions of all leakage paths are considered.

Using either fit testing or filtration data to assess the overall respirator performance is not sufficient. The assessment of respiratory protection has frequently been conducted using the heads of mannequins [18] instead of human subjects, disregarding that human factors—such as facial dimensions [19] and breathing patterns and flow [13]—may interfere with protection provided by respirators.

This study aimed to investigate (1) the overall protection performance of disposable DFHFRs with different categories against particles of different sizes using the TIL test and (2) the relationship between protection factors and fit factors. We tested FFP1, FFP2, and FFP3 respirators from two manufacturers and three models of SMs to particle size-selectively assess respiratory protection with human subjects, because there is lack of information on the protection performance. A personal sampling system, which was modified according to the system developed by Lee et al. (2004) [20], was used to assess the protection provided by respirators. In order to control environmental factors, the experiment was conducted in a subject test chamber where the particle concentrations could be controlled. Furthermore, in order to particle size-selectively assess respiratory protection, this research carried out real-time particle measurement by using an electrical, low-pressure impactor (ELPI).

## 2. Methods

*2.1. Description of the Personal Sampling System for Evaluation of Respiratory Protection.* The assessment of the protection level of a respirator should collect samples from both outside and inside the respirator—the ratio of which is identified as the protection factor. Therefore, a personal sampling system assessing the protection of respirators requires two sampling lines (ambient and in-facepiece sampling lines) to collect samples outside and inside the respirators and also to connect the particle measuring equipment with the test respirator. In addition, because the sampling line inside the respirator contains nearly 100% relative humidity (RH)—which may affect particle measurement—the sampling system requires a dryer to reduce the moisture content of exhaled air. Based on the design concept, we modified the sampling system developed by Lee et al. (2008, 2004) [6, 20] to establish the system—presented in Figure 1. The sampling system had two sampling lines that collected the particles inside and outside the respirator. Each sampling line consisted of a sampling probe (adaptor kit 8025-N95, TSI Inc., St. Paul, MN, USA) and 1/2″ Tygon tubing (Tygon tubing, Fisher Scientific, Pittsburgh, PA, USA), which were both connected with a three-way valve (Legris Inc., France), a Nafion dryer (HPMS PD-50T-12, Perma Pure LLC, NJ, USA), and an electrical low-pressure impactor (ELPI, Dekati Ltd., Finland). The sampling probe used in fit testing was used to collect samples inside the mask because it was easily mounted on the respirator's surface. A helmet with a copper tubing frame was used to fix two sampling lines to reduce face seal leaks due to the movement of the test system. The ambient sampling line was located on the top of the helmet, while the in-facepiece sampling line was placed above the shoulder. The length of the ambient sampling line was 136.9 cm, and the length of

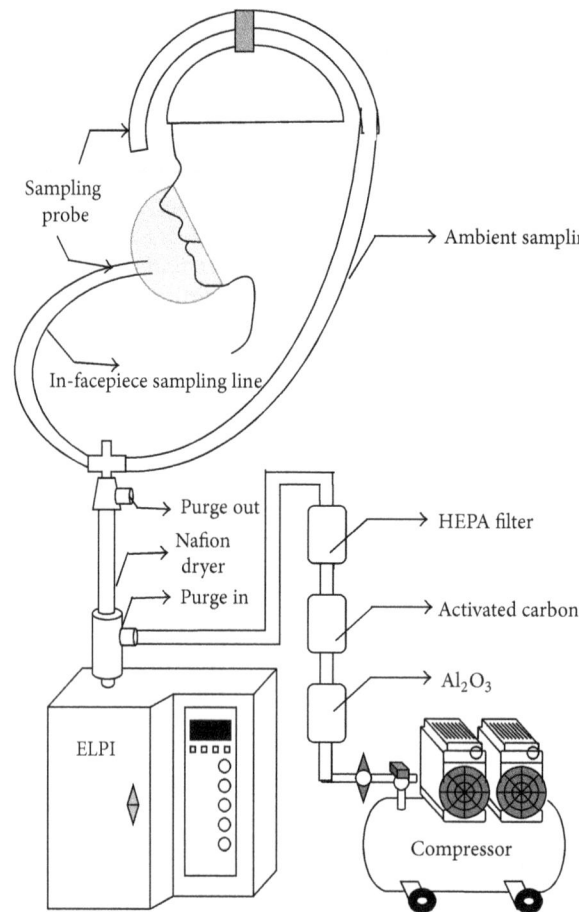

FiɢuʀE 1: Personal sampling system for assessing respirator protection factors. This system was modified based on the system developed by Lee et al. (2008, 2004) [6, 20].

the in-facepiece sampling line was 122.6 cm. Two sampling lines were connected with the ELPI by using the three-way valve. The Nafion dryer was installed between the three-way valve and the ELPI to reduce to the RH of exhaled air down to 50–60%, which is about the same RH range as the indoor environment and can prevent bias in particle measurement. The additional dry air was introduced to create a humidity gradient during the operation of the Nafion dryer. This dry air was generated using a compressor equipped with an $Al_2O_3$ dehumidifier, activated carbon, and a HEPA filter (PN 12144, Pall Corporation, Bourne, MA, USA). The RH of the generated dry air was between 20% and 30%. In order to achieve efficient drying, the flow of dry air had to be 2-3 times greater than the sampling flow.

*2.2. Establishment of the Subject Test Chamber.* Because the ELPI is costly, we only had one ELPI to serve two sampling lines. The stability of particle concentrations in the test environment was important when the PF was determined by a ratio of concentrations outside the respirator to those inside the respirator. The experiment was conducted in a subject test chamber with a ventilation system, which was located in the Laboratory for Industrial Hygiene and Safety in Feng Chia University in Taichung, Taiwan. The schematic design of the

subject test chamber is shown in Figure 2. The total size of the subject test chamber was 19.5 m³ (3.6 m (length) × 2.1 m (width) × 2.58 m (height)), which represents the size of the typical residential room in Taiwan. The subject test chamber was enclosed with four vertical side walls and one ceiling, which were made of cleanroom aluminum honeycomb panels, and the floor was epoxy. An airtight door was installed to prevent contamination from outside of the chamber.

We used two high-pressure direct-drive blowers (1 HP, maximum airflow 27 m³/min, static pressure 24 mm $H_2O$, TECO Electric & Machinery Co., Taipei, Taiwan) connected with HEPA air-purifying units to provide exhaust air and supply air to the subject test chamber. Each of the two HEPA air-purifying units consisted of a prefilter (35% filtration efficiency) and a HEPA filtration unit (99.97% filtration efficiency). The air was transported using 4- and 6-inch ducts. A total of 22 slot gates (14 gates for the air supply and 8 gates for the air exhaust) were installed on the vertical walls and ceiling of the test chamber. The left-side (airtight door side) and right-side walls had six supply gates: three pairs at 0.43, 1.29, and 2.15 meters, respectively, above the floor. The ceiling had two supply gates, which were located in the center of ceiling. The front wall, which was adjacent to the airtight door, had a pair of exhaust gates at 0.43 meters above the floor.

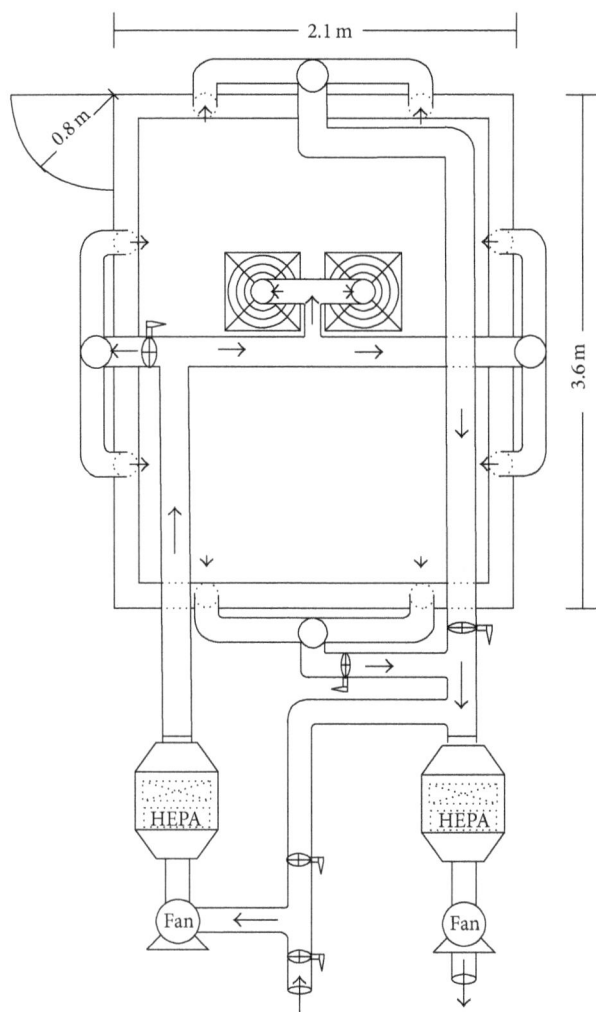

FIGURE 2: Schematic design of the subject test chamber.

a six-hole Collison nebulizer (BGI Inc., Waltham, MA, USA). A flow rate of 12 L/min of NaCl particle-laden air was then mixed with a 16 L/min of diluted dry air. Since laboratory-generated particles might carry high electrical charges, the entire airflow of 28 L/min was directed through a charge equilibrator (3.6 $\mu$Ci Am 241) to achieve the Boltzmann charge equilibrium. An air circulation fan (with a flow rate of about 900 CFM) located at the outlet of the aerosol generation system distributed the aerosolized particles within the test chamber. The particle concentrations inside the test chamber could be stably controlled at $(0.1\sim1) \times 10^5$ particles/cm$^3$.

*2.4. Requirement and Characteristics of Human Subjects.* To test the respirators and surgical masks, 30 students aged 18 to 24 were recruited from Feng Chia University (15 men and 15 women). Values for the distance from the Menton process to the top of the head were 13.0 to 25.6 cm ($21.8\pm2.4$ cm); for the bitragion breadth, they were 12.5 to 16.2 cm ($14.4 \pm 1.0$ cm); and for the lip width, they were 3.7 to 6.0 cm ($4.8 \pm 0.5$ cm). All subjects were nonsmokers and inexperienced respirator users. Human testing in this study had been approved by the Institutional Review Board of China Medical University Hospital, Taichung, Taiwan, through the approval number DMR99-IRB-165—and each test subject provided written informed consent. A researcher informed the subjects that they could demand suspension of the experiment if they experienced any discomfort.

For the total inward leakage (TIL) test carried out in the laboratory, each subject had to be free of allergies and any cardiovascular or respiratory tract diseases. Each subject was not permitted to drink or smoke half an hour before the test, and male subjects were required to be clean-shaven [21]. A researcher taught subjects how to properly don the respirator and implemented the fit testing. All participants had to undergo the fit test before the TIL experiment was carried out.

The back wall had six exhaust gates, which were paired at each of the same three heights of two-side walls. Each slot gate could be operated independently of the others in the open or closed position. This allowed for the chamber to be operating using any possible combination of slots, thus creating various directions of air current in the chamber.

The air exchange rate could be controlled from 0 to 60 air exchanges per hour. The pressure of the test chamber was monitored in real time by a Magnehelic pressure gage (Model 2300-20MM, Dwyer Instrument, Inc., USA). The VelociCalc air velocity meter (Model 9535, TSI Inc., USA) and the inclined-vertical manometer (Model MARK II MM-80, Dwyer Instrument, Inc., USA) measured the velocity of the slot gates and the pressure drop of the HEPA air-purifying unit, in order to evaluate the air exchange rate of the test chamber and the performance of the HEPA air-purifying unit. The relative humidity and temperature of the test chamber could be maintained at $25 \pm 3°$C and 40–60% by the air conditioner and dehumidifier.

*2.3. Aerosol Generation in the Subject Test Chamber.* NaCl solution (1.5 g/100 mL) was aerosolized in the test chamber by

*2.5. Selection of the FFP Respirators and Surgical Masks.* In order to evaluate the protection performance of similar DFHFR (the same appearance, shape, materials, etc.) with different categories against particles of different sizes, we selected cone shaped FFP1, FFP2, and FFP3 respirators from two different companies (A and B represented two companies in text, tables, and figures), comprising the same classes of respirators and one single size, yet with different filtration efficiencies. In addition, flat shaped surgical masks—C, D, and E—from three different manufacturers were chosen for testing.

*2.6. Experimental Protocol.* Before the fit testing and TIL test, each subject was trained to wear the tested respirator by guidance from a researcher. A user seal check was performed to ensure that an adequate seal was achieved when the respirator was put on the subject's face. Subjects performed the US's Occupational Health and Safety Association's (OSHA) fit testing exercises, including normal breathing, deep breathing, turning head side to side, moving head up and down, talking, grimace, bending over, and returning to normal breathing [21]. The fit factor for each exercise was recorded using a

PortaCount Plus (TSI Inc., St. Paul, MN, USA). The overall fit factor (FF) is calculated as follows:

$$FF = \frac{\text{Number of exercises}}{1/ff_1 + 1/ff_2 + 1/ff_3 + 1/ff_4 + 1/ff_5 + 1/ff_6 + 1/ff_7 + 1/ff_8}, \quad (1)$$

where $ff_1$, $ff_2$, $ff_3$, and so forth are the fit factors for Exercises 1, 2, 3, and so forth (grimace (Exercise #6) is excluded).

For the TIL test, the numerical concentrations of NaCl particles were size-selectively measured using the ELPI with a sampling flow of 10 L/min. The ELPI measures the numerical concentration of particles in an aerodynamic size, ranging from $D_a$ = 0.028 to 10.01 $\mu$m, in 12 channels. In this study, we used six channels with geometric mean (GM) diameters of 0.121, 0.203, 0.318, 0.486, 0.766, and 1.238 $\mu$m, in the particle size range of 0.093–1.61 $\mu$m. Particle sizes between 0.093 and 1.61 $\mu$m were measured because viral and bacterial particles fall within this range. When the particle concentrations were stable in the test chamber, the subjects equipped with the personal system donned the test respirators and performed the OSHA fit testing exercises. Each exercise was performed for two minutes and the particle concentrations inside the respirator were averaged over the second minute. The concentration inside the respirator ($C_{in}$) for the entire test was averaged over all the exercises, excluding the grimace maneuver. The particle concentrations outside the respirator ($C_{out}$) were measured before and after the subject performed the exercises. The average of these concentrations was used as the concentration outside the respirator for each test. The protection factor (PF) was calculated by dividing the particle concentrations outside the respirator with those inside the respirator:

$$PF = \frac{C_{out}}{C_{in}}. \quad (2)$$

Each subject was tested on the FFP1, FFP2, and FFP3 respirators of manufacturer A and manufacturer B and on the three models of surgical masks (C, D, and E).

The particle losses in the sampling line have been addressed in our previous study [20], where we found that a difference in the penetration efficiencies of particles between the two sampling lines was due to slightly different configurations. Therefore, all PFs presented in this paper were corrected by a ratio of concentrations measured in the two sampling lines when no respirator was attached in the system. These ratios varied from 0.97 to 1.04, depending on the particle size.

*2.7. Data Analysis.* Data were organized and managed using Microsoft Excel 2013, and the plots were made by SigmaPlot 10.0. The data analysis was performed using ANOVA test, t-test, and the Pearson correlation model provided by SPSS 12.0 for Windows (SPSS Inc., USA) software. All data were log-transformed before conducting statistical testing. $p$ values of <0.05 were considered significant. The difference in fit factors and PFs among FFP respirators was examined by the ANOVA test followed by a pairwise comparison using

Tukey's Studentized Range test. This test method was also used to examine the effect of particle size on PFs. The Pearson correlation coefficients were obtained to examine the association between protection factors and fit factors.

## 3. Results

*3.1. Fit Testing Results.* Before we carried out human tests to assess actual respirator performance, the subjects were first required to undergo quantitative fit testing that was conducted using a PortaCount Plus, not the N95 Companion. There are three reasons for not using the N95 Companion in this study: (1) Generally, only FFP2 respirators use the N95 Companion for fit testing, whereas this type of mask fit tester is unnecessary in conducting fit tests for FFP respirators and surgical masks—which are the focus of this study. (2) The original concept developed by the N95 Companion for fit testing respirators is to measure the amount of particulate getting through the face seal only. However, Rengasamy et al. (2012) have shown that negatively charged particles between 0.04 and 0.06 $\mu$m are small enough to penetrate not only the face seals of these respirators, but also their filters [22]—ultimately skewing test results and making this type of fit testing inaccurate. (3) In order to establish the relationship between PFs and fit factors in assessing protection against particles, the wider-sized range of the PortaCount Plus covering the size of tested particles was favorable and comparable. The fit testing results are shown in Table 1. The highest percentage of subjects passing FFP fit testing was 93.3% for FFP1_A and FFP2_B. No subjects passed fit testing with SMs. The nine respirators are listed in descending order of the geometric mean as follows: FFP2_B (174.2) > FFP1_A (171.6) > FFP3_B (138.4) > FFP3_B (112.4) > FFP3_A (103.2) > FFP1_B (138.4) > SM_E (3.1) > SM_C (3.0) > SM_D (2.1).

*3.2. Protection Factors of Tested Respirators.* After fit testing, all 30 subjects underwent respirator and surgical mask testing. Each subject was required to don nine DFHFRs to assess the protection of the respirators. The experimental results were plotted for PFs versus particle size in a boxplot chart. The results of nine DFHFRs are presented in Figures 3–5 and Table 2. Figures 3 and 4 show the PFs of FFP respirators, respectively, for manufacturers A and B in the particle size range of 0.093–1.61 $\mu$m and represent the range of viral and bacterial sizes. Regardless of the fit testing results, the overall GM of PFs was 19.6 for PPF1 respirators, 27.1 for FFP2 respirators, and 26.7 for FFP3 respirators. The respective GMs for subjects passing the fit testing were 25.5, 30.9, and 37.6. Thus, on average, the PFs were 1.1–1.4 (30.9/27.1–37.6/26.7) times greater when only data for those who passed the fit testing were included. The differences were not statistically significant ($p$ > 0.05), nor were the PFs statistically significantly different among FFP classes ($p$ > 0.05) for both data sets (all subjects and subjects passing the fit testing). The lowest PFs occurred between particle sizes of 0.263 and 0.384 $\mu$m. PFs were not significantly different among different particle sizes in the size range of 0.093–1.61 $\mu$m ($p$ > 0.05) for both data sets (all subjects and subjects passing the fit testing). The assigned protection factor

TABLE 1: Fit factors of 6 FFP respirators and 3 surgical masks (SMs). Total observations are 30 (30 subjects).

|  | FFP1_A | FFP2_A | FFP3_A | FFP1_B | FFP2_B | FFP3_B | SM_C | SM_D | SM_E |
|---|---|---|---|---|---|---|---|---|---|
| Percentage of fit factors > 100 (%) | 93.3 | 80.0 | 73.3 | 60.0 | 93.3 | 76.7 | 0 | 0 | 0 |
| Geometric mean | 171.6 | 112.4 | 103.2 | 75.0 | 174.2 | 138.4 | 3.0 | 2.1 | 3.1 |
| Geometric standard deviation | 1.7 | 2.2 | 3.0 | 2.9 | 2.5 | 4.9 | 1.7 | 1.6 | 1.8 |

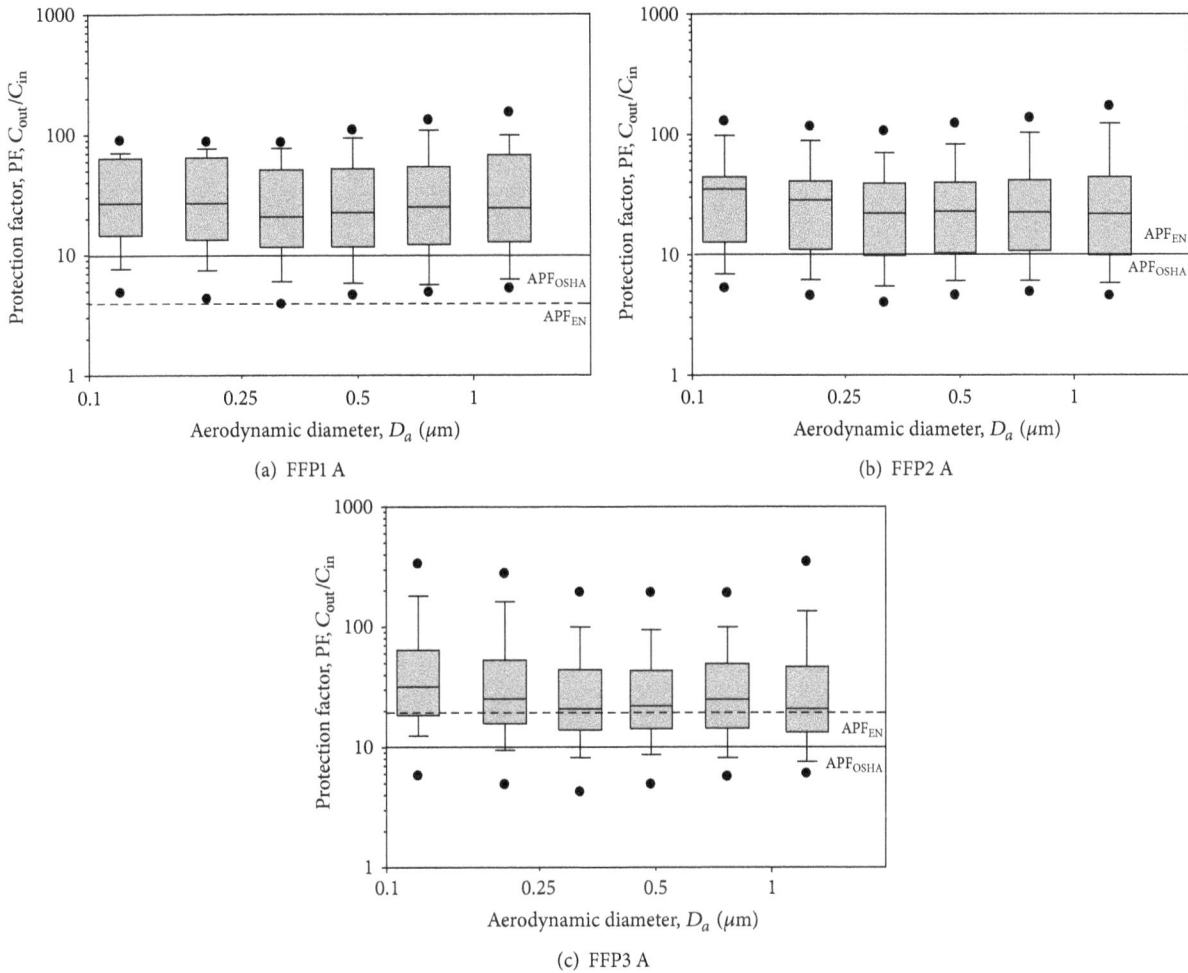

(a) FFP1 A

(b) FFP2 A

(c) FFP3 A

FIGURE 3: PF-values against particles in size range of 0.093–1.61 $\mu$m for FFP1, FFP2, and FFP3 respirators manufactured by company A. The tests were performed when the FFP respirators were donned on human subjects. Total observations are 30 (30 subjects). The boxplots show the following: dots (from bottom) represent 5% and 95% percentiles; horizontal lines (from bottom) represent 10%, 25%, 50%, 75%, and 90% percentiles. APF refers to the assigned protection factor for that particular mask.

(APF) of 10 for N95 FFRs [23] is shown by a horizontal solid line, denoted as 4, 10, and 20, respectively, for FFP1, FFP2, and FFP3 respirators (which are represented by a short dashed line in the figures). The APF value represents the level of protection that a properly functioning respirator is expected to provide for adequately fitted and trained users in a respiratory protection program in the workplace. Among the 60 tested FFP1 respirators (30 subjects × 2 manufacturers), PFs below 4, 10, and 20 were found for 5.0%, 28.3%, and 53.3% of the respirators, respectively. The respective percentages for PFs of FFP2 respirators were 1.7%, 18.3%, and 35.0%, while they were 1.7%, 20.0%, and 41.7% for FFP3 respirators. The respective percentages for subjects passing the fit testing were

2.5%, 17.5%, and 40.0% for FFP1 respirators, 0.0%, 10.9%, and 30.4% for FFP2 respirators, and 0.0%, 12.8%, and 28.2% for FFP3 respirators. The percentages significantly decreased after fit testing ($p < 0.05$).

PFs for the three models of SMs are shown in Figure 5 and Table 2. The overall geometric mean of PFs was 1.7. The minimum numbers of the PFs were also found to be approximately between 0.263 and 0.384 $\mu$m particle size for SMs C, D, and E. It was found that PFs were not significantly different among different particle sizes in the size range of 0.093–1.61 $\mu$m ($p > 0.05$) for SMs C and E, while the particle size was found to significantly affect PFs for SM D. We found that PFs for particles > 0.616 $\mu$m were significantly greater

TABLE 2: Protection factors of 6 FFP respirators and 3 surgical masks (SMs). Total observations are 30 (30 subjects).

| | FFP1_A | FFP2_A | FFP3_A | FFP1_B | FFP2_B | FFP3_B | SM_C | SM_D | SM_E | Total FFP1 | Total FFP2 | Total FFP3 | Total SM |
|---|---|---|---|---|---|---|---|---|---|---|---|---|---|
| The fifth percentile* | 5.0 | 6.5 | 13.5 | 6.4 | 8.1 | 6.1 | 1.2 | 1.3 | 1.3 | 5.3 | 6.7 | 6.1 | 1.2 |
| GM ± GSD (all subjects) | 24.1 ± 2.5 | 23.4 ± 2.5 | 31.9 ± 3.0 | 15.9 ± 2.4 | 31.4 ± 2.8 | 22.6 ± 3.1 | 1.7 ± 1.3 | 1.5 ± 1.2 | 1.8 ± 1.3 | 19.6 ± 2.5 | 27.1 ± 2.7 | 26.7 ± 3.1 | 1.7 ± 1.3 |
| GM ± GSD (pass fit test) | 26.6 ± 2.5 | 30.0 ± 2.3 | 46.5 ± 3.1 | 23.7 ± 2.4 | 31.6 ± 2.7 | 30.8 ± 3.0 | | | | 25.5 ± 2.5 | 30.9 ± 2.5 | 37.6 ± 3.1 | |

*The fifth percentile was calculated only for subjects passing the fit test with FFP respirators. Because no subjects passed the fit test for surgical masks, the fifth percentile was calculated for all subjects wearing surgical masks ($n = 30$). GM refers to the geometric mean of PF data; GSD refers to the geometric standard deviation of PF data.

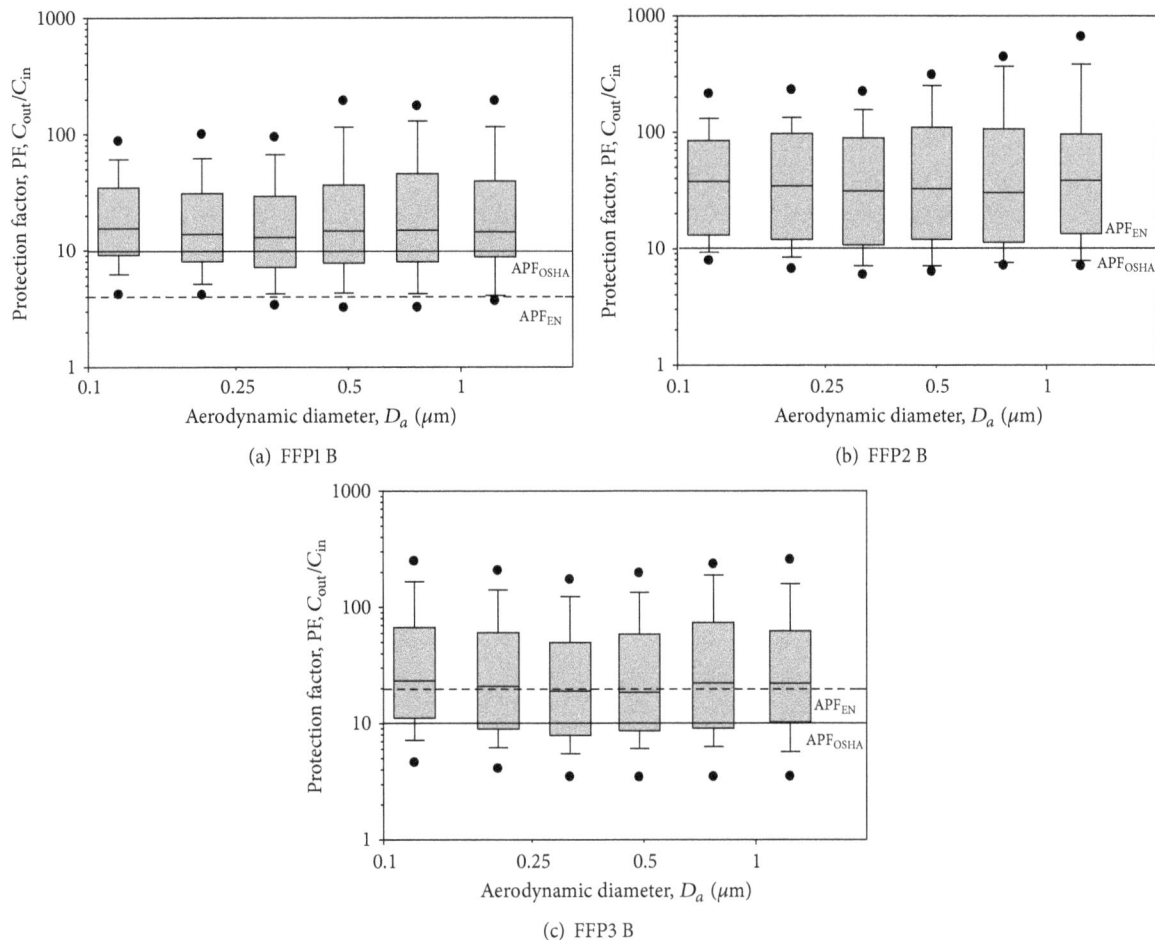

FIGURE 4: PF-values against particles in size range of 0.093–1.61 $\mu$m for FFP1, FFP2, and FFP3 respirators manufactured by company B. The tests were performed when the FFP respirators were donned on human subjects. Total observations are 30 (30 subjects). The boxplots show the same as in Figure 3. AFF refers to the assigned protection factor for that particular mask.

than the minimum PFs for SM D ($p < 0.05$). None of the tested SMs had PFs > 4. With respect to the geometric mean of PFs, the overall PF provided by SMs was 11.5 times less than that for FFP1 respirators, 15.9 times less than that for FFP2 respirators, and 15.7 times less than that for FFP3 respirators ($p < 0.05$).

*3.3. Association between Fit Factors and Protection Factors.* Figure 6 presents the regression plots for the associations between fit factors and PFs. We found that the correlation coefficients were 0.378 for FFP respirators and 0.482 for SMs. These values were in the middle of weak ($r = 0.3$) and moderate ($r = 0.5$) positive linear relationships and were statistically significant ($p < 0.05$). When the data for FFP respirators and SMs were combined, the correlation coefficient increased to 0.835 ($p < 0.05$), which presented a significantly strong positive association between fit factors and PFs.

## 4. Discussion

Current guidance issued by the Centers for Disease Control and Prevention (CDC) and the Health and Safety Executive

(HSE) recommends the use of N95 or higher respirators and FFP3 respirators against airborne infectious diseases in healthcare settings. When these certified DHFFRs are in short supply or not available, SMs may be an alternative. No previous investigations have utilized human subjects to investigate the protection provided by FFP respirators against particles in the size of 0.093–1.61 $\mu$m, representing bacterial and viral size ranges.

We found the minimum PF for both FFP respirators and SMs appeared for particle sizes between 0.263 and 0.384 $\mu$m. When particles pass through face seal leaks and filter materials, diffusion causes deposition of smaller particles on the surface, while impaction and interception dominate deposition of larger particles. This is why we had minimum protection for particle sizes between 0.263 and 0.384 $\mu$m. However, the protection provided by both FFP respirators and SMs was not significantly affected by the particle size ranging from 0.093 to 1.61 $\mu$m. In a recent study [24], we found that particle penetration through face seal leaks was greater than that through filter material (SMs were ~4 to 8 times greater, and FFP respirators were ~1.5–6.7 times greater). This finding is similar to the results published by Grinshpun et al. (2009) for N95 FFRs

(a) Surgical mask C

(b) Surgical mask D

(c) Surgical mask E

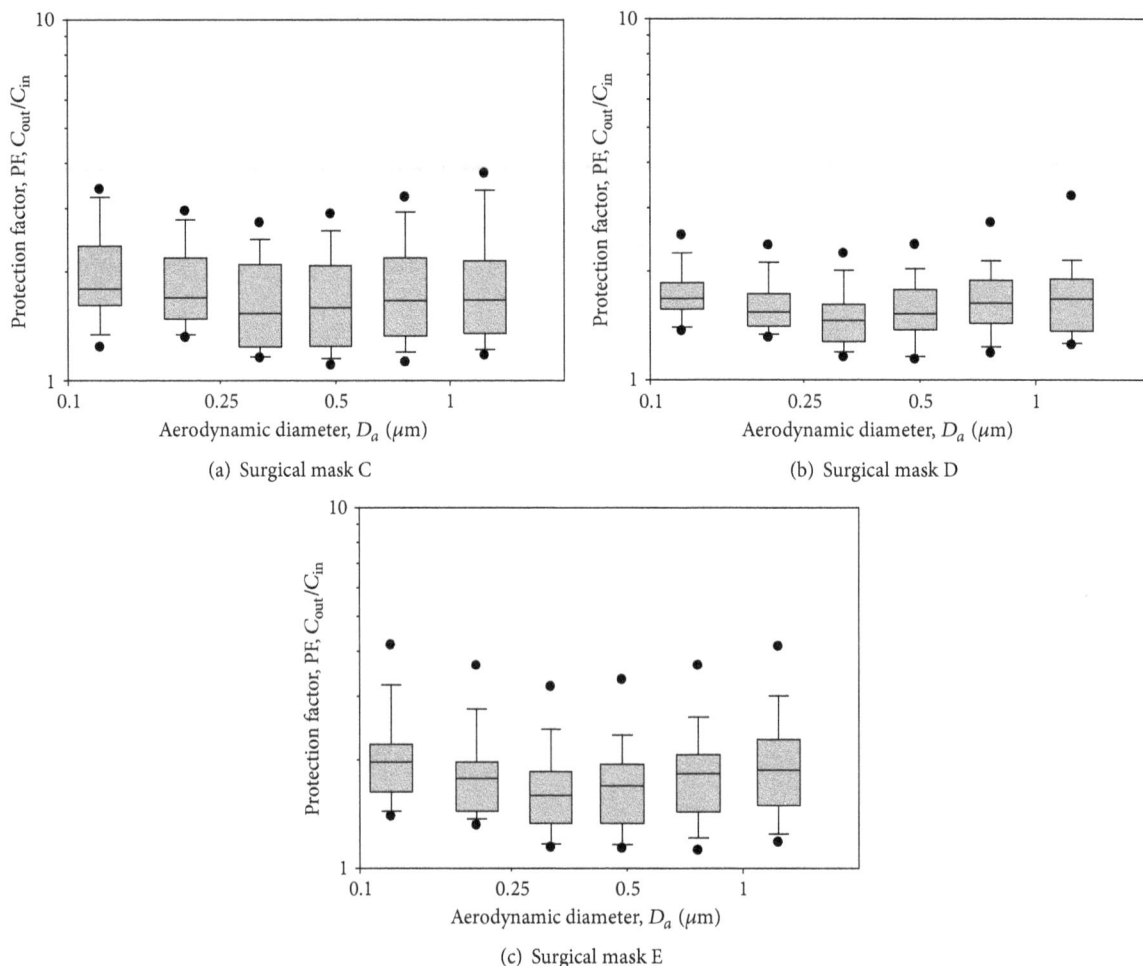

FIGURE 5: PF-values against particles in size range of 0.093–1.61 $\mu$m for three models of surgical masks: C, D, and E. The boxplots show the same as in Figure 3. The tests were performed when the surgical masks were donned on human subjects. Total observations are 30 (30 subjects).

and SMs [12]. The subjects' average breathing rate measured was between 8.4 and 16.9 L/min during fit testing exercises. The leak flow through face seal leaks was laminar at these flow rates [25], resulting in PFs independent of particle size. The size ranges of viral and bacterial particles fall into this size range, and they are expected to have similar PFs. In contrast, Lee et al. (2008) and Grinshpun et al. (2009) show that PFs are significantly size-dependent for N95 filtering facepiece respirators in a similar size range [6, 12]. However, Grinshpun et al. (2009) have found that the particle penetration through face seal leaks is not significantly size-dependent [12]. Our recent study has shown that face seal leaks contribute more particle concentrations inside the respirator than does filter penetration [24] and indicates that characteristics of face seal leaks (including shape, size, etc.) might affect particle penetration inside the respirator, resulting in size-independent PFs.

For subjects passing the fit testing, the percentage of the respirators that had PFs greater than 4 was greater than 95% for FFP respirators. However, the corresponding percentages for PFs greater than 10 and 20, respectively, were 82.5% and 60.0% for FFP1 respirators, 89.1% and 69.6% for FFP2

respirators, and 87.2% and 71.8% for FFP3 respirators. This is interesting in that the FFP3 respirators performed the same or worse than the FFP2 respirators. This also happened for the fit testing results where subjects donning FFP3 respirators did not have the highest fit testing pass rates, which indicates that respirators with the highest filtration efficiencies are not necessary for having the best fit factors and PFs. FFP3 respirators generally have a greater packing density and pressure drop in respirator filters than do FFP2 respirators, which results in a more pronounced particle penetration through face leaks than with filter materials. Face seal leaks do not perform like filters to prevent particles from entering the respirator, which results in FFP3 respirators not being equal to or better than FFP2 respirators, as was expected. This study also shows that the PFs for FFP respirators increased when subjects who did not pass the fit testing were excluded from the analysis, which further demonstrates the power of fit testing to improve respirator protection.

The APF is the ratio of pollutant outside the device to that inside the device and is defined by British Standard BS EN 529:2005 as the level of respiratory protection that can

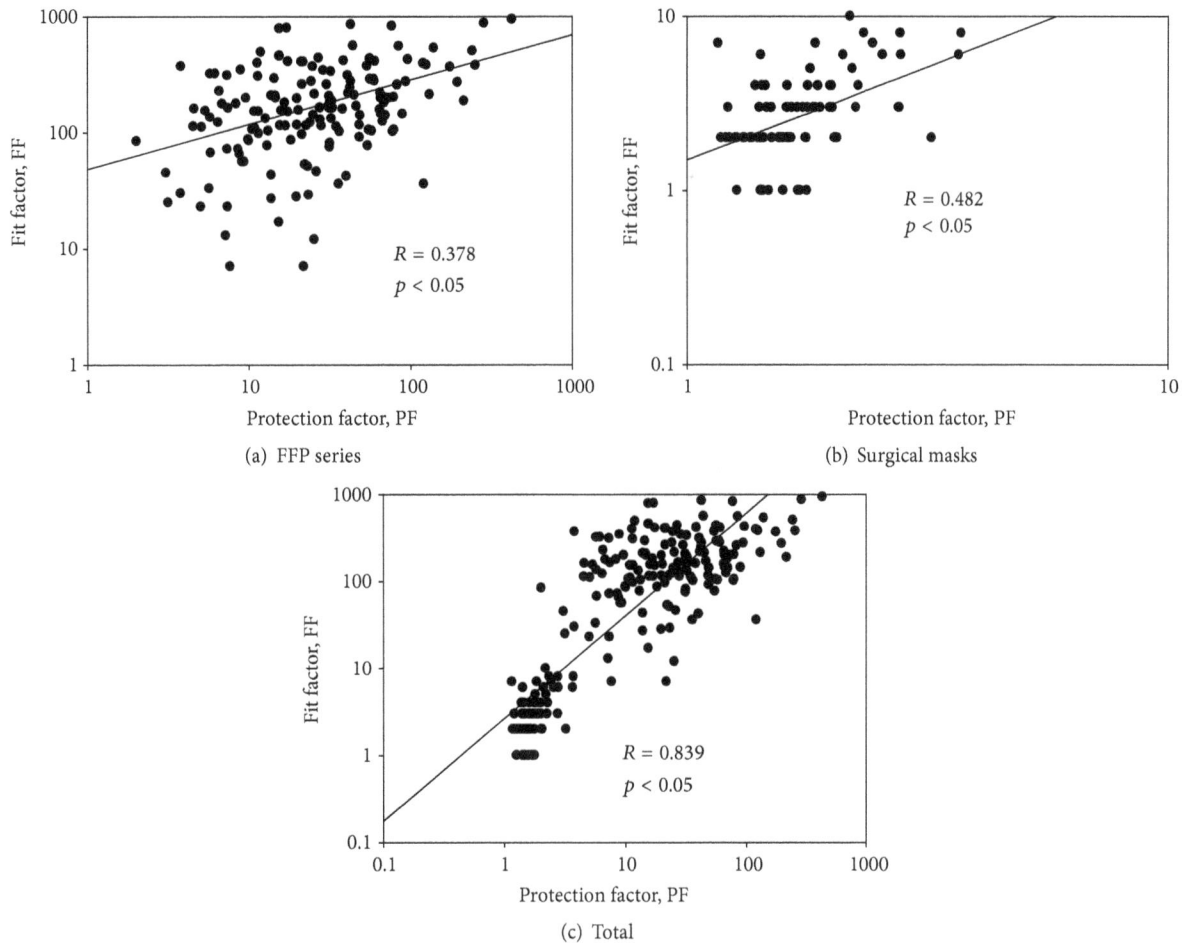

FIGURE 6: The association between fit factors and protection factors. The associations for FFP respirators, surgical masks, and total (all respirators combined) are presented, respectively, in (a), (b), and (c).

realistically be expected to be achieved in the workplace by 95% of adequately trained and supervised wearers using a properly functioning and correctly fitted respiratory protective device and is based on the 5th percentile of the Workplace Protection Factor (WPF) data. In the US, the APF is 10 for half masks, while they are 4, 10, and 20, respectively, for FFP1, FFP2, and FFP3 respirators in the UK. The fifth percentile of PFs obtained in this study was 5.3 for FFP1 respirators, 6.7 for FFP2 respirators, and 6.1 for FFP3 respirators. Only the APF result for FFP1 respirators fit the European standard, indicating that APF standards for FFP2 and FFP3 respirators should be considered for revision. This finding is similar to previous results for N95 filtering facepiece respirators [6, 10, 26, 27]. In addition, the fifth percentile values of FFP respirators were close to each other, whereas the APF standard for FFP respirators could be one number. Based on the results obtained in our study, we recommend the APF value of 5 for FFP respirators. Although there were no significant difference in PFs among FFP respirators, FFP2 respirators and above are recommended in healthcare settings against infectious diseases. This is because the overall performance of FFP1 respirators is somewhat inferior to FFP2 and FFP3 respirators. Regardless of fit testing, the overall PF provided by SMs was,

significantly, 11.5 times less than that for FFP1 respirators, 15.9 times less than that for FFP2 respirators, and 15.7 times less than that for FFP3 respirators. This suggests that SMs are not a good substitute for FFP respirators when concerns exist about airborne transmission of viral or bacterial pathogens.

For tight-fitting respirators with higher filtration efficiencies such as N95 respirators and FFP respirators, Coffey et al. (2004) found that subjects failing a fit test also received adequate protection, resulting in high alpha errors [26]. High alpha errors could result in subjects erroneously failing a particular fit test with a higher level of protection than those subjects correctly passing the fit test. For loose-fitting respirators with lower filtration efficiencies, the FFs and PFs are too small to demarcate any difference detected by the measurement devices, which is why we had weak association between FFs and PFs for FFP respirators and SMs. However, the difference in FFs and PFs between FFP respirators and SMs is very large. Therefore, we had greater FFs corresponding to greater PFs for FFP respirators, while we had smaller FFs corresponding to smaller PFs for SMs. This resulted in an increase in the $r$ value when the two data were combined. Zhuang et al. (2003) also found that the association between PFs and FFs decreased when subjects who failed the fit testing were excluded but increased when all subjects were included in the analysis [28]. Although the fit factors are meant to assess the face seal leaks rather than overall leaks evaluated by the PFs, our results indicate that the PFs of respirators against particles can be assessed by fit factors. Considerable time, labor, and expense could therefore be saved by assessing PFs of respirators against particles. However, there are clear differences in FFP respirators and surgical masks, and SMs do not fall under OSHA fit test requirements. It is recommended that the protection of FFP respirators and SMs should be investigated separately when fit factors are used to assess actual respirator performance.

The study was conducted in a test chamber instead of a real work environment. Due to restrictions within the test environment, the data interpretation extending to other work environments may be limited. Also, because the subjects were selected only from a younger population in Taiwan and the number of subjects was small, there is a limitation for data interpretation extending to all workers and other races. In addition, we only tested FFP1, FFP2, and FFP3 respirators manufactured by two companies, and three models of SMs. More respirators are needed for further studies to confirm our results.

## 5. Conclusion

The tested FFP respirators and SMs in this study were observed to have the worst protection against particles between 0.263 and 0.384 $\mu$m. The protection factors of FFP respirators against particles in the size range of 0.093–1.61 $\mu$m were not size dependent. The size ranges of viral and bacterial particles fall into this size range, and they are expected to have similar PFs. The FFP respirators provided about 11.5 to 15.9 times better protection than the SMs, suggesting that SMs are not a good substitute for FFP respirators when concerns exist about airborne transmission of bacterial and viral pathogens. About 18.3% of the tested FFP2 respirators had PFs <10, and ~41.7% of the tested FFP3 respirators had PFs <20, indicating that the European standard for APF of 10 for FFP2 respirators and 20 for FFP3 respirators may overestimate the actual protection offered by these respirators against particles in the size range of 0.093–1.61 $\mu$m. PFs among FFP respirator classes were not significantly different, indicating the APF value for FFP respirators could possibly be revised to one value rather than three for FFP1, FFP2, and FFP3 respirators. Fit factors could be used as an indicator to assess the protection provided by FFP respirators and SMs.

## Conflict of Interests

The authors declare that there is no conflict of interests.

## Acknowledgments

This research was supported by the Executive Yuan's Ministry of Labor, Institute of Labor, and Occupational Safety and Health through the Research Grant no. IOSH99-H311. The authors are also thankful to the students who volunteered to be human subjects in the study.

## References

[1] D.-H. Han, K. Willeke, and C. E. Colton, "Quantitative fit testing techniques and regulations for tight-fitting respirators: current methods measuring aerosol or air leakage, and new developments," *American Industrial Hygiene Association Journal*, vol. 58, no. 3, pp. 219–228, 1997.

[2] W. Popendorf, J. A. Merchant, S. Leonard, L. F. Burmeister, and S. A. Olenchock, "Respirator protection and acceptability among agricultural workers," *Applied Occupational and Environmental Hygiene*, vol. 10, no. 7, pp. 595–605, 1995.

[3] Centers for Disease Control and Prevention (CDC), *Guidance on Personal Protective Equipment (PPE) To Be Used By Healthcare Workers during Management of Patients with Confirmed Ebola or Persons under Investigation (PUIs) for Ebola who are Clinically Unstable or Have Bleeding, Vomiting, or Diarrhea in U.S. Hospitals, Including Procedures for Donning and Doffing PPE*, Centers for Disease Control and Prevention, U.S. Department of Health and Human Services, Atlanta, Ga, USA, 2015, http://www.cdc.gov/vhf/ebola/healthcare-us/ppe/guidance.html.

[4] National Institute for Occupational Safety and Hygiene (NIOSH), *NIOSH Guide to the Selection and Use of Particulate Respirators Certified Under 42 CFR 84*, DHHS (NIOSH) Publication no. 96-101, National Institute for Occupational Safety and Hygiene (NIOSH), Cincinnati, Ohio, USA, 1996.

[5] J. E. Coia, L. Ritchie, A. Adisesh et al., "Guidance on the use of respiratory and facial protection equipment," *Journal of Hospital Infection*, vol. 85, no. 3, pp. 170–182, 2013.

[6] S.-A. Lee, S. A. Grinshpun, and T. Reponen, "Respiratory performance offered by N95 respirators and surgical masks: human subject evaluation with NaCl aerosol representing bacterial and viral particle size range," *Annals of Occupational Hygiene*, vol. 52, no. 3, pp. 177–185, 2008.

[7] M. Loeb, N. Dafoe, J. Mahony et al., "Surgical mask vs N95 respirator for preventing influenza among health care workers: a randomized trial," *The Journal of the American Medical Association*, vol. 302, no. 17, pp. 1865–1871, 2009.

[8] Medicines and Healthcare Products Regulatory Agency, *Medical Devices Directive*, Medicines and Healthcare Products Regulatory Agency, London, UK, 2010.

[9] UK Government, "Personal protective equipment regulations 2002," Statutory Instrument 1144, HMSO, London, UK, 2002.

[10] S.-A. Lee, A. Adhikari, S. A. Grinshpun et al., "Respiratory protection provided by N95 filtering facepiece respirators against airborne dust and microorganisms in agricultural farms," *Journal of Occupational and Environmental Hygiene*, vol. 2, no. 11, pp. 577–585, 2005.

[11] A. Bałazy, M. Toivola, T. Reponen, A. Podgórski, A. Zimmer, and S. A. Grinshpun, "Manikin-based performance evaluation of N95 filtering-facepiece respirators challenged with nanoparticles," *Annals of Occupational Hygiene*, vol. 50, no. 3, pp. 259–269, 2006.

[12] S. A. Grinshpun, H. Haruta, R. M. Eninger, T. Reponen, R. T. McKay, and S.-A. Lee, "Performance of an N95 filtering facepiece particulate respirator and a surgical mask during human breathing: Two pathways for particle penetration," *Journal of Occupational and Environmental Hygiene*, vol. 6, no. 10, pp. 593–603, 2009.

[13] S.-A. Lee, S. A. Grinshpun, A. Adhikari et al., "Laboratory and field evaluation of a new personal sampling system for assessing the protection provided by the N95 filtering facepiece

respirators against particles," *Annals of Occupational Hygiene*, vol. 49, no. 3, pp. 245–257, 2005.

[14] T. Reponen, S.-A. Lee, S. A. Grinshpun, E. Johnson, and R. McKay, "Effect of fit testing on the protection offered by N95 filtering facepiece respirators against fine particles in a laboratory setting," *Annals of Occupational Hygiene*, vol. 55, no. 3, pp. 264–271, 2011.

[15] K. Lee, A. Slavcev, and M. Nicas, "Respiratory protection against *Mycobacterium tuberculosis*: quantitative fit test outcomes for five type N95 filtering-facepiece respirators," *Journal of Occupational and Environmental Hygiene*, vol. 1, no. 1, pp. 22–28, 2004.

[16] A. Penconek, P. Drayk, and A. Moskal, "Penetration of diesel exhaust particles through commercially available dust half masks," *Annals of Occupational Hygiene*, vol. 57, no. 3, pp. 360–373, 2013.

[17] National Institute for Occupational Safety and Health (NIOSH), *Standard Development: Program Concept for Total Inward Leakage (TIL) Performance Requirements and Test Methods*, US Department of Health and Human Services, Centers for Disease Control and Prevention, Atlanta, Ga, USA, 2004, http://www.cdc.gov/niosh/npptl/standardsdev/til/.

[18] S. Rengasamy, B. C. Eimer, and J. Szalajda, "A quantitative assessment of the total inward leakage of nacl aerosol representing submicron-size bioaerosol through N95 filtering facepiece respirators and surgical masks," *Journal of Occupational and Environmental Hygiene*, vol. 11, no. 6, pp. 388–396, 2014.

[19] Z. Q. Zhuang, C. C. Coffey, and R. B. Ann, "The effect of subject characteristics and respirator features on respirator fit," *Journal of Occupational and Environmental Hygiene*, vol. 2, no. 12, pp. 641–649, 2005.

[20] S. A. Lee, T. Reponen, W. Li, M. Trunov, K. Willeke, and S. A. Grinshpun, "Development of a new method for measuring the protection provided by respirators against dust and microorganisms," *Aerosol and Air Quality Research*, vol. 4, no. 1, pp. 56–73, 2004.

[21] Department of Labor-Occupational Safety and Health Administration (OSHA), *29 CFR Parts 1910.134 Appendix A Fit Testing Procedures (Mandatory)*, Department of Labor, Occupational Safety and Health Administration (OSHA), Washington, DC, USA, 1998.

[22] S. Rengasamy, B. C. Eimer, and R. E. Shaffer, "Evaluation of the performance of the N95-companion: effects of filter penetration and comparison with other aerosol instruments," *Journal of Occupational and Environmental Hygiene*, vol. 9, no. 7, pp. 417–426, 2012.

[23] Department of Labor-Occupational Safety and Health Administration (OSHA), *29 CFR Parts 1910, 1915, and 1926 Assigned Protection Factors; Final Rule—71:50121-50192. Federal Register 71:164*, Department of Labor-Occupational Safety and Health Administration (OSHA), Washington, DC, USA, 2006.

[24] S. A. Lee, H. Y. Li, C. F. Tsai, C. W. Chen, and C. L. Wu, "The effect of filter and faceseal leakage on the protection performance of disposable masks," *Journal of Labor, Occupational Safety and Health*, vol. 23, pp. 179–190, 2015.

[25] C. C. Chen and K. Willeke, "Characteristics of face seal leakage in filtering facepieces," *American Industrial Hygiene Association Journal*, vol. 53, no. 9, pp. 533–539, 1992.

[26] C. C. Coffey, R. B. Lawrence, D. L. Campbell, Z. Zhuang, C. A. Calvert, and P. A. Jensen, "Fitting characteristics of eighteen N95 filtering-facepiece respirators," *Journal of Occupational and Environmental Hygiene*, vol. 1, no. 4, pp. 262–271, 2004.

[27] M. G. Duling, R. B. Lawrence, J. E. Slaven, and C. C. Coffey, "Simulated workplace protection factors for half-facepiece respiratory protective devices," *Journal of Occupational and Environmental Hygiene*, vol. 4, no. 6, pp. 420–431, 2007.

[28] Z. Zhuang, C. C. Coffey, P. A. Jensen, D. L. Campbell, R. B. Lawrence, and W. R. Myers, "Correlation between quantitative fit factors and workplace protection factors measured in actual workplace environments at a steel foundry," *American Industrial Hygiene Association Journal*, vol. 64, no. 6, pp. 730–738, 2003.

# Permissions

The contributors of this book come from diverse backgrounds, making this book a truly international effort. This book will bring forth new frontiers with its revolutionizing research information and detailed analysis of the nascent developments around the world.

We would like to thank all the contributing authors for lending their expertise to make the book truly unique. They have played a crucial role in the development of this book. Without their invaluable contributions this book wouldn't have been possible. They have made vital efforts to compile up to date information on the varied aspects of this subject to make this book a valuable addition to the collection of many professionals and students.

This book was conceptualized with the vision of imparting up-to-date information and advanced data in this field. To ensure the same, a matchless editorial board was set up. Every individual on the board went through rigorous rounds of assessment to prove their worth. After which they invested a large part of their time researching and compiling the most relevant data for our readers.

The editorial board has been involved in producing this book since its inception. They have spent rigorous hours researching and exploring the diverse topics which have resulted in the successful publishing of this book. They have passed on their knowledge of decades through this book. To expedite this challenging task, the publisher supported the team at every step. A small team of assistant editors was also appointed to further simplify the editing procedure and attain best results for the readers.

Apart from the editorial board, the designing team has also invested a significant amount of their time in understanding the subject and creating the most relevant covers. They scrutinized every image to scout for the most suitable representation of the subject and create an appropriate cover for the book.

The publishing team has been an ardent support to the editorial, designing and production team. Their endless efforts to recruit the best for this project, has resulted in the accomplishment of this book. They are a veteran in the field of academics and their pool of knowledge is as vast as their experience in printing. Their expertise and guidance has proved useful at every step. Their uncompromising quality standards have made this book an exceptional effort. Their encouragement from time to time has been an inspiration for everyone.

The publisher and the editorial board hope that this book will prove to be a valuable piece of knowledge for researchers, students, practitioners and scholars across the globe.

# List of Contributors

**Yiannis Koumpouros**
Technological Educational Institute of Athens, Department of Informatics, Agiou Spyridonos, Aigaleo, 12243 Athens, Greece

**Jori Reijula**
Finnish Institute of Occupational Health, Neulaniementie 4, 70210 Kuopio, Finland

**Sauli Karvonen**
SKA-Research Oy, Teollisuustie 9, 02880 Veikkola, Finland

**Hanna Petäjä and Liisa Lehtonen**
Turku University Hospital, Kiinamyllynkatu 4-8, 20520 Turku, Finland

**Kari Reijula**
University of Helsinki, Yliopistonkatu 4, 00100 Helsinki, Finland

**Mario Salai, István Vassányi and István Kósa**
Medical Informatics R&D Centre, University of Pannonia, Egyetem Utca 10, Veszpŕem 8200, Hungary

**A. G. González**
School of Design Engineering, Department of Mechanical, Energy, and Materials Engineering, University of Extremadura, 06800 Mérida, Spain

**J. García-Sanz-Calcedo**
Department of Projects, University of Extremadura, 06007 Badajoz, Spain

**D. R. Salgado**
School of Industrial Engineering, Department of Mechanical, Energy, and Materials Engineering, University of Extremadura, 06007 Badajoz, Spain

**A. Mena**
School of Industrial Engineering, Department of Engineering Design and Projects, University of Huelva, 21003 Huelva, Spain

**Pei-Fang (Jennifer) Tsai, Po-Chia Chen, Yen-You Chen and Hao-Yuan Song**
Department of Industrial Engineering and Management, National Taipei University of Technology, Taipei 10608, Taiwan

**Hsiu-Mei Lin**
Division of Health Insurance, Mackay Memorial Hospital, Taipei 10449, Taiwan

**Fu-Man Lin**
Medical Affairs Department, Mackay Memorial Hospital, Taipei 10449, Taiwan

**Qiou-Pieng Huang**
Registration and Admitting, Mackay Memorial Hospital, Taipei 10449, Taiwan

**Roman Melecky, Vladimir Socha, Patrik Kutilek, Lenka Hanakova and Jakub Schlenker**
Faculty of Biomedical Engineering, Czech Technical University in Prague, 272 01 Kladno, Czech Republic

**Peter Takac**
Department of Rehabilitation and Spa Medicine, Faculty of Medicine, P. J. Šafárik University in Košice, 040 01 Košice, Slovakia

**Zdenek Svoboda**
Palacky University of Olomouc, Faculty of Physical Culture, 771 11 Olomouc, Czech Republic

**Yang-chun Wu, Wei Zuo, Yan Yu, Jian-jie Wang, Li-ming Cheng and Zhi-li Zeng**
Spine Division of Orthopaedic Department, Tongji Hospital, Tongji University School of Medicine, 389 Xincun Road, Shanghai 200065, China

**Rui Zhu**
Department of Histology and Embryology, Tongji University School of Medicine, 1239 Siping Road, Shanghai 200092, China

**Nathan Huynh and Omor Sharif**
Civil & Environmental Engineering, University of South Carolina, Columbia, SC 29208, USA

**Rita Snyder**
College of Nursing, University of Arizona, Tucson, AZ 85721, USA

**José M. Vidal and Bridgette Parsons**
Computer Science and Engineering, University of South Carolina, Columbia, SC 29208, USA

**Bo Cai**
Epidemiology and Biostatistics, University of South Carolina, Columbia, SC 29208, USA

**Kevin Bennett**
School of Medicine, University of South Carolina, Columbia, SC 29208, USA

**Lisa Bürgermeister**
Fraunhofer Institute for Laser Technology, Steinbachstrasse 15, 52074 Aachen, Germany

**Marcus Hermann**
Nonlinear Dynamics of Laser Processing, RWTH Aachen University, Steinbachstrasse 15, 52074 Aachen, Germany

**Katalin Fehér**
Institute of Textile Technology, RWTH Aachen University, Otto-Blumenthal-Strasse 1, 52074 Aachen, Germany

**Catalina Molano Lopez and Andrij Pich**
Functional and Interactive Polymers, DWI, RWTH Aachen University, Forckenbeckstrasse 50, 52074 Aachen, Germany

**Julian Hannen**
Innovation, Strategy and Organization Group, RWTH Aachen University, Kackertstrasse 7, 52072 Aachen, Germany

**Felix Vogt**
Department of Cardiology, RWTH Aachen University, Pauwelstrasse 30, 52074 Aachen, Germany

**Wolfgang Schulz**
Fraunhofer Institute for Laser Technology, Steinbachstrasse 15, 52074 Aachen, Germany
Nonlinear Dynamics of Laser Processing, RWTH Aachen University, Steinbachstrasse 15, 52074 Aachen, Germany

**Hiromi Matsumoto and Mari Osaki**
Rehabilitation Division, Tottori University Hospital, Nishi-cho 36-1, Yonago, Tottori 683-8504, Japan

**Masaru Ueki, Kazutake Uehara and Nobuko Nozawa**
Center for Promoting Next-Generation Highly Advanced Medicine, Tottori University Hospital, Nishi-cho 36-1, Yonago, Tottori 683-8504, Japan

**Hisashi Noma**
Department of Data Science,The Institute of Statistical Mathematics, Midori-cho 10- 3, Tachikawa, Tokyo 190-8562, Japan

**Hiroshi Hagino**
Rehabilitation Division, Tottori University Hospital, Nishi-cho 36-1, Yonago, Tottori 683-8504, Japan
School of Health Science, Faculty of Medicine, Tottori University, Nishi-cho 86, Yonago, Tottori 683-8503, Japan

**Tiina M. Seppänen and Tapio Seppänen**
Center for Machine Vision and Signal Analysis, University of Oulu, Oulu, Finland
Medical Research Center Oulu, Oulu University Hospital and University of Oulu, Oulu, Finland

**Olli-Pekka Alho**
Medical Research Center Oulu, Oulu University Hospital and University of Oulu, Oulu, Finland
Department of Otorhinolaryngology, Oulu University Hospital, Oulu, Finland
Research Unit of Otorhinolaryngology and Ophthalmology, University of Oulu, Oulu, Finland

**Jeng-Chung Woo**
Department of Product Design, Sanming University, Sanming City, Fujian, China

**Yi-Ling Lin**
Department of Arts and Plastic Design, Taipei University of Education, Taipei City, Taiwan

**Funda Samanlioglu and Ayse Humeyra Bilge**
Faculty of Engineering and Natural Sciences, Kadir Has University, 34083 Istanbul, Turkey

**Tonia C. Carter**
Center for Human Genetics, Marshfield Clinic Research Foundation, Marshfield, WI 54449, USA

**Max M. He**
Center for Human Genetics, Marshfield Clinic Research Foundation, Marshfield, WI 54449, USA
Biomedical Informatics Research Center, Marshfield Clinic Research Foundation, Marshfield, WI 54449, USA
Computation and Informatics in Biology and Medicine, University of Wisconsin-Madison, Madison, WI 53706, USA

**Mana Sezdi**
Department of Biomedical Device Technology, Istanbul University, 34320 Istanbul, Turkey

**Cholada Kittipittayakorn**
Graduate Institute of Industrial and Business Management, National Taipei University of Technology, No. 1, Section 3, Zhongxiao E. Road, Taipei 10608, Taiwan

**Kuo-Ching Ying**
Department of Industrial Engineering and Management, National Taipei University of Technology, No. 1, Section 3, Zhongxiao E. Road, Taipei 10608, Taiwan

**Juan Manuel Carrillo-de-Gea, Ginés García-Mateos and José Luis Fernández-Alemán**
Computer Science and Systems Department, Faculty of Computer Science, University of Murcia, 30100 Murcia, Spain

**José Luis Hernández-Hernández**
Academic Unit of Engineering, Autonomous University of Guerrero, 39087 Chilpancingo, GRO, Mexico

**Ju Hwan Lee**
Department of Medical Devices Industry, Dongguk University-Seoul, 26 Pil-dong 3-ga, Jung-gu, Seoul 04620, Republic of Korea

**Yoo Na Hwang and Ga Young Kim**
Department of Medical Biotechnology, Dongguk University-Bio Medi Campus, 32 Dongguk-ro, Ilsandong-gu, Goyang-si, Gyeonggi-do 10326, Republic of Korea

**Eun Seok Shin**
Department of Cardiology, Ulsan University Hospital, University of Ulsan College of Medicine, 877 Bangeojinsunhwando-ro, Dong-gu, Ulsan 44033, Republic of Korea

**Sung Min Kim**
Department of Medical Devices Industry, Dongguk University-Seoul, 26 Pil-dong 3-ga, Jung-gu, Seoul 04620, Republic of Korea
Department of Medical Biotechnology, Dongguk University-Bio Medi Campus, 32 Dongguk-ro, Ilsandong-gu, Goyang-si, Gyeonggi-do 10326, Republic of Korea

**Shu-An Lee, Dong-Chir Hwang, He-Yi Li and Chieh-Fu Tsai**
Department of Environmental Engineering and Science, Feng Chia University, Taichung 40724, Taiwan

**Chun-Wan Chen**
Division of Occupational Hygiene, Institute of Labor, Occupational Safety and Health, Ministry of Labor, New Taipei City 22143, Taiwan

**Jen-Kun Chen**
Institute of Biomedical Engineering and Nanomedicine, National Health Research Institutes, Miaoli 35053, Taiwan

# Index

www.ingramcontent.com/pod-product-compliance
Lightning Source LLC
Chambersburg PA
CBHW050449200326
41458CB00014B/5114